3rd Edition

Study Guide and Workbook for

Understanding Pathophysiology

Sue E. Huether
Kathryn L. McCance

Prepared by

Clayton F. Parkinson

Professor Emeritus
College of Health Sciences
Weber State University
Ogden, Utah

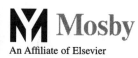
Mosby
An Affiliate of Elsevier

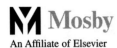

An Affiliate of Elsevier

11830 Westline Industrial Drive
St. Louis, Missouri 63146

STUDY GUIDE AND WORKBOOK FOR UNDERSTANDING PATHOPHYSIOLOGY
Copyright © 2004, Mosby, Inc. All rights reserved.

NOTICE

Pathophysiology is an ever-changing field. Standard safety precautions must be followed, but as new
research and clinical experience broaden our knowledge, changes in treatment and drug therapy may
become necessary or appropriate. Readers are advised to check the most current product information
provided by the manufacturer of each drug to be administered to verify the recommended dose, the method
and duration of administration, and contraindications. It is the responsibility of the licensed prescriber,
relying on experience and knowledge of the patient, to determine dosages and the best treatment for each
individual patient. Neither the publisher nor the editor assumes any liability for any injury and/or damage
to persons or property arising from this publication.

Previous edition copyrighted 2000.

International Standard Book Number 0-323-02846-2

Acquisitions Editor: Darlene Como
Managing Editor: Brian Dennison
Editorial Assistant: Courtney R. Adkins
Publishing Services Manager: Deborah L. Vogel
Senior Project Manager: Ann E. Rogers
Book Design Manager: Kathi Gosche
Cover Art: Anne Wolfer

Printed in the United States of America.
Last digit is the print number: 9 8 7 6 5 4 3 2 1

Preface

The study of pathophysiology is complex, ever expanding, and challenging. It provides correlations between normal anatomy and physiology and the processes resulting in the manifestations of disease.

This *Study Guide and Workbook* is designed for students as an adjunct to *Understanding Pathophysiology*, third edition, by Sue E. Huether and Kathryn L. McCance. It is intended to encourage an understanding of the consequences of pathologic processes on the structure and function of the human body.

The *Study Guide and Workbook* contains 40 chapters, each following the organization of the textbook. The *Guide's* chapters have two different formats—one for normal anatomy and physiology and another for anatomic and physiologic alterations.

For the normal anatomy and physiology chapters, it is assumed that the student possesses foundational knowledge of anatomy and physiology.

- These chapters direct review of information, principles, and concepts that are essential for understanding the specific diseases that follow.
- Each chapter has a practice examination to give students an opportunity to assess their understanding of normality.

The chapters on alterations direct the learner's study of abnormal anatomy and physiology.

- These chapters include foundational objectives and study objectives with both narrative and charts.
- Each chapter has a practice examination requiring factual and conceptual knowledge related to disease mechanisms.
- Each chapter includes a case study linking fact and concept to reality.

The objectives for all chapters are referenced to corresponding pages in the third edition of *Understanding Pathophysiology*. Huether and McCance's philosophy that students need to grasp basic laws and principles to understand how alterations occur led them to develop an understandable and conceptually integrated textbook.

I enjoyed working with Mosby, particularly with Courtney Adkins, Brian Dennison, and Ann Rogers. All of Mosby's staff ensured that my efforts were developed into a creative, professional, and pleasing style for student learners. Without Klaus Gurgel, a sales representative for Mosby who encouraged me, the joint effort between Mosby and me would not have happened.

I wish to dedicate my efforts during the preparation of this *Study Guide and Workbook* to eager students who made teaching pleasurable and inspired me to search for truth and a better way to convey it to students.

Clayton F. Parkinson

Reviewers

Jacqueline Rosenjack Burchum, DNSc, APRN, BC
Assistant Professor
The University of Memphis
Loewenberg School of Nursing
Memphis, Tennessee

Margaret M. Gingrich, RN, MSN
Instructor
Harrisburg Area Community College
Harrisburg, Pennsylvania

Cynthia Taylor Smith, RN, MSN
Associate Professor
Middle Georgia College
Cochran, Georgia

Contents

Cellular Biology

1

Objectives

After reviewing this chapter, the learner will be able to do the following:

1. **State the functions of a typical eukaryotic cell.**
   Review page 2.

2. **Describe the structure and function of the nucleus and identify the cytoplasmic organelles.**
   Review pages 2-3; refer to Figures 1-1 and 1-2 and Table 1-1.

3. **Describe the structure and function of the plasma membrane.**
   Review pages 3, 4, 6, and 8; refer to Figures 1-3 through 1-5 and Tables 1-2 and 1-3.

4. **Describe cellular receptors.**
   Review pages 8-9; refer to Figure 1-6.

5. **Describe cellular catabolism and the transfer of energy to accomplish other cellular processes.**
   Refer to Figures 1-7 through 1-9.

6. **Differentiate between mediated and active transport and passive transport, between endocytosis and exocytosis, and between phagocytosis and pinocytosis.**
   Refer to Figures 1-10 through 1-16 and Table 1-3.

7. **Describe the changes in the plasma membrane that result in an action potential.**
   Review pages 17-18; refer to Figure 1-17.

8. **Identify the phases of mitosis and cytokinesis.**
   Review pages 19-20; refer to Figure 1-18.

9. **Describe the stimulation of cell proliferation by growth factors.**
   Review page 20; refer to Figure 1-19 and Table 1-4.

10. **Identify the three mechanisms that bind cells together.**
    Review pages 21-22; refer to Figures 1-20 and 1-21.

11. **Describe the primary modes of chemical signaling.**
    Review pages 22-24; refer to Figures 1-22 through 1-24 and Table 1-5.

12. **Characterize pattern formation.**
    Review page 24.

13. **Identify the location and a major function for each type of tissue: epithelial, connective, muscle, and nervous.**
    Refer to Figure 1-25 and Boxes 1-1 through 1-3.

Practice Examination

1. Which are principal parts of a eukaryotic cell?
   a. fat, carbohydrate, and protein
   b. minerals and water
   c. organelles
   d. phospholipids and protein
   e. protoplasm and nucleus

2. The cell membrane is described as a fluid mosaic. Proteins have a degree of mobility within the lipid bilayer. (More than one answer may be correct.)
   a. The first sentence is true.
   b. The first sentence is false.
   c. The second sentence is true.
   d. The second sentence is false.
   e. The second sentence is relevant to the first.
   f. The second sentence is irrelevant to the first.

3. Which particle can penetrate cell membranes most easily?
   a. lipid-soluble, transport protein present
   b. neutral charge, water-soluble
   c. smaller, water-soluble
   d. uncharged, larger
   e. All of the above are correct.

4. In order for a cell to engage in active transport processes, it requires:
   a. mitochondria.
   b. appropriate fuel.
   c. ATP.
   d. enzymes.
   e. All of the above are correct.

5. Which is *inconsistent* with the others?
   a. diffusion
   b. osmosis
   c. filtration
   d. phagocytosis
   e. facilitated diffusion

6. Which can transport substances "uphill" against the concentration gradient?
   a. active transport
   b. osmosis
   c. dialysis
   d. facilitated diffusion
   e. none of the above

7. Caveolae:
   a. serve as repositories for some receptors.
   b. provide a route for transport into a cell.
   c. relay signals into cells.
   d. All of the above are correct.

8. Which statement is true for cytoplasm?
   a. It is located outside the nucleus.
   b. It provides support for organelles.
   c. It is mostly water.
   d. a, b, and c
   e. a and b

Match the term with its descriptor.

_____ 9. anaphase   a. 75%-90% H_2O, lipids, and protein

_____10. chromatin   b. within the nucleus, stored RNA

_____11. metaphase   c. compartmentalizes cellular activity

_____12. mitochondria   d. single strand of DNA, nondividing cell

_____13. prophase   e. "generation plant" for ATP

_____14. ribosome   f. centriole migration

                                 g. chromatid pair alignment

                                 h. chromatid migration

                                 i. daughter nuclei

                                 j. protein synthesis site

---

15. The retinoblastoma (Rb) protein:
     a. is a brake on the progress of the cell cycle.
     b. binds to gene regulatory proteins.
     c. slows cell proliferation.
     d. a and c
     e. a, b, and c

16. A major function of connective tissue is:
     a. to form glands.
     b. support and binding.
     c. covering and lining.
     d. movement.
     e. to conduct nerve impulses.

17. Which are characteristic of epithelial tissue? (More than one answer may be correct.)
     a. elasticity
     b. protection
     c. fills spaces between organs
     d. secretion

Match the location with the tissue type found.

_____18. lining of the kidney tubules   a. simple squamous

_____19. lining of the upper respiratory tract   b. simple cuboidal

                                                     c. simple columnar, ciliated

                                                     d. stratified squamous

                                                     e. transitional

20. Signaling molecules cause all of the following *except:*
    a. acceleration/initiative of intracellular protein kinases.
    b. arrest of cellular growth.
    c. apoptosis.
    d. conversion of an intracellular signal into an extracellular response.

21. Ligands that bind with membrane receptors include which of the following? (More than one answer may be correct.)
    a. hormones
    b. antigens
    c. neurotransmitters
    d. drugs
    e. infectious agents

22. The products from the metabolism of glucose include which of the following? (More than one answer may be correct.)
    a. kilocalories
    b. CO_2
    c. H_2O
    d. ATP

23. Identify the correct sequence of events for initiation and conduction of a nerve impulse.
    1. Sodium moves inside.   a. 1, 3, 2, 5, 4
    2. Potassium leaves cell.   b. 3, 1, 5, 2, 4
    3. Sodium permeability changes.   c. 5, 2, 3, 1, 4
    4. Resting potential is reestablished. d. 4, 5, 2, 3, 1
    5. Potassium permeability changes.

24. Increased cytoplasmic calcium:
    a. causes one cell to adhere to another.
    b. increases permeability at the junctional complex.
    c. decreases permeability at the junctional complex.
    d. None of the above is correct.

25. Cell junctions:
    a. coordinate activities of cells within tissues.
    b. are an impermeable part of the plasma membrane.
    c. hold cells together.
    d. Both a and c are correct.
    e. Both b and c are correct.

Genes and Genetic Diseases

a. **Describe the interrelationships of DNA, RNA, and proteins.**
   Review pages 38-40; refer to Figures 2-1 through 2-5.

MEMORY CHECK!

- The gene consists of a particular sequence of nucleotides in the deoxyribonucleic acid (DNA) of the chromosome. The sequence of nucleotides in a gene determines which proteins are found in a cell, and these proteins determine both the form and function of the cell.

- Genetic information flows from DNA to RNA to proteins. Three major processes are involved in the preservation and transmission of genetic information. The first is replication, or the copying of DNA to form identical daughter molecules. The second is transcription, in which the genetic message encoded within DNA is transcribed into RNA and is carried to the ribosomes, the sites of protein synthesis. The third is translation, in which the genetic message is decoded and converted into the 20-letter alphabet of protein structure. Because the sequence of nucleotides in the DNA bears a linear correspondence to the sequence of amino acids in the formed proteins, genetic information is preserved and transmitted to progeny.

b. **Define general genetic terms.**
   Review pages 41-42, 44, and 46-49.

MEMORY CHECK!

Genetic Term	Definition
Progeny	Offspring
Chromosomes	Structures in the nucleus that contain DNA, which transmits genetic information; each chromosome is composed of many genes arranged in linear order
Gene	DNA, the basic unit of heredity, located at a particular locus on the chromosome
Locus	The position each gene occupies along a chromosome
Allele	One of two or more alternative genes that contain specific inheritable characteristics (such as eye color) and occupy corresponding positions on paired, homologous chromosomes—one gene from each parent; a different version of the same paired gene
Homozygous	A trait of an organism produced by identical or nearly identical alleles
Heterozygous	Possessing different alleles at a given chromosomal location

Continued.

MEMORY CHECK!—cont'd

Genetic Term	Definition
Karyotype	A display of human chromosomes based on their length and the location of the centromere
Genotype	The basic combination of genes of an organism
Phenotype	The expression of the gene or trait in an individual (e.g., physical appearance, such as eye color)
Carrier	An individual who has a gene for disease but is phenotypically normal
Dominant traits	Traits for which one of a pair of alleles is necessary for expression (e.g., brown eyes)
Recessive traits	Traits for which two alleles of a pair are necessary for expression (e.g., blue eyes, a recessive gene on the male's X chromosome, will be expressed because the gene is not matched by a corresponding gene on the Y chromosome)
Pedigree chart	A schematic method for classifying genetic data
Penetrance	The percentage of individuals with a specific genotype who exhibit the expected phenotype
Expressivity	The extent of variation in phenotype for a particular genotype
Genetic imprinting	Imprinted genes are normally inactive.

Single-gene disorders are known to be caused by mutation in a single gene. The mutated gene may be present on one or both chromosomes of a gene pair.

Multifactorial disorders result when small variations in genes combine with environmental factors to produce serious defects. Multifactorial disorders tend to cluster in families.

Objectives

After studying this chapter, the learner will be able to do the following:

1. **Characterize chromosome disorders.**
   Study pages 42, 44, and 46-49; refer to Figures 2-10, 2-15, and 2-17.

In **chromosome disorders,** the defect is due to an abnormality in chromosome number or structure. The structure of the genes in chromosome disorders may be normal, but the genes may be present in multiple copies or be situated on a different chromosome.

Normal somatic cells having two sets of 23 chromosomes are **diploid** (double), or 2N. Gametes with a single set of 23 chromosomes are **haploid** (single), or N. A cell with an exact multiple of the haploid number is **euploid.** Euploid numbers may be 2N, 3N (triploid), or 4N (tetraploid). Chromosome numbers that are exact multiples of N but greater than 2N are called **triploid, polyploid. Aneuploidy** refers to a chromosome complement that is abnormal in number but is not an exact multiple of N. An aneuploid cell may be **trisomic** (2N + 1 chromosome) or **monosomic** (2N – 1 chromosome).

Disjunction is the normal separation and migration of chromosomes during cell division. Failure of the process, or **nondisjunction,** in a meiotic division results in one daughter cell receiving both homologous chromosomes and the other receiving neither. It is the primary cause of aneuploidy. If this deviation in normal processes occurs during the first meiotic division, half of the gametes will contain 22 chromosomes and half will contain 24. If joined with a normal gamete, a gamete produced in this manner will produce either a monosomic (2N – 1) or trisomic (2N + 1) zygote.

Deviations in the normal structure of chromosomes result from the chromosome material breaking and reassembling in an abnormal arrangement. Structural abnormalities include deletion, duplication, inversion, or translocation.

In **deletion,** or loss of a portion of a chromosome, the missing segment may be a terminal portion of the chromosome resulting from a single break or an internal section resulting from two breaks. **Cri-du-chat syndrome** is such a deletion and is manifested by the "cry of the cat" in an affected child.

Duplication is the presence of a repeated gene or gene sequence. A deleted segment of one chromosome may become incorporated into its homologous chromosome.

Inversion is the reversal of gene order. The linear arrangement of genes on a chromosome is broken, and the order of a portion of the gene complement is reversed in the process of reattachment.

Translocation is the transfer of part of one chromosome to a nonhomologous chromosome. This occurs when two chromosomes break and the segments are rejoined in an abnormal arrangement.

2. Cite examples of chromosome disorders.
  Refer to Figures 2-11 through 2-14 and 2-16 and
  Table 2-1.

A common example of an autosomal aneuploidy disorder that results from an abnormality of chromosome number is trisomy 21, or **Down syndrome.** This disorder can result when nondisjunction of chromosome 21 occurs at meiosis, producing one gamete with an extra chromosome 21 and one gamete with no chromosome 21. Union of the extra chromosome female gamete with a normal sperm produces a 47 chromosome zygote, or trisomy 21.

The overall incidence of Down syndrome is 1 per 800 live births. The incidence increases with increasing maternal age. Clinical diagnosis of trisomy 21 is often based on facial appearance. A low nasal bridge, epicanthal folds, protruding tongue, and low-set ears are common. Mental retardation is consistent in children with Down syndrome, but its degree may vary. The average IQ is approximately 50.

Two sex chromosome aneuploidy disorders are **Turner syndrome** (female) and **Klinefelter syndrome** (male). The most common karyotype showing female phenotype is 45, X; the male karyotype is 47, XXY.

The diagnosis of Turner syndrome is suggested in the newborn by the presence of redundant neck skin and peripheral lymphedema. Later, the presence of short stature is suggestive.

Klinefelter syndrome is a common cause of infertility in men. Other manifestations include long lower extremities, sparse body hair with female distribution, and female breast development in about 50 percent of the cases. A moderate degree of mental impairment may be present.

3. Characterize single-gene disorders.
  Study pages 50-56; refer to Figures 2-19 and 2-24
  through 2-28.

An inherited gene may be present on one or both chromosomes of a pair. The pedigree patterns of inherited traits are dependent on whether the gene is located on an autosomal chromosome, any chromosome other than a sex chromosome, or the X chromosome and

whether the gene is dominant or recessive. These factors allow four basic patterns of inheritance for single-gene traits, whether normal or abnormal: autosomal dominant, autosomal recessive, X-linked dominant, and X-linked recessive.

In **autosomal dominant** inheritance of genetic defects, the abnormal allele is dominant and the normal allele is recessive. The phenotype is the same whether the allele is present in either a homozygous or heterozygous state.

Principles of autosomal dominant inheritance are (1) affected persons have an affected parent, (2) affected persons mating with normal persons have affected and unaffected offspring in equal proportion, and (3) males and females are equally affected.

In **autosomal recessive** disorders, the abnormal allele is recessive. For the trait to be expressed, a person must be homozygous for the abnormal allele. Because the dominant or normal allele masks the trait, most persons who are heterozygous for an autosomal recessive allele are phenotypically normal. When two heterozygous individuals mate and an offspring receives the recessive allele from each parent, the trait is expressed.

Characteristics of autosomal recessive inheritance are (1) the trait usually appears in siblings only, not in the parents; (2) males and females are equally likely to be affected; (3) for parents of one affected child, the recurrence risk is one in four for every subsequent birth; (4) both parents of an affected child carry the recessive allele; and (5) the parents of the affected child may be consanguineous or blood relatives.

Unlike the 44 autosomes that can be arranged in 22 homologous pairs, the two sex chromosomes in the female are XX and in the male are XY. Because the ovum must contain an X chromosome, if it is fertilized by a sperm containing an X chromosome, the progeny will be a female (XX). If the sperm contributes a Y chromosome, the progeny will be male (XY).

Traits determined by either dominant or recessive **X-linked genes** are expressed in the male. The genes on the X chromosome cannot be transmitted from father to son (fathers contribute a Y chromosome to sons) but are transmitted from father to all daughters through one X chromosome. Recessive abnormal genes on the X chromosome of a female may not be expressed because they are matched by normal genes inherited with the other X chromosome.

X-linked dominant disorders are rare. The main characteristic of this inheritance pattern is that an affected male transmits the gene to all of his daughters and to none of his sons. The affected female may transmit the gene to offspring of either sex.

In **X-linked recessive** disorders, the recessive gene located on the one X chromosome of the male is not balanced by the dominant allele on the Y chromosome and is thus expressed. Only matings between an affected male and a carrier or affected female should result in an affected female.

Males affected with an X-linked recessive disorder cannot transmit the gene to sons but transmit it to all daughters. An unaffected female who is heterozygous (a carrier) for the recessive gene transmits it to 50% of her sons and daughters.

Principles of the X-linked recessive inheritance are (1) males are predominantly affected, (2) affected males cannot transmit the gene to sons but do transmit the gene to all daughters, (3) sons of female carriers have a 50% risk of being affected, and (4) daughters of female carriers have a 50% risk of being carriers.

4. **Cite examples of single-gene disorders.**
   Study pages 51-55; refer to Figures 2-20 through 2-22 and 2-29 and Table 2-2.

One of the best-known autosomal dominant diseases is **Huntington disease,** a neurologic disorder that exhibits progressive dementia and increasingly uncontrollable movements of the limbs. A key feature of this disease is that its symptoms are not usually seen until after age 40. Thus, those who develop the disease often have had children before they are aware that they have the gene.

The severity of an autosomal dominant disease can vary greatly. An example of variable expressivity in an autosomal dominant disease is type 1 **neurofibromatosis,** or von Recklinghausen disease, which has been mapped to the long arm of chromosome 17. The expression of this gene can vary from a few harmless "cafe au lait" spots on the skin to numerous malignant neurofibromas, scoliosis, seizures, gliomas, neuromas, hypertension, and mental retardation.

The **cystic fibrosis** gene, the cause of an autosomal recessive disease, has been mapped to the long arm of chromosome 7. In this disease, defective transport of chloride ion leads to a salt imbalance that results in secretions of abnormally thick, dehydrated mucus. Some of the digestive organs, particularly the pancreas, become obstructed with mucus, resulting in malnutrition. The lung airways tend to become clogged with mucus, making them highly susceptible to bacterial infections.

The most common and severe of all X-linked recessive disorders is **Duchenne muscular dystrophy,** which affects males. This disorder is characterized by progressive muscle degeneration; individuals are usually unable to walk by age 10 or 12. The disease also affects the heart and respiratory muscles, and death because of respiratory or cardiac failure may occur before age 20. These cases are due to an absence of dystrophin, without which the muscle cell cannot survive, and muscle deterioration follows.

5. **Characterize multifactorial inheritance and cite examples.**
   Study pages 58-60; refer to Figures 2-30 and 2-31.

Not all traits are produced by single genes; some traits are the result of several genes acting together. When several genes act together, the trait is referred to as **polygenic.** When environmental factors also influence the expression of the trait, the term **multifactorial inheritance** is used. Both genes and environment contribute to variation in traits. Multifactorial disorders tend to cluster in families.

Although both height and IQ are determined by genes, they are also influenced by environment. For example, height has increased by 5 to 10 cm since the turn of the century because of improvements in nutrition and health care. Also, IQ scores can be improved by exposing children to enriched learning environments.

A number of diseases do not follow the bell-shaped distribution of polygenic and multifactorial traits. Instead, a certain threshold of liability must be crossed before the disease is expressed. A well-known example of a threshold trait is pyloric stenosis, a disorder characterized by narrowing or obstruction of the pylorus. Chronic vomiting, constipation, weight loss, and electrolyte imbalance can result from this condition. Pyloric stenosis is much more common in males than in females. The reason for this difference is that the threshold of liability is much lower in males than in females. Thus, fewer defective alleles are required to generate the disorder in males. This also means that the offspring of affected females are more likely to have pyloric stenosis because affected females carry more disease-causing alleles than do most affected males.

Other multifactorial diseases include cleft lip and/or cleft palate, neural tube defects, clubfeet, and some forms of congenital heart disease. Hypertensive heart disease and diabetes mellitus likely can be grouped in the category of multifactorial disorders.

Practice Examination

1. Which genetic disease is caused by an abnormal karyotype?
   a. Down syndrome
   b. Huntington disease
   c. PKU
   d. neurofibromatosis
   e. cystic fibrosis

2. Which is *not* characteristic of Down syndrome?
   a. It is an autosomal aneuploidy.
   b. It is a genetic error of metabolism.
   c. Mental retardation is consistently expressed.
   d. Clinical diagnosis can be suggested by facial appearance.
   e. The karyotype is 47, XY + 21.

3. Cri-du-chat syndrome is an abnormality of chromosomal structure involving:
   a. translocation.
   b. an inversion.
   c. duplication.
   d. deletion.

4. An individual's karyotype lacks a homologous X chromosome and has only a single X chromosome present. Which statement is *not* true?
   a. The karyotype is 45, X.
   b. Features include ribbed neck and short stature.
   c. The karyotype is 46, XY.
   d. The disorder is a sex chromosome aneuploidy.

5. If homologous chromosomes fail to separate during meiosis, the disorder is:
   a. polyploidy.
   b. aneuploidy.
   c. disjunction.
   d. nondisjunction.
   e. translocation.

6. Cystic fibrosis has been mapped to chromosome:
   a. 17.
   b. 7.
   c. X.
   d. 16.

7. In autosomal dominant inherited disorders:
   a. affected individuals do not have an affected parent.
   b. affected persons mating with normal persons have a 50% risk of having an affected offspring.
   c. male offspring are most often affected.
   d. unaffected children born to affected parents will have affected children.

8. In X-linked recessive inherited disorders:
   a. affected males have normal sons.
   b. affected males have affected daughters.
   c. sons of female carriers have a 50% risk of being affected.
   d. the affected female may transmit the gene to both sons and daughters.

9. Which is *not* an autosomal dominant disease?
   a. Huntington disease
   b. neurofibromatosis
   c. Duchenne muscular dystrophy
   d. von Recklinghausen disease
   e. pyloric stenosis

10. When environmental influences cause varied phenotypic expressions of genotypes, the result is a/an:
    a. multifactorial trait.
    b. threshold liability.
    c. autosomal dominant trait.
    d. X-linked recessive trait.

11. Which likely is *not* a multifactorial inherited disorder?
    a. cleft palate
    b. hypertension
    c. diabetes mellitus
    d. cystic fibrosis
    e. heart disease

Match the term with the circumstance.

_____12. recessive disorder

_____13. multifactorial inheritance

_____14. aneuploidy

_____15. chromosomal aberration

_____16. phenotype

_____17. pedigree

_____18. autosomal recessive inheritance

a. due to numerical or structural aberrations

b. many genes are common

c. two or more cell lines with different karyotypes

d. individual is homozygous for a gene

e. failure of homologous chromosomes to separate during meiosis or mitosis

f. outward appearance of an individual

g. a probability of .25

h. summarizes family relationships

Match the term with the circumstance.

_____19. expressivity

_____20. X-linked

_____21. inversion

_____22. dominant trait

_____23. allele

_____24. 47, XXY

_____25. karyotype

a. a probability of .5

b. females are unlikely to be affected

c. species chromosomal morphology

d. expressed by one allele

e. Turner syndrome

f. different version of the same paired gene

g. Klinefelter syndrome

h. no loss or gain of genetic material, reversed order

i. extent of phenotypic variation of a particular genotype

3

Altered Cellular and Tissue Biology

Foundational Objective

a. **Describe processes of cellular intake and output.**
Review pages 10-15 and 17.

MEMORY CHECK!

- The intact, normally functioning plasma membrane is selectively or differentially permeable to substances; it allows some substances to pass while excluding others. Water and small, uncharged substances move through pores of the lipid bilayer by passive transport, which requires no expenditure of energy. This process is driven by the forces of osmosis, hydrostatic pressure, and diffusion. Larger molecules and molecular complexes are moved into the cell by active transport, which requires the expenditure of energy or ATP by the cell. In active transport, materials move from low concentrations to high concentrations. The largest molecules and fluids are ingested by endocytosis (from the extracellular medium) and expelled by exocytosis (into the extracellular medium) after cellular synthesis of smaller building blocks. When the plasma membrane is injured, it becomes permeable to virtually everything, and substances move into and out of the cells in an unrestricted manner. Notably, such substances may affect (1) the nucleus and its genetic information or (2) the cytoplasmic organelles and their varied functions. Then, there is altered cellular physiology and pathology.

Objectives

After studying this chapter, the learner will be able to do the following:

1. **Describe the cellular adaptations occurring in atrophy, hypertrophy, hyperplasia, dysplasia, and metaplasia. Identify the conditions under which each can occur.**
   Study pages 66 and 68-69; refer to Figures 3-1 through 3-3.

When confronted with environmental stresses that disrupt normal structure and function, the cell undergoes adaptive changes that permit survival and maintain function. An adapted cell is neither normal nor injured—rather, it is somewhere between these two states. These changes may lead to atrophy, hypertrophy, hyperplasia, dysplasia, or metaplasia.

Cellular atrophy decreases the cell substance and results in cell shrinkage. Causes of atrophy include disuse, denervation, decreased endocrine stimulation, decreased nutrition, and ischemia. These can cause decreased protein synthesis, increased protein catabolism, or both. Atrophy commonly is seen in muscles that are not used or innervated.

Hypertrophy increases cell size. Hypertrophy is commonly seen in cardiac and skeletal muscle tissue. The increase in cell components is related to an increased rate of protein synthesis. Mechanical signals, such as stretch; and trophic signals, such as growth factors, hormones, and vasoactive agents, are triggers for hypertrophy. Physiologic hypertrophy is observed in uterine tissue and mammary glands during pregnancy.

Hyperplasia is an increase in the number of cells of a tissue or organ. It occurs in tissues where cells are capable of mitotic division. Breast and uterine enlargement during pregnancy are examples of physiologic hyperplasia and hypertrophy that are hormonally regulated. A pathologic hyperplasia occurs when the endometrium enlarges because of excessive estrogen production. Then, the abnormally thickened uterine layer may bleed excessively and frequently. Compensatory hyperplasia enables certain organs, such as the liver, to regenerate after loss of substance. Hyperplasia and hypertrophy often occur together if cells can synthesize DNA; however, in nondividing cells, only hypertrophy occurs.

Dysplasia is deranged cell growth that results in cells that vary in size, shape, and appearance as compared to mature cells and is related to hyperplasia. Dysplasia occurs in association with chronic irritation or inflammation in the uterine cervix, oral cavity, gallbladder, and respiratory passages. Dysplasia is potentially reversible once the irritating cause has been removed. However, dysplastic changes may progress to neoplastic disease.

Metaplasia is a reversible conversion from one adult cell type to another adult cell type. It allows for replacement with cells that are better able to tolerate environmental stresses. In metaplasia, one type of cell may be converted to another type of cell within its tissue class. An example of metaplasia is the substitution of stratified squamous epithelial cells for ciliated columnar epithelial cells in the airways of an individual who is a habitual cigarette smoker.

2. **Identify the mechanism of cellular injury from hypoxia, free radicals, chemicals, unintentional and intentional injuries, infectious agents, immunologic and inflammatory responses, and genetic factors.**
Study pages 69-74 and 76-84; refer to Figures 3-4 through 3-18 and Tables 3-1 through 3-7.

Hypoxia deprives the cell of oxygen and interrupts oxidative metabolism and the generation of ATP. As oxygen tension within the cell falls, oxidative metabolism ceases and the cell reverts to anaerobic metabolism. One of the earliest effects of reduced ATP is acute cellular swelling caused by failure of the sodium-potassium membrane pump. With impaired function of this pump, intracellular potassium levels decrease and sodium and water accumulate within the cell. As fluid and ions move into the cell, there is dilation of the endoplasmic reticulum, increased membrane permeability, and decreased mitochondrial function as extracellular calcium accumulates in the mitochondria. If the oxygen supply is not restored, there is continued loss of essential enzymes, proteins, and ribonucleic acid through the very permeable

membrane of the cell. Hypoxia can result from inadequate oxygen in the air, respiratory disease, decreased blood flow due to circulatory disease, anemia, or inability of the cells to utilize oxygen. Restoration of oxygen, however, can cause **reperfusion injury.** Reperfusion injury results from the generation of high reactive oxygen intermediates, including hydroxyl radical, superoxide, and hydrogen peroxide; these are known as free radicals.

An important mechanism of membrane damage is caused by **free radicals,** especially by activated oxygen species. A free radical is an atom or group of atoms with an unpaired electron. The unpaired electron makes the atom or group unstable. To gain stability, the radical gives up an electron to another molecule or steals an electron. These radicals can bond with proteins, lipids, and carbohydrates, which are key molecules in membranes and nucleic acids. These reactive species cause injury by (1) lipid peroxidation, which destroys unsaturated fatty acids, (2) fragmentation of polypeptide chains within proteins, and (3) alteration of DNA by breakage of single strands. Free radicals are difficult to control, and they initiate chain reactions. Free radicals may be initiated within cells by the absorption of ultraviolet light or x-rays, oxidative reactions that occur during normal metabolism, and enzymatic metabolism of exogenous chemicals or drugs.

Antioxidants can decrease the damage done by free radicals by inactivating them. Effective antioxidants include superoxide dismutase present in peroxisomes of cells and the nutrient vitamins C and E and beta carotene, a precursor to vitamin A.

Toxic chemical agents can injure the cell membrane and cell structures, block enzymatic pathways, coagulate cell proteins, and disrupt the osmotic and ionic balance of cells. Chemicals may injure cells during the process of metabolism or elimination. Carbon tetrachloride, for example, causes little damage until it is metabolized by liver enzymes to highly reactive free radicals, and then it is extremely toxic to liver cells. Carbon monoxide has a special affinity for the hemoglobin molecule and reduces hemoglobin's ability to carry oxygen.

Alcohol (ethanol) is the favorite mood-altering drug in the United States. Liver disease, nutritional disorders, and CNS impairment are serious consequences of alcohol abuse. The hepatic changes, initiated by ethanol conversion to acetaldehyde, include deposition of fat, enlargement of the liver, interruption of transport of proteins and their secretion, increase in intracellular water, depression of fatty acid oxidation, increased membrane rigidity, and acute liver cell necrosis. In the CNS, alcohol is a depressant, initially affecting subcortical structures. Consequently, motor and intellectual activity become disoriented. At high blood alcohol levels, respiratory medullary centers become depressed.

Unintentional and intentional injuries are important health issues in the United States affecting more men than women and more blacks than whites or other racial groups. Injuries by blunt force result from mechanical energy applied to the body. A contusion—bleeding in skin or underlying tissue—and an abrasion—removal of skin—are consequences of blunt blows. Contusions and abrasions exhibit a patterned appearance that mirrors the shape and features of an injuring object. Asphyxial injuries are caused by a failure of cells to receive or use oxygen; thus, injuries can be categorized as suffocation, strangulation, chemical, and drowning.

Infectious agents that survive and proliferate in the body may produce substances that injure cells and tissues. They also produce toxins and damaging hypersensitivity reactions.

Immunologic and inflammatory injury are important causes of cellular injury. Cellular membranes are injured by direct contact with cellular and chemical components of the immune and inflammatory responses. Such mediators are lymphocytes and macrophages and chemicals such as histamine, antibodies, lymphokines, complement, and proteases. Complement, a serum protein, is responsible for many of the membrane alterations that occur during immunologic injury. Membrane alterations are associated with rapid leakage of potassium out of the cell and rapid influx of water. Antibodies can interfere with membrane function by binding to and occupying receptor molecules on the plasma membrane. (Later chapters will deal with these injurious consequences as well as with hypersensitivity and autoimmune disease.)

Genetic disorders may alter the cell's nucleus and the plasma membrane's structure, shape, receptors, or transport mechanisms. (Mechanisms causing genetic abnormalities are discussed in Chapter 2.)

3. **Identify various cellular accumulations occurring in response to injury and the subsequent manifestations of cellular damage.**
   Study pages 85-88 and 90; refer to Figures 3-19 through 3-23 and Table 3-8.

Cellular accumulations or infiltrations occur whenever normal substances are produced in excess, normal and abnormal substances are ineffectively catabolized, or harmful exogenous materials accumulate intracellularly. (See box on page 14 of *Workbook*.)

4. **Identify the major types of cellular necrosis and cite examples of the tissues involved in each type. Compare necrosis to apoptosis.**
   Study pages 90-93; refer to Figures 3-24 through 3-29.

Necrosis is local cell death and involves the process of cellular self-digestion known as *autodigestion* or *autolysis*. As necrosis progresses, most organelles are disrupted and *karyolysis*, nuclear dissolution from the action of hydrolytic enzymes, becomes evident. The process of the nucleus fragmenting into "nuclear dust" is known as *karyohexis*. There are four major types of necrosis: coagulative, liquefactive, caseous, and fatty. Gangrenous necrosis is not a distinctive type of cell death but instead refers to large areas of tissue death.

Coagulative necrosis occurs primarily in the kidneys, heart, and adrenal glands and usually results from hypoxia caused by severe ischemia. Protein denaturation causes coagulation.

Liquefactive necrosis is common following ischemic injury to neurons and glial cells in the brain. Because brain cells are rich in digestive hydrolytic enzymes and lipids, the brain cells are digested by their own hydrolases. The brain tissue becomes soft, liquefies, and is walled off from healthy tissue to form cysts. Bacterial infections are causes of liquefactive necrosis.

Caseous necrosis is commonly seen in tuberculous pulmonary infection and is a combination of coagulative and liquefactive necrosis. The necrotic debris is not digested completely by hydrolases, so tissues appear soft and granular and resemble clumped cheese. A granulomatous inflammatory wall may enclose the central areas of caseous necrosis.

The **fatty necrosis** found in the breast, pancreas, and other abdominal structures is a specific cellular dissolution caused by lipases. Lipases break down triglycerides and release free fatty acids, which then combine with calcium, magnesium, and sodium ions to create soaps, or saponification. The necrotic tissue appears opaque and chalk white.

Gangrenous necrosis refers to death of tissue, usually in considerable mass and with putrefaction. It results from severe hypoxic injury subsequent to arteriosclerosis or blockage of major arteries followed by bacterial invasion. Dry gangrene is usually due to a coagulative necrosis, whereas wet gangrene develops when neutrophils invade the site and cause liquefactive necrosis. Gas gangrene, a special type of gangrene, is due to bacterial infection of injured tissue by species of *Clostridium*. These anaerobic bacteria produce hydrolytic enzymes and toxins that destroy connective tissue and cellular membrane; bubbles of gas likely form in muscle cells.

Apoptosis is an important, distinct type of cell death that differs from necrosis. It is an active process of cellular self-destruction in both normal and pathologic tissue changes. Apoptosis likely plays a role in deletion of cells during embryonic development and in endocrine-

Cellular Accumulations

Accumulation	Causes	Injury
H_2O	Extracellular H_2O shifts into cell, reduced ATP and ATPase, sodium accumulates in cell	Cellular swelling, vacuolation, oncosis
Lipids, carbohydrates	Imbalance in production, utilization, or mobilization of lipids or carbohydrates	Vacuolation, displaced nucleus and organelles; leads to fibrosis and scarring
Glycogen	Genetic disorders, diabetes mellitus	Cytoplasmic vacuolation
Proteins	Enzymes digest cellular organelles, renal disorders, plasma cell tumors	Disrupted function and intracellular communication, displaced cellular organelles
Pigments	Exogenous particle ingestion, UV light stimulates melanin production, malignancy, loss of hormonal feedback, genetic defects, bruising and hemorrhage increases hemosiderin, liver dysfunction	Membrane injury, disrupted cellular metabolism
Calcium	Altered membrane permeability, influx of extracellular calcium, excretion of H^+ leading to more OH^-, which precipitates Ca^{++}, endocrine disturbances	Hardening of cellular structure, interferes with function
Urate	Absence of enzymes	Crystal deposition, inflammation

dependent tissues that are undergoing atrophic change. It may occur spontaneously in malignant tumors and in normal, rapidly proliferating cells treated with cancer chemotherapeutic agents and ionizing radiation. Unlike necrosis, apoptosis affects scattered, single cells and results in shrinkage of a cell, whereas in necrosis, cells swell and lyse. Apoptotic cell antigens have been identified as targets of autoantibodies in autoimmune diseases such as systemic lupus erythematosus.

5. **Compare the different theories of aging.**
   Study pages 94 and 98-99; refer to Figure 3-30 and Table 3-11.

   There are two general theories of aging: (1) aging is caused by the accumulations of injurious events, which are sometimes called **damage-accumulation theories,** or (2) aging is the result of a **genetically controlled developmental program.** In support of these two categories, three suggested mechanisms of aging have emerged: (1) genetic, environmental, and behavioral factors produce cellular aging change; (2) changes in regulatory mechanisms, especially in the cells of the endocrine, immune, and central nervous systems, are responsible for aging; and (3) degenerative extracellular and vascular alterations cause aging.

   Regardless of injurious environmental factors, some believe that **each cell may have a finite life span** during which it can replicate. Fibroblasts have been demon-

strated to be limited to 40 to 60 cell doublings. Alternatively, an **intrinsic program within the human genome progressively slows or shuts down mitosis.**

   Alterations of **cellular control mechanisms** include increased hormonal degradations, decreased hormonal synthesis and secretion, and decreased receptors for hormones and neuromodulators. This suggests that a genetic program for aging is encoded in the brain and relayed through hormonal and neural agents because of shared, common receptors within these systems.

   Immune function declines with age and the number of autoantibodies that attack body tissues increases with age; these observations implicate the immune system in the aging process.

   A **degenerative extracellular change** that affects the aging process is collagen cross-linking, which makes collagen more rigid and results in decreased cell permeability to nutrients. It is believed that **free radicals** of oxygen damage tissues as they age. These reactive species not only permanently damage cells but also may lead to cell death. Damage accumulates over time and reduces the body's ability to maintain a steady state. There is new support for the theory that reactive species damage of the DNA in mitochondria is greater than that occurring in nuclear DNA. Superoxide radicals react with mitochondrial nitric oxide to produce damaging peroxynitrite.

6. **Characterize somatic death and its manifestations.**
   Study page 99.

Somatic death is death of the entire organism. Unlike the changes that follow cellular death in a viable body, somatic death is diffuse and does not involve components of the inflammatory response, a vascular response to injury. The most notable manifestations of somatic death are that there is *complete cessation of respiration and circulation,* the surface of the skin usually becomes pale and yellowish, and body temperature falls gradually until, after 24 hours, body temperature equals that of the environment.

Within 6 hours after death, depletion of ATP interferes with ATP-dependent detachment of the contractile proteins, and muscle stiffening or rigor mortis develops. Within 12 to 14 hours, rigor mortis usually affects the entire body. Rigor mortis gradually diminishes as the body becomes flaccid due to the release of enzymes and lytic dissolution.

Practice Examination

1. A cellular adaptation observable in uterine cervical epithelium is:
   a. atrophy.
   b. hyperplasia.
   c. hypertrophy.
   d. dysplasia.
   e. metaplasia.

2. What are the consequences when a cell is forced into anaerobic glycolysis? (More than one answer may be correct.)
   a. insufficient glucose production
   b. excessive pyruvic acid retention
   c. increased lactic acid
   d. inadequate ATP production
   e. excessive CO_2 production

Match the descriptor with the term.

_____ 3. reduced oxygen tension

_____ 4. bleeding in skin or underlying tissue

a. anoxia

b. melanin

c. lipids

d. hypoxia

e. contusion

5. What is the probable cause of cellular swelling in the early stages of cell injury?
   a. fat inclusion
   b. loss of genetic integrity
   c. hydrolytic enzyme activation
   d. Na-K pump fails to remove intracellular Na^+.
   e. None of the above is correct.

Match the process with its cause.

_____ 6. lipid peroxidation

_____ 7. neurotransmitter interference

_____ 8. asphyxiation

_____ 9. depressed fatty acid oxidation

_____10. depressed protein synthesis

a. carbon monoxide

b. oxygen-derived free radicals

c. ethanol

d. lead

e. detached ribosomes

f. increased lactate

g. lysosomal edema

---

11. Dystrophic calcification:
    a. occurs in dying or dead tissues.
    b. is the result of excess calcium in the blood.
    c. is observed in chronic lesions.
    d. Both a and c are correct.
    e. a, b, and c are correct.

12. Cellular swelling is:
    a. irreversible.
    b. evident early in all types of cellular injury.
    c. manifested by decreased intracellular sodium.
    d. None of the above is correct.
    e. Both b and c are correct

13. Which is *not* reversible?
    a. karyolysis
    b. fatty infiltration
    c. oncosis
    d. All of the above are reversible.

14. Aging:
    a. is easy to distinguish from pathology.
    b. does not have a genetic relationship.
    c. is more advanced in primitive societies.
    d. None of the above is correct.
    e. a, b, and c are correct.

15. In aging, cross-linking implies that:
    a. the life span and number of times a cell can replicate are programmed.
    b. the number of cell doublings is limited.
    c. there is oxygen toxicity.
    d. cell permeability decreases.
    e. Both a and b are correct.

Match the manifestation with the condition.

_____16. necrosis caused by *Clostridia*

_____17. rigidity of muscles after somatic death

_____18. increased cell numbers

_____19. necrosis resulting from lysosomal release

_____20. replacement of one cell type with another, more suitable type

a. liquefactive

b. rigor mortis

c. gas gangrene

d. hyperplasia

e. metaplasia

f. cloudy swelling

g. coagulation

Match the circumstance with the condition.

_____21. decreased cell size

_____22. pancreatic necrosis

_____23. coagulative and liquefactive necrosis

_____24. tissue death

_____25. normal and pathologic cellular self-destruction

a. fatty necrosis

b. gangrene

c. atrophy

d. caseous necrosis

e. apoptosis

f. algor mortis

g. hypertrophy

4

Fluids and Electrolytes, Acids and Bases

Review pages 118 and 120-121; refer to Figure 4-8 and Tables 4-10 and 4-11.

Foundational Objectives

a. **Describe the different compartments for body fluids and identify the fluid distribution changes occurring with age.**
   Review page 106; refer to Tables 4-1 through 4-3.

b. **Describe the factors that affect water movement.**
   Review page 107; refer to Figure 4-2.

c. **Identify the distribution of electrolytes in body compartments.**
   Refer to Table 4-4.

MEMORY CHECK!

- $mEq/L = \dfrac{\text{milligrams of ion per liter of solution} \times \text{number of charges of one ion}}{\text{atomic weight of ion}}$

- mEq/L expresses the concentration of chemicals dissolved in body fluids; they relate to chemical activity.

d. **Identify the role of ADH, aldosterone, and natriuretic hormone in water and electrolyte balance.**
   Review pages 109-111; refer to Figures 4-4 through 4-6.

e. **Identify body mechanisms to buffer excessive hydrogen ion/acid and explain the mechanics of the most important buffer. Distinguish between short-term and long-term adjustments.**

MEMORY CHECK!

- Pulmonary acid/base regulation of blood involves CO_2 and is rapid.

$$CO_2 + H_2O \leftrightarrow H_2CO_3 \leftrightarrow H^+ + HCO_3^-$$

An increase in CO_2 tension liberates hydrogen ions; thus, the pH decreases. A decrease in CO_2 tension results in fewer hydrogen ions; thus, the pH increases.

- Renal acid/base regulation of blood is slow and involves HCO_3^- conservation with H^+ and NH_3 excretion. This process essentially secretes H^+ into the urine and returns HCO_3^- to the blood plasma.

Objectives

After studying this chapter, the learner will be able to do the following:

1. **Identify the mechanisms causing edema.**
   Study pages 107-109; refer to Figure 4-3.

   Edema is the accumulation of fluid within interstitial spaces. It may be excess or sequestered fluid.
   Edema may be localized or generalized. Localized edema appears confined to traumatized tissues or within

organ systems. Generalized edema exhibits a uniform distribution of fluid in the interstitial spaces.

Fluid movement can be explained by the following formula:

$$Q = \frac{(BHP + IFOP)}{[\text{from vessel}]} - \frac{(IFHP + BOP)}{[\text{to vessel}]}$$

where Q = fluid movement, BHP = blood hydrostatic pressure, IFOP = interstitial fluid osmotic pressure, IFHP = interstitial fluid hydrostatic pressure, and BOP = blood osmotic pressure.

Fluids move from where there is more to where there is less (in this way fluids can dilute the solutes), or the fluids remain where there are solutes.

2. **Define isotonic, hypertonic, and hypotonic water and solute alterations.**
Study pages 111-113; refer to Tables 4-5 through 4-7. (See flow chart on this page.)

Isotonic Imbalances—Extracellular fluid loss or gain is accompanied by proportional changes of electrolytes in these alterations. Losses are seen in hemorrhage or excessive sweating. Gains occur in administration of intravenous normal saline or renal retention of sodium and water. Cells do not shrink or swell in isotonic fluids.

Hypertonic Imbalances—Water loss or solute gain occurs in these changes. These alterations are seen in administration of hypertonic saline solutions, hyperaldosteronism, Cushing syndrome, diabetes, diarrhea, or insufficient water intake. Cells shrink in hypertonic fluids.

Hypotonic Imbalances—Water gain or solute loss occurs in these changes. These alterations may be caused ing, or renal failure to excrete water. Cells swell in hypotonic fluids.

3. **Identify the major consequences of abnormal levels of sodium, potassium, calcium, phosphate, and magnesium. Define the terms associated with excess or deficit of each electrolyte.**
Study pages 113-118; refer to Figure 4-7 and Table 4-8. (See box on page 20 of *Workbook*.)

4. **Differentiate between metabolic/respiratory acidosis and metabolic/respiratory alkalosis.**
Study pages 121-124; refer to Figures 4-9 through 4-13.

Important values include the following: pH = 7.35–7.45, K^+ = 5 mEq/L, Na^+ = 142 mEq/L, Cl^- = 104 mEq/L, HCO_3^- = 24 mEq/L, pCO_2 = 35–45 mm Hg, and CO_2 = 28 mEq/L.

Essentially, acidosis causes nervous system depression, and alkalosis causes nervous system irritability. The manifestations vary with the degree of alteration. (See box on page 21 of *Workbook*.)

5. **Describe what is meant by the "anion gap" and explain the significance of an abnormal anion gap in metabolic acidosis.**
Study Box 4-1 on p. 123 and Table 4-12.

The blood and cellular electrolytes must maintain osmotic neutrality; that is, the number of cations must equal the number of anions present. Routine measurement of serum electrolytes usually involves only Na^+ and K^+ cations and the anions of Cl^- and HCO_3^- as total CO_2. There are about 12 mEq/L of other anions present in the

Mechanisms of Edema Formation

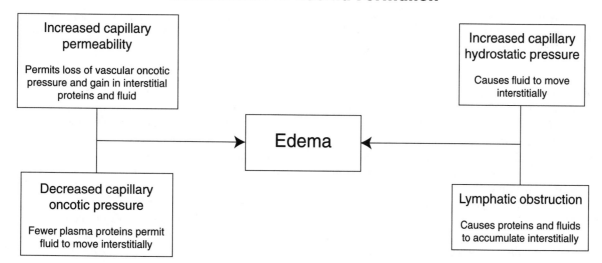

Clinical Manifestations of Excess and Deficit States of Major Electrolytes

Excess	Deficit
Sodium	
Hypernatremia	*Hyponatremia*
>147 mEq/L	*<135 mEq/L*
Cellular shrinking due to hypertonic extracellular fluid; may cause central nervous system irritability, convulsions, tachycardia, dry and flushed skin, pulmonary edema, hypertension, thirst, elevated temperature, rapid pulse, weight loss, oliguria, anuria	Cellular swelling; may cause cerebral edema, headache, stupor, coma, peripheral edema, polyuria, absence of thirst, decreased body temperature, rapid pulse, hypotension, nausea, vomiting
Potassium	
Hypokalemia	*Hyperkalemia*
>5.5 mEq/L	*<3.5 mEq/L*
Depressed conductivity in heart, muscle cramping, paresthesias, nausea, diarrhea; associated with metabolic acidosis	Cardiac irritability, dysrhythmias, vomiting, paralytic ileus, thirst; associated with metabolic alkalosis, inability to concentrate urine
Calcium	
Hypercalcemia	*Hypocalcemia*
>12 mg/dl	*<8.5 mg/dl*
Decreased neuromuscular excitability, muscle weakness, central nervous system depression, stupor to coma, increased risk of bone fracture, vomiting, constipation, kidney stones	Increased neuromuscular excitability, skeletal muscle cramps, tetany, laryngospasm, asphyxiation, death
Phosphate	
Hyperphosphatemia	*Hypophosphatemia*
>4.5 mg/dl	*<2.0 mg/dl*
See Hypocalcemia	Anorexia, weakness, osteomalacia, muscle weakness, tremors, seizures, coma, anemia, bleeding disorders, leukocytic alterations
Magnesium	
Hypermagnesemia	*Hypomagnesemia*
>2.5 mEq/L	*<1.5 mEq/L*
Skeletal muscle depression, muscle weakness, hypotension, bradycardia, respiratory depression	Hypocalcemia and hypokalemia, neuromuscular irritability, tetany, convulsions, tachycardia, hypertension

blood that are not routinely measured; that is, phosphates, sulfates, and protein anions. Therefore, assuming that no abnormal anions are present, an individual's serum sodium and potassium should equal the chloride + bicarbonate + 12 mEq/L of unmeasured, normal anions. If this is true, then the individual would have a normal **anion gap.** This may be expressed by the following formula:

$$Na^+ + K^+ = Cl^- + HCO_3^- + 12 \text{ mEq/L of unmeasured anions}$$

In metabolic acidosis, a normal anion gap is related to bicarbonate loss and retention of chloride to maintain an ionic balance. This is described as hyperchloremic metabolic acidosis.

The significance of an abnormally large anion gap is that an abnormal anion is present in the blood from lactic acid, ketone bodies, salicylates, etc. When this is the case, the individual will have a low bicarbonate level, but there is not a corresponding increase in chloride. The anion gap will be greater than 12 mEq/L. If the anion gap is normal but the Cl^- has increased and the HCO_3^- is low, the metabolic acidosis may be due to diarrhea, ammonium chloride ingestion, or renal dysfunction.

Comparison of Common Acid-Base Disturbances

Disturbance	Primary Disturbance	Correction/Compensation	Usual Causes
Metabolic acidosis $HCO_3^- < 24$ mEq/L	Excess endogenous acid depletes bicarbonate or bicarbonate is lost by kidneys	Hyperventilation (respiratory compensation) lowers pCO_2; kidneys (renal correction) excrete more hydrogen ions and retain more bicarbonate	Renal failure, ketosis, aspirin poisoning, overproduction of lactic acid
Respiratory acidosis ($pCO_2 > 45$ mm Hg)	Inefficient excretion of carbon dioxide by lungs	Additional bicarbonate retention and H^+ excretion by kidneys (renal compensation)	Chronic pulmonary disease, drug depression of respiratory center
Metabolic alkalosis ($HCO_3^- > 26$ mEq/L)	Excess plasma bicarbonate	Hypoventilation (respiratory compensation) raises pCO_2 to acidify blood; kidneys (renal correction) increase H^+ retention and excrete HCO_3^-	Loss of gastric juice, chloride depletion, excess corticosteroid hormones, ingestion of excessive bicarbonate or other antacids
Respiratory alkalosis ($pCO_2 < 35$ mm Hg)	Hyperventilation lowers pCO_2	Increased excretion of bicarbonate and retention of H^+ by kidneys (renal compensation)	Severe anxiety with hyperventilation, central nervous system disease, hypoxia, pulmonary imbalances

Practice Examination

1. The total water loss per day in the adult is approximately:
   a. 0.8 liter.
   b. 1.2 liters.
   c. 1.8 liters.
   d. 2.2 liters.
   e. 2.8 liters.

2. Of the 60% of the body weight made up of water, about two-thirds is:
   a. extracellular water.
   b. intracellular water.
   c. intravascular water.
   d. interstitial water.
   e. None of the above is correct.

3. Sodium is responsible for:
   a. ICF osmotic balance.
   b. ECF osmotic balance.
   c. TBW osmolality.
   d. osmotic equilibrium.

4. A milliequivalent is a unit of:
   a. mass.
   b. physical activity.
   c. chemical activity.
   d. osmotic concentration.

5. Which statement is true?
   a. The number of ions and anions in the body must be equal.
   b. Intravascular molecules of protein are without charge.
   c. The sodium ions must be united with chloride ions.
   d. The positive and negative charges in blood plasma must be equal to each other.

6. Aldosterone controls ECF volume by:
   a. carbohydrate, fat, and protein catabolism.
   b. sodium reabsorption.
   c. potassium reabsorption.
   d. water reabsorption.
   e. Both b and d are correct.

7. The release of ADH is *not* stimulated by:
   a. stress.
   b. hyponatremia.
   c. hypernatremia.
   d. an increase in plasma osmolality.
   e. a decrease in plasma volume.

Match the term with its definition.

_____ 8. hydrostatic pressure

_____ 9. oncotic pressure

a. water-pulling effect of plasma proteins

b. pressure of blood within the capillaries

c. mechanism to move fluid to lymph glands

d. movement of fluid through semipermeable membranes

---

10. Laboratory studies of an adult reveal the following:
    Plasma sodium = 110 mEq/L
    Plasma chloride = 85 mEq/L
    Plasma potassium = 4.8 mEq/L
    Plasma calcium = 5.2 mEq/L
    Plasma bicarbonate = 26 mEq/L
    The most likely alteration is:
    a. base bicarbonate deficit (metabolic acidosis).
    b. hypokalemia.
    c. hyponatremia.
    d. base bicarbonate excess (metabolic alkalosis).
    e. calcium deficit.

11. An individual suffers from weakness, dizziness, irritability, and intestinal cramps. Laboratory studies reveal the following:
    Plasma sodium = 138 mEq/L
    Plasma potassium = 6.8 mEq/L
    Blood pH = 7.38
    Plasma bicarbonate = 25 mEq/L
    An EKG with tall, peaked T wave but otherwise normal
    The individual is suffering from:
    a. hypernatremia.
    b. hyponatremia.
    c. hypercalcemia.
    d. hyperkalemia.
    e. hypokalemia.

12. An acid is:
    a. an anion.
    b. a cation.
    c. a substance/chemical that combines with a hydrogen ion to lower pH.
    d. a substance/chemical that donates a hydrogen ion or a proton to the solution.

13. Strong acids (more than one answer may be correct):
    a. include phosphoric acid.
    b. contribute many H^+ to the solution.
    c. have a pH of 7.
    d. have a pH of 14.
    e. are eliminated by the renal tubules.
    f. are good buffers.

14. The blood pH is maintained near 7.4 by buffering systems. The sequence from the fastest acting to the slowest acting system is:
    a. lungs, kidneys, blood buffers.
    b. blood buffers, lungs, kidneys.
    c. blood buffers, kidneys, lungs.
    d. lungs, blood buffers, kidneys.

15. The pH of saliva is about 7 and the pH of gastric juice is about 2. How many times more concentrated is the hydrogen ion in gastric juice than in saliva?
    a. 5
    b. 50
    c. 100
    d. 10,000
    e. 100,000

16. Which would *not* shift the blood pH toward alkalosis?
    a. hydrogen ion secretion into urine
    b. exhalation of carbon dioxide
    c. bicarbonate ion secretion into urine
    d. All of the above would shift the blood pH toward alkalosis.
    e. None of the above would do so.

17. A young female became quite agitated and apprehensive and eventually lost consciousness. At the hospital emergency room, the following laboratory values were obtained:
    Plasma sodium = 137 mEq/L
    Plasma potassium = 5.0 mEq/L
    Blood pH = 7.53
    Serum CO_2 = 22 mm Hg
    Plasma bicarbonate = 24 mEq/L
    Her immediate diagnosis was:
    a. hypokalemia.
    b. metabolic acidosis.
    c. metabolic alkalosis.
    d. respiratory acidosis.
    e. respiratory alkalosis.

18. As HCO_3^- shifts from the red blood cell to the blood plasma, it is expected that the plasma:
    a. Na^+ increases.
    b. Cl^- shifts into the red blood cell.
    c. K^+ increases.
    d. pH decreases.

Match the acid-base imbalance with the probable cause.

_____19. respiratory acidosis

_____20. respiratory alkalosis

_____21. metabolic alkalosis

a. severe anxiety

b. diabetes

c. chronic diarrhea

d. emphysema

e. excessive baking soda ingestion

Match the acid-base imbalance with the compensatory mechanism.

_____22. respiratory acidosis

_____23. respiratory alkalosis

_____24. metabolic acidosis

a. kidneys retain H^+ and excrete HCO_3^-

b. kidneys excrete H^+ and retain HCO_3^-

c. respirations increase, more CO_2 is eliminated

d. respirations decrease, more CO_2 is retained

25. An elevated anion gap is associated with an accumulation of:
    a. chloride anions.
    b. lactate anion.
    c. Both a and b are correct.
    d. Neither a nor b is correct.

Immunity

5

Objectives

After reviewing this chapter, the learner will be able to do the following:

1. **Distinguish between natural and acquired immunity between humoral and cell-mediated immunity, and between central and peripheral lymphoid organs.**
   Review pages 127 and 129-130; refer to Figures 5-1 through 5-5 and 5-8, and Table 5-1.

2. **Distinguish among the HLA complex, the ABO system, and the Rh system.**
   Review pages 133-135; refer to Figures 5-6 and 5-7.

3. **Describe the role of the B cell in humoral immunity.**
   Review pages 135 and 140; refer to Figures 5-5 and 5-8.

4. **Identify the structure and an important role for each of the five classes of immunoglobulins.**
   Review pages 135-138 and 140-141; refer to Figures 5-9 through 5-12 and Tables 5-2 and 5-3.

5. **Describe the secretory immune system.**
   Review page 142 and Figure 5-4.

6. **Describe the role of the T cell in cellular immunity.**
   Review pages 142-144; refer to Figures 5-14 and 5-15 and Table 5-4.

7. **Distinguish between primary and secondary immune responses.**
   Review page 144; refer to Figure 5-13.

8. **Characterize the interactions within the immune response; describe the cytokines.**
   Review pages 144-145 and 147-150; refer to Figures 5-16 through 5-19 and Table 5-5.

9. **Compare pediatric immune function to immune function in the elderly.**
   Review pages 149-150.

Practice Examination

Match the term with its definition or characteristic.

_____ 1. phagocytosis

_____ 2. specific immunity

_____ 3. macrophage

_____ 4. nonspecific immunity

_____ 5. antigen

a. immunoglobulins, lymphokines

b. lymphocyte that attacks antibodies directly

c. ingestion and destruction

d. phagocytic, agranular leukocyte of the immune system

e. resistant to a large variety of antigens

f. macromolecular pattern for antibody production

g. protein produced by T cells

h. exclusively thymus-dependent

6. Antigenicity depends on:
   a. chemical structure.
   b. foreignness.
   c. complexity.
   d. Both b and c are correct.
   e. a, b, and c are correct.

7. The HLA complex:
   a. has both A and B antibodies.
   b. antigens are found on the surfaces of most cells except erythrocytes.
   c. is an antigen system found on erythrocytes.
   d. None of the above is correct.

8. When antigen binds to its appropriate antibody:
   a. agglutination may occur.
   b. phagocytosis may occur.
   c. antigen neutralization may occur.
   d. All of the above are correct.
   e. None of the above is correct.

9. Antibodies are produced by:
   a. B cells.
   b. T cells.
   c. helper cells.
   d. plasma cells.
   e. memory cells.

10. An immunoglobulin contains:
    a. two heavy and two light polypeptide chains.
    b. four heavy and four light polypeptide chains.
    c. two heavy and four light polypeptide chains.
    d. four heavy and two light polypeptide chains.

11. The antibody class having the highest concentration in the blood is:
    a. IgA.
    b. IgD.
    c. IgE.
    d. IgG.
    e. IgM.

12. Which antibody is matched with its appropriate role?
    a. IgA/allergic reactions
    b. IgD/found in respiratory secretions
    c. IgE/found in gastric secretions
    d. IgG/first to challenge the antigen
    e. IgM/first to challenge the antigen

13. The primary immune response involves:
    a. a rapid plasma cell response with peak antibody by 3 days.
    b. macrophage production of antibodies.
    c. T cell production of antibodies.
    d. a latent period followed by peak antibody production.

14. Which cells are phagocytic?
    a. B cells
    b. T cells
    c. T suppressors
    d. T killers
    e. macrophages

15. When a child develops measles and acquires an immunity to subsequent infections, the immunity is:
    a. acquired.
    b. active.
    c. natural.
    d. Both a and b are correct.

Match the term with its descriptor.

_____16. superantigens

_____17. epitopes

_____18. monoclonal antibodies

_____19. mucous membrane

_____20. memory cell

a. antigenic determinants

b. useful for diagnosis

c. first line of defense

d. increased activation signal and immune response

e. secretes antibodies

f. long-term immunity

g. produced after initial contact with an antigen

h. predominant antibody of secondary response

Match the lymphocytic activity with the involvement.

_____21. capable of forming clones

_____22. produces lymphokines

_____23. helper and suppressor cells

_____24. antibody formation

_____25. cell-mediated response

a. T cell involvement

b. B cell involvement

c. both T cell and B cell involvement

6

Inflammation

After reviewing this chapter, the learner will be able to do the following:

1. **Describe inflammation and contrast it to immunity.**
   Review pages 153-154; refer to Figures 6-1 through 6-3.

2. **Indicate the causes of mast cell degranulation and the effects of vasoactive amines and chemotactic factors.**
   Review pages 155 and 157; refer to Figures 6-4 and 6-5.

3. **State the effects of the synthetic products of the mast cell.**
   Review page 157; refer to Figure 6-4.

4. **Identify the plasma protein systems and their interactions in inflammation.**
   Review pages 158-162; refer to Figures 6-6 through 6-13.

5. **Identify a role for neutrophils, monocytes, macrophages, and eosinophils in the inflammatory process.**
   Review pages 164-167; refer to Figures 6-14 through 6-18.

6. **State the roles for inflammatory cytokines; note their relationships within the immune system.**
   Review pages 168-170; refer to Figures 6-19 and 6-20.

7. **Name and describe the local and systemic manifestations of inflammation.**
   Review pages 170-171; refer to Table 6-1.

8. **Characterize chronic inflammation.**
   Review pages 171-172; refer to Figure 6-21.

9. **Differentiate between the resolution and repair processes; identify the adverse factors affecting wound healing.**
   Review pages 173 and 175-177; refer to Figures 6-22 through 6-24.

10. **Compare pediatric to aging self-defense mechanisms.**
    Review page 177.

Practice Examination

1. Inflammation:
   a. destroys injurious agents.
   b. confines injurious agents.
   c. stimulates and enhances immunity.
   d. promotes healing.
   e. All of the above are correct.

2. Inflammatory microcirculation changes involve all of the following *except:*
   a. vasodilation.
   b. days to develop.
   c. increased vascular permeability.
   d. exudation of leukocytes to injury site.

3. A phagocyte's role begins with an inflammatory response. The sequence for phagocytosis is:
   a. margination or pavementing, recognition of the target, adherence or binding, fusion with lysosomes inside the phagocyte.
   b. diapedesis, margination or pavementing, phagosome formation, recognition of the target, fusion with lysosomes inside the phagocyte.
   c. recognition of the target, margination or pavementing, destruction of the target by lysosomal enzymes.
   d. margination, diapedesis, recognition, adherence, ingestion, fusion with lysosomes inside the phagocyte, destruction of the target.

4. Chemotactic factors for phagocytes include all of the following *except:*
   a. complement components.
   b. streptolysins.
   c. plasminogen activator.
   d. prostaglandins.
   e. mast cell degranulation products.

5. Which is *not* a local manifestation of inflammation?
   a. swelling
   b. pain
   c. heat
   d. leukocytosis
   e. redness

6. Complement is:
   a. a series of proteins in the blood.
   b. an antibody.
   c. a hormone.
   d. a lymphokine.

7. Diapedesis is a process in which:
   a. neutrophils migrate from the bloodstream to an injured tissue site.
   b. phagocytes stick to capillary and venule walls.
   c. bacteria are "coated" with an opsonin.
   d. there is oxygen-dependent killing of cells.

8. Interferon:
   a. interferes with the ability of bacteria to cause disease.
   b. prevents viruses from infecting healthy host cells.
   c. inhibits macrophage migration from inflamed sites.
   d. increases the phagocytic activity of macrophages.
   e. increases the number of circulating neutrophils.

9. The complement system can be activated by:
   a. the binding of complement 1 to a complement binding site of an antibody.
   b. components of other plasma protein systems.
   c. the binding of complement 3 to bacteria.
   d. Both a and c are correct.
   e. a, b, and c are correct.

10. Which is *not* a systemic manifestation of inflammation?
    a. leukocytosis
    b. fever
    c. increased acute-phase reactants
    d. exudation

11. The inflammatory response:
    a. prevents blood from entering the injured tissue.
    b. elevates body temperature to prevent spread of infection.
    c. prevents formation of abscesses.
    d. minimizes injury and promotes healing.

12. Scar tissue is:
    a. nonfunctional collagenous and fibrotic tissue.
    b. functional tissue that follows wound healing.
    c. regenerated tissue formed in the area of injury.
    d. fibrinogen that has entrapped phagocytes and neurons.

13. Repair involves processes that:
    a. fill in the wound.
    b. cover or seal the wound.
    c. shrink the wound.
    d. Both a and b are correct.
    e. a, b, and c are correct.

14. Swelling during acute inflammation is caused by:
    a. collagenase.
    b. fluid and cellular exudation.
    c. lymphocytic margination.
    d. neutrophilic margination.
    e. anaerobic glycolysis.

15. Which is *not* released from mast cells during degranulation?
    a. chemotactic factors
    b. histamine
    c. complement
    d. vasoactive amines

16. Chronic inflammation is characterized by:
    a. hypertrophy.
    b. metaplasia.
    c. neutrophilic infiltration.
    d. lymphocytic and macrophagic infiltration.
    e. All of the above are correct.

17. Which is synthesized by mast cells?
    a. histamine
    b. serotonin
    c. neutrophil chemotactic factor
    d. leukotrienes
    e. eosinophil chemotactic factor

18. Primary intention healing:
    a. involves collagen synthesis.
    b. requires little wound contraction.
    c. requires little wound epithelialization.
    d. Both b and c are correct.
    e. a, b, and c are correct.

19. Interleukins:
    a. provide messages between leukocytes.
    b. are produced in response to tissue injury.
    c. stimulate cells to produce antiviral substances.
    d. increase antibody production and populations of
       T cells.
    e. All of the above are correct.

20. Eosinophils:
    a. are agranulocytes.
    b. control the vascular effects of serotonin and hist-
       amine by lysosomal mediators.
    c. have a lysosomal protein that can dissolve the
       surface membranes of parasites.
    d. All of the above are correct.
    e. Both b and c are correct.

Match the term with its definition or characteristic.

_____21. resolution

_____22. bradykinin

_____23. granulation tissue

_____24. IL-10

_____25. scar

a. increases the phagocytic activity of macrophages

b. original structure and physiologic function

c. inhibits macrophage migration from the inflamed area

d. increases vascular permeability

e. new capillaries, fibroblasts, and macrophages

f. avascular

g. inhibits production of pro-inflammatory cytokines

h. proliferates antigen-specific clones of B and T cells

7

Hypersensitivities, Infection, and Immunodeficiencies

a. **Chart the development and activities of specific immunity.**
   Review pages 127 and 129-130; refer to Figures 5-1 through 5-6 and 5-8.

MEMORY CHECK!

Bone marrow

↓

Lymphocyte stem cell

Thymus   Human bursal equivalent

↓   ↓

Immunocompetent T cell   Immunocompetent B cell
(Receptor generation)   (Receptor generation)

↓   ↓

Lymphoid tissue ◄——— Antigenic challenge ———► Lymphoid tissue
                     Macrophage processing

↓   ↓

Specific cellular immunity   **Specific humoral immunity**
Clonal selection   **Clonal selection**

- Memory cells   - Memory cells
- T suppressors   - IgG producers
- T cytotoxic (killer)   - IgM producers
- T helpers   - IgA producers
- T lymphokine producers   - IgE producers

                        Antigens neutralized

- Fungi   - Bacteria toxins
- Parasites   - Viruses
- Intracellular viruses
- Neoplastic cells
- Transplanted cells

                        Antigenic destruction/removal

- Cell membrane perforation   - Phagocytosis
- Recruitment and activation of macrophage mechanisms

30

b. **Compare innate (nonspecific) defenses to acquired (specific) immunity.**
    Review pages 127 and 153 and Summary Reviews on pages 150-151 and 178.

MEMORY CHECK!

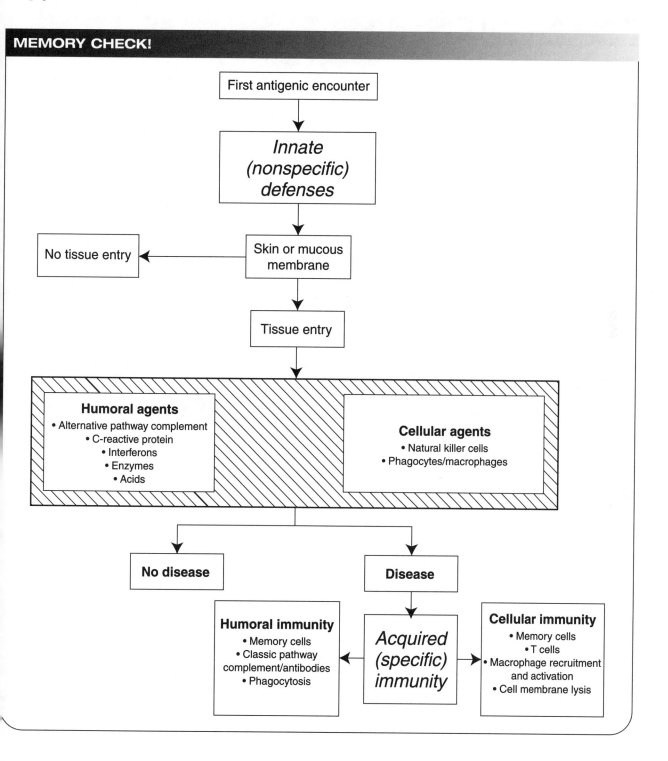

c. **Identify the source and function of the major cytokines.**
   Review Table 5-5.

MEMORY CHECK!

Memory Check!

Types	Sources	Function
Interleukins (ILs) IL-1	Macrophages	Increase inflammatory and immune responses
IL-2	Helper T cells	Increase T cells and NK cells
IL-3	T cells, mast cells, NK cells	Growth factor for immature hematopoietic cells
IL-4	T cells, mast cells	Increase immune and chronic inflammatory responses
IL-5 through IL-17	Various cells	Increase B and T cells; modify activity of other cytokines; elevate inflammatory responses
Interferons (IFNs)	B and T cells, macrophages, fibroblasts, epithelial cells	Antiviral protection; decrease neoplastic growth; regulate interleukins
Tumor necrosis factors (TNFs)	T cells, macrophages	Tumor cytotoxicity; increase inflammatory and immune responses
Colony-stimulating factors (CSFs)	Various cells	Myelocytic stem cell growth factor; macrophage growth factor
Transforming growth factor (TGF)	Lymphocytes, macrophages, platelets, bone	Macrophage chemotaxis; stimulate fibroblasts

d. **Diagram the interrelationships between cell-mediated immunity and humoral immunity.**
   Refer to Figures 5-16 through 5-18 and Table 5-5.

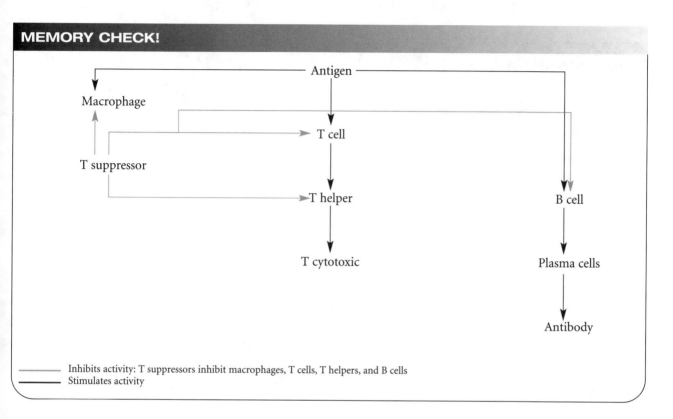

MEMORY CHECK!

_____ Inhibits activity: T suppressors inhibit macrophages, T cells, T helpers, and B cells
━━━━━━ Stimulates activity

e. **Diagram the interaction between lymphocytes and phagocytes.**
   Refer to Figure 5-17.

MEMORY CHECK!

Note: There is interaction between specific and nonspecific areas of the immune system. The phagocytes cannot specifically recognize antigens but process and present them to the lymphocytes. Lymphocytes specifically recognize and produce antibodies or lymphokines, which help the phagocytes combat the antigen.

f. **Diagram a scheme for complement's role in the amplification of the immune response. Relate opsonization, inflammation, and cytolysis to the components of complement.**
  Review pages 158-160; refer to Figures 6-6 and 6-8.

MEMORY CHECK!

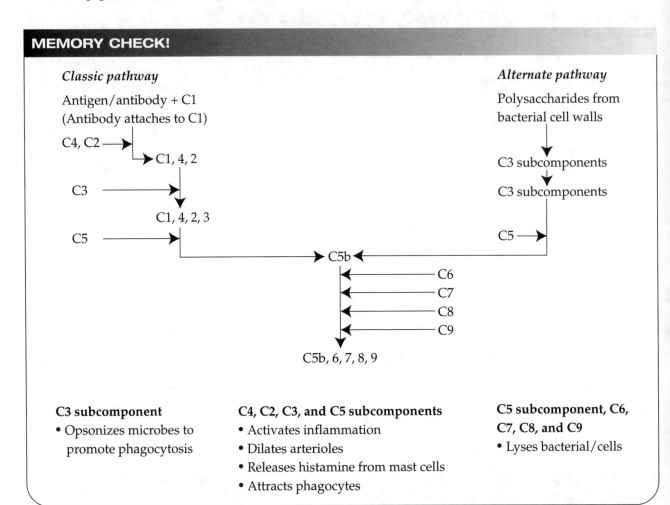

C3 subcomponent
• Opsonizes microbes to promote phagocytosis

C4, C2, C3, and C5 subcomponents
• Activates inflammation
• Dilates arterioles
• Releases histamine from mast cells
• Attracts phagocytes

C5 subcomponent, C6, C7, C8, and C9
• Lyses bacterial/cells

g. **Diagram the consequences of the acute inflammatory process.**
   Review page 154; refer to Figure 6-2.

MEMORY CHECK!

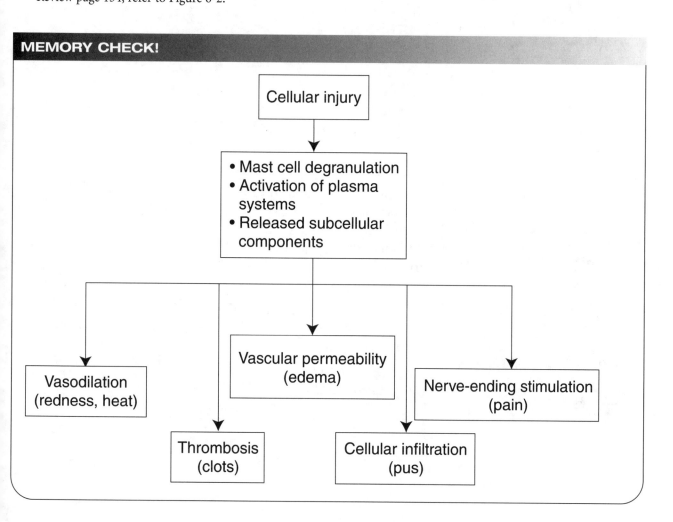

h. Diagram the consequences of the chronic inflammatory process.
   Review pages 171-172; refer to Figure 6-21.

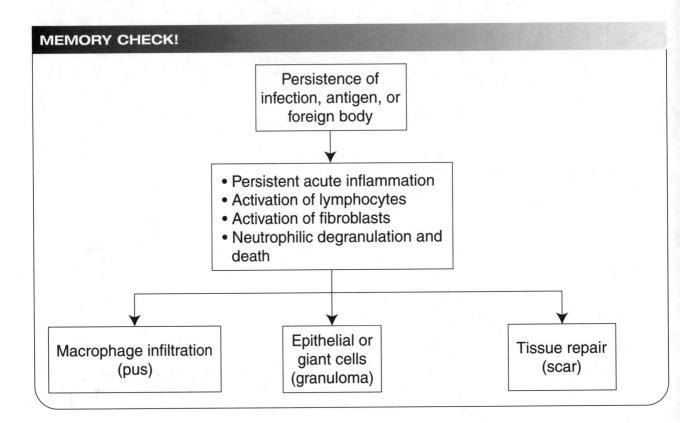

i. Diagram the difference between regeneration and repair.
   Review pages 173 and 175-177.

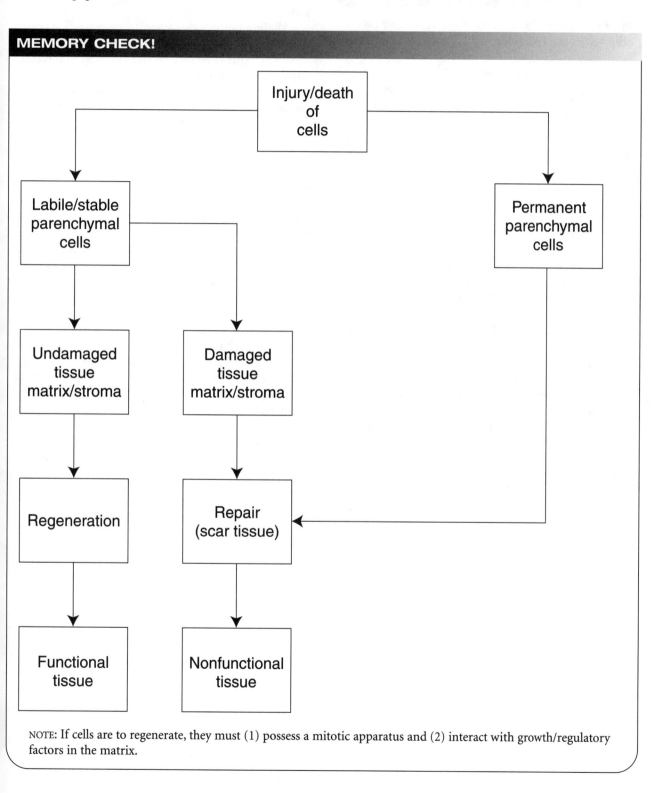

NOTE: If cells are to regenerate, they must (1) possess a mitotic apparatus and (2) interact with growth/regulatory factors in the matrix.

Objectives

After studying this chapter, the learner will be able to do the following:

1. **Compare the four hypersensitivities.**
   Study pages 182 and 184-190; refer to Figures 7-1 through 7-7 and Tables 7-1 and 7-3 through 7-5.

   Hypersensitivity is an excessive immunologic reaction to an antigen that results in a pathologic response after reexposure to the same antigen. Allergy, autoimmunity, and alloimmunity are all hypersensitivity responses. The difference is the source of the antigen to which the hypersensitivity is directed.
   (See box on page 30 of *Workbook*.)

2. **Describe the likely causes of autoimmune and alloimmune diseases; cite examples.**
   Study pages 190-192; refer to Tables 7-2 and 7-6.

   Self-antigens are usually tolerated by the host's own immune system. This immunologic tolerance develops in humans during the embryonic period. Autoreactive lymphocytes are either eliminated or suppressed. **Autoimmunity** is a breakdown of tolerance in which the body's immune system begins to recognize self-antigens as foreign. The mechanisms of breakdown of tolerance are varied and often unknown. Mechanisms implicated in the development of autoimmunity include alterations of self-antigenic markers by infectious diseases and genetic factors associated with the products of the HLA locus or the histocompatibility-complex-linked immune response genes.

   Alloimmunity occurs when an individual's immune system reacts against antigens of the tissues of other members of the same species. Two examples of this reactivity are transient neonatal diseases and transplant rejection and transfusion reactions. Because a fetus has mother and father antigens, fetal paternal antigens different from maternal antigens can cross the placenta and elicit an immune response in the mother. Maternally produced antibody may be transported into the fetal circulation to produce alloimmune disease in the fetus. Examples of diseases that can affect the fetus, neonate, or child include Graves disease, myasthenia gravis, systemic lupus erythematosus, immune thrombocytopenic purpura, and erythroblastosis fetalis.

   Transplantation of organs is commonly complicated by an immune response against donor antigens. The primary mechanism of the rejection of transplanted organs is a Type IV, cell-mediated reaction. HLA antigens are the principal targets of the rejection reaction.

   Transplant rejection is classified as hyperacute, acute, or chronic depending on the amount of time that elapses between transplantation and rejection. Hyperacute rejection usually occurs in recipients having preexisting IgG or IgM antibody to antigens in the graft. As circulation to the graft is reestablished, antibody binds to the grafted tissue and activates the inflammatory response. This response initiates the coagulation or blood-clotting cascade, which results in cessation of blood flow into the graft.

Comparison of Hypersensitivity Disorders

Hypersensitivity	Immunity/Response Time	Effectors	Examples
Type I IgE-mediated Anaphylactic	Humoral/immediate	*Antigen* reacts with IgE bound to mast *cells, histamine* release, histamine effects	Allergy Allergic rhinitis asthma, urticaria, food allergies, anaphylactic shock

Type II
Cytotoxic
Tissue-specific
	Humoral/immediate	*IgG* or *IgM* reacts with *antigen* on cell's membrane, *complement* is activated, lysis or phagocytosis of cells, cell-mediated cytolysis, antibody binding to receptors	Allergy
			  Immediate drug reaction
			Autoimmunity
			  Hemolytic anemia, Graves disease
			Alloimmunity
			  Transfused blood cells, hemolytic disease of the newborn

Type III
Immune complex
	Humoral/immediate	*IgG* or *IgM* unites with *antigen* to form a complex that is deposited in vessel walls or tissues, neutrophil attraction, *complement* activation, *lysosomal enzymes* injure tissue	Allergy
			  Arthus reaction, allergic alveolitis
			Autoimmunity
			  Serum sickness, celiac disease, glomerulonephritis, systemic lupus erythematosus

Type IV
Cell-mediated
	Cellular/delayed	Reaction of sensitized *T lymphocytes with antigen* leads to *lymphokine* release, recruitment of *macrophages* and subsequent *lysosomal release*	Allergy
			  Contact dermatitis
			Autoimmunity
			  Hashimoto thyroiditis, rheumatoid arthritis
			Alloimmunity
			  Graft rejection, tuberculin reaction

NOTE: Rarely is a particular disorder associated with a single mechanism.

Acute rejection is a cell-mediated immune response that occurs approximately 2 weeks after the transplantation. The recipient develops an immune response against unmatched HLA antigens and shows an infiltration of lymphocytes and macrophages characteristic of Type IV hypersensitivity reactions.

Chronic rejection may occur after months or years of normal function. It is characterized by slow, progressive organ failure. Chronic rejection may be caused by inflammatory damage to endothelial cells lining blood vessels. It is likely a result of a weak immunologic reaction against minor histocompatibility antigens on the grafted tissue.

3. **Describe the relationships between humans and infectious agents.**
   Study pages 192-197; refer to Figures 7-8 through 7-10 and Tables 7-9 and 7-10.

Many microbes grow and flourish in our bodies. Symbiosis, mutualism, commensalism, and pathogenicity are relationships between hosts and microorganisms. **Symbiosis** benefits the human without harming the microbe. **Mutualism** benefits both host and microbe. **Commensalism** benefits the microorganism without harming the human host. **Pathogenicity** benefits the microbe while harming the human host.

Pathogens injure cells and tissue because they circumvent the defensive barriers, the inflammatory system, and the immune system of the host. Pathogenic microbes directly damage cells, interfere with cellular metabolism, and render the cell dysfunctional because of their increased numbers.

A bacterial pathogen's **virulence** or ability to cause disease is increased by enzymes and either exotoxins or endotoxins. Some bacteria produce thick capsules of carbohydrate or protein that are antiphagocytic. Viral pathogens bypass many defense mechanisms because they develop intracellularly; thus they avoid inflammatory or immune responses.

The first line of human host defense against infectious organisms is the intact skin and mucous membranes. The digestive, respiratory, and genitourinary tracts form a closed barrier between the internal organs and external environment. The second and third lines of defense are the inflammatory response and immune system including the lymphatic system. The lymphatic system provides a network for internal defensive products to circulate throughout the body.

4. **Describe the mechanisms of infection and cellular injury by bacteria, viruses, and fungi.**
   Study pages 197-199 and 201-202; refer to Figures 7-13 and 7-15 and Tables 7-11 through 7-13.

Bacteria are prokaryotes lacking discrete nuclei; they are relatively small. Their survival and growth depend on the effectiveness of the host's defense mechanisms and on the bacterium's ability to resist these defenses. Some bacteria have coatings that protect them from phagocytosis. These coatings include polysaccharide coverings for the pneumococcus, the waxy capsule surrounding the tubercle bacillus, and the M protein cell wall of the streptococcus.

Other bacteria survive and proliferate in the body by producing hemolysins, leukocidins, coagulases, exotoxins, and endotoxins that injure cells and tissues. **Exotoxins** are metabolic proteins released into the environment primarily from gram-positive bacteria during bacterial growth. These proteins have highly specific effects on host cells. **Endotoxins** are lipopolysaccharides contained in the cell walls of gram-negative bacteria that are released from cell walls during lysis or destruction of the bacteria. Their effects are generalized. Endotoxins can be released from the bacterial membrane during treatment with antibiotics. Therefore, antibiotics cannot prevent the toxic effects of endotoxins. Once in the host's blood, endotoxins cause the release of vasoactive peptides that produce vasodilation. This, in turn, reduces blood pressure, decreases oxygen delivery, and can result in cardiovascular shock.

Viruses are intracellular parasites that take over the genetic and metabolic machinery of host cells and use them for their own survival and replication. Viruses contain genetic information in either DNA or RNA. This genetic material is protected by a protein coat that must be removed in the cytoplasm of the host cell if the virus is to replicate. Viruses are incapable of independent reproduction; replication depends totally on their ability to infect a **permissive** host cell—a cell unable to resist viral invasion and replication. Infection with a virus requires its binding to a **specific receptor** on the plasma membrane of the host cell. Viral replication depends on absorption, penetration, uncoating, replication, assembly, and release of new virions.

Once inside the host cell, virions have many harmful effects, including the following: (1) cell protein synthesis cessation, (2) disruption of lysosomal membranes resulting in release of enzymes that can kill the host cell, (3) fusion of host cells, (4) alteration of antigenic properties causing the immune system to attack the host cell as if it were foreign, and (5) transformation of host cells into cancerous cells. Cells damaged by viruses may enable secondary bacterial infections to develop.

Fungi are relatively large organisms with thick walls that grow as either single-celled yeasts or multicelled molds. Molds are aerobic, and yeasts are facultative anaerobes. Pathogenic fungi release mycotoxins and enzymes that damage connective tissues.

Diseases caused by fungi are called **mycoses.** Most fungi grow as parasites on or near skin or mucous membranes and usually produce mild and superficial disease. Injury to tissue can lead to secondary bacterial infection.

Fungi causing deep infection enter the body through inhalation or through open wounds. Deep infections are most common in association with other diseases or as opportunistic infections in immunosuppressed individuals. Some fungi are part of the normal body flora and become pathogenic when antibiotics kill bacteria that normally compete for nutrients and preclude fungal growth. For example, yeasts in the vagina may undergo rapid proliferation when vaginal bacteria are killed by antibiotics.

5. **Characterize immunodeficiencies; describe examples of congenital or primary diseases.**
   Study pages 206-209; refer to Figure 7-16 and Table 7-17.

Immune deficiencies occur because of impaired function of one or more components of the immune or inflammatory response. B cells, T cells, phagocytic cells, or complement may be involved. The clinical manifestation of immune deficiency is a tendency to develop unusual or recurrent severe infections. Deficiencies in T cell immune responses are suspected when recurrent infections are caused by certain viruses, fungi, and yeasts or certain atypical organisms. B cell deficiencies are suspected if the individual has recurrent infections with encapsulated bacteria or viruses against which humoral immunity is normally effective.

It may be unsafe to administer conventional immunizing agents or blood products to many immunologically compromised individuals because of the risk that the immunizing agent will cause an uncontrolled infection. Uncontrolled infection is a problem particularly when attenuated vaccines that contain live, but weakened, microorganisms are used. Vaccinia virus used for immunization against smallpox is an example of such a vaccine.

Although the virus is attenuated enough to be destroyed by a normal immune system, it can survive, multiply, and cause severe disease in an immunodeficient recipient.

Individuals with immune deficiencies are also at risk for graft-versus-host disease. This occurs if T cells in transfused blood are mature and capable of the cell-mediated destruction of tissues in the graft recipient. The grafted T cells are controlled by normal immune systems and no tissue destruction occurs. If the recipient's immune system is deficient, the grafted T cells will attack the recipient's tissue.

Congenital or primary immune deficiency occurs if lymphocyte development is disturbed in the fetus or embryo or if there is a genetic anomaly. Some diseases are primarily caused by a defect in one or the other of the cell lines, although both T and B cell lines may be partially deficient.

Severe combined immune deficiencies (SCID) occur when a common stem cell for all white blood cells is absent. Therefore, T cells, B cells, and phagocytic cells never develop. Most children with SCID caused by reticular dysgenesis, the most severe SCID form, die in utero or very soon after birth. Many individuals with SCID are deficient only in a stem cell for lymphocyte development rather than for all white blood cells, as in reticular dysgenesis, and therefore have normal numbers of all other white cells. T and B lymphocytes are few or totally absent in the circulation, the spleen, and the lymph nodes. The thymus is usually underdeveloped. IgM and IgA immunoglobulin levels are absent or greatly reduced; however, IgG levels may be almost normal because of the presence of maternal antibodies. Other forms of SCID are caused by autosomal recessive enzymatic defects that result in the accumulation of toxic metabolites to rapidly dividing lymphocytes.

DiGeorge syndrome is the complete lack or, more commonly, partial lack of the thymus. This thymus deficiency causes lymphopenia and greatly decreased T cell numbers and function. **Bruton agammaglobulinemia** is caused by failure of B cell precursors to become mature B cells because of the lack of normal bursal-equivalent tissue. There are few or no circulating B cells, though T cell number and function are normal.

Some immune deficiencies involve a defect that results in depressed development of a small portion of the immune system. An example is **Wiskott-Aldrich syndrome,** an X-linked recessive disorder, in which IgM antibody production is greatly depressed. Therefore, antibody responses against polysaccharide antigens from bacterial cell walls are deficient.

Another common defect in which a particular class of antibody is affected is selective IgA deficiency. Individuals with selective **IgA deficiency** are able to produce other classes of immunoglobulin but fail to produce IgA. Individuals with IgA deficiency often present with chronic intestinal candidiasis. IgA may normally prevent the uptake of allergens from the environment. Therefore, IgA deficiency may lead to increased allergen uptake and a more intense challenge to the immune system because of prolonged exposure to environmental antigens.

6. **Cite causes and consequences of acquired or secondary immune deficiencies.**
   Study pages 209-210.

Acquired or secondary immune and inflammatory deficiency develops after birth and is not related to genetic defects. **Nutritional deficits** in calorie or protein intake can lead to deficiencies in T cell function and numbers. The humoral immune response is less affected by starvation, although complement activity, neutrophilic chemotaxis, and bacterial killing by neutrophils are often depressed. Enzyme cofactors, such as zinc and vitamins, may result in severe depressions of both B and T cell function.

Iatrogenic disorders are caused by some form of medical treatment. Cancer chemotherapeutic agents suppress blood cell formation in the bone marrow. Immunosuppressive corticosteroids for treatment of individuals with transplants or autoimmune diseases depress B and T cell formation. The consequence of these therapies for cancer and immunosuppression is manifested as a progressive increase in infections with opportunistic microorganisms.

Trauma in burn victims makes these individuals more susceptible to severe bacterial infections because of decreased neutrophil function and complement levels. Burn victims also have increased suppressor cell function, which may increase antigen-specific suppression.

A relationship between **emotional stress** and depressed immune function seems to exist. Many lymphoid organs are innervated and can be affected by nerve stimulation. Also, lymphocytes have receptors for many hormones such as neurotransmitters and can respond to changing levels of these chemicals with increased or decreased function.

7. **Describe acquired immune deficiency syndrome (AIDS).**
   Study pages 210-211, 213, and 215-217; refer to Figures 7-17 through 7-22.

AIDS is caused by a virus currently named human immunodeficiency virus, or HIV. The virus was isolated by researchers at the National Institutes of Health as the human T-lymphotropic virus type III, or HLV-III, and earlier by the Pasteur Institute as the lymphadenopathy/AIDS virus, or LAV. At least one other AIDS virus (HIV-2) has been identified.

HIV is a retrovirus carrying genetic information in RNA rather than DNA. Retroviruses infect cells by binding a target cell through a surface receptor and inserting their RNA into the target cell. A viral enzyme, reverse transcriptase, converts the viral RNA to DNA and inserts that DNA into the infected cell's genetic material. Viral proliferation may occur, resulting in the lysis and death of the infected cell. If, however, the cell remains relatively dormant rather than active, the viral genetic material integrated into the infected cell's DNA may remain latent for years, if not for the life of the individual.

CD4 is an antigen on the surface of cells that acts as a receptor for the HIV. The virus primarily infects CD4–positive T helper lymphocytes, but it may also infect and lyse various other cells that express the CD4 antigen.

At the time of diagnosis, the individual may manifest one of four different conditions: serologically negative, serologically positive but asymptomatic, early stages of HIV disease, or AIDS. The currently accepted Centers for Disease Control definition of AIDS relies on both laboratory tests and clinical symptoms. The most common laboratory test is for antibodies against HIV. Without a positive test for antibodies, individuals can be diagnosed as having AIDS if they have a lymphoma of the brain and are less than 60 years of age or if they have lymphoid interstitial pneumonitis and are less than 13 years of age. If they are seropositive, the diagnosis of AIDS is made in association with a variety of clinical symptoms. These include disseminated coccidioidomycosis or histoplasmosis, extrapulmonary tuberculosis, persistent isosporiasis, recurrent salmonella septicemia, recurrent bacterial infections, HIV encephalopathy, HIV wasting syndrome, lymphoma of the brain at any age, non-Hodgkin lymphoma, and uterine cervical cancer. Other clinical symptoms of AIDS include persistent lymphadenopathy, weight loss, recurrent fevers, neurologic abnormalities with dementia in late stages, recurrent pulmonary infiltrates, and the development of opportunistic infections such as *Pneumocystis carinii* pneumonia and other atypical malignancies such as Kaposi sarcoma.

The major immunologic finding in AIDS is the striking decrease of T helper cells or CD4-positive cells. Suppressor cells that have the CD8 antigen are usually normal or slightly elevated. This results in a reversal of the normal helper-to-suppressor T cell ratio, which is about 1:9 (19 helpers to 10 suppressors). Most individuals with AIDS have ratios much lower than 0:9 (9 helpers to 10 suppressors). In contrast, B cell numbers are usually normal.

The presence of circulating antibody against the AIDS virus apparently indicates infection by the virus. Antibody appears soon after infection through blood products, usually within 4 to 7 weeks. After sexual exposure, the individual can be infected yet seronegative for 6 to 14 months. In the late stages of the disease, some individuals become seronegative because of a deficient immune system. The period between infection and the appearance of antibody is referred to as the window period. Although the patient may not have antibody, he or she may be viremic and infectious to others within 2 weeks of being infected.

Several antimicrobials have been tried in an effort to prevent viral replication. Reverse transcriptase inhibitors prevent conversion of the viral RNA into double-stranded DNA. Although most are effective in preventing AIDS virus replication in vitro, their efficacy in individuals generally has not been good. In addition, reverse transcriptase has a very high mutation rate that makes it rapidly become resistant to these antibiotics.

Protease inhibitors block the viral protease and prevent the production of proteins needed for viral replication. Resistant variants to multiple protease inhibitors have been identified, suggesting resistance to one may result in multiple resistance. Trials with protease inhibitors combined with reverse transcriptase inhibitors have yielded highly promising results. The current recommendations are for initial therapy with a combination of two different nucleoside reverse transcriptase inhibitors with one or two protease inhibitors.

The newest drugs to be considered are integrase inhibitors. Retroviruses integrate their genetic information into the infected cell's chromosomes using a viral enzyme, an integrase. Integrase inhibitors prevent that step of the infection. Without integration, HIV cannot make copies of itself and infect other cells.

Drug therapy for AIDS is difficult because the AIDS retrovirus incorporates into the genetic material of the host and may never be removed by antiviral therapy. Therefore, drug administration may have to continue for the lifetime of the individual.

The development of an effective AIDS vaccine has been slowed by several major difficulties. The AIDS virus is genetically and antigenically variable. Thus a vaccine created against one variant may not provide protection against another variant. This is a real problem, because as many as 30 to 40 different genetic variants have been isolated from the same individual during the progression of the disease. Many of these may coexist in the individual. Although individuals with AIDS have high levels of circulating antibodies against the virus, these antibodies do not appear to be protective. The AIDS virus is transmitted from cell to cell and may initially enter the body in an infected cell that is not susceptible to circulating antibody. Also, HIV-infected cells tend to fuse with other cells, so infection can spread to uninfected cells without viral particles being produced.

Finally, the only good model for AIDS experimentation is the chimpanzee, which is a protected animal species and relatively unavailable for medical research. Thus efficacy and toxicity of possible vaccines cannot easily be evaluated.

8. Describe some laboratory tests and replacement therapies for immunodeficiencies.
Study page 217; refer to Table 7-18.

Immunodeficiency syndromes usually are treated using replacement therapy. Deficient antibody production is treated by replacement of missing immunoglobulins with commercial gamma (γ) globulin preparations. Lymphocyte deficiencies are treated with the replacement of host lymphocytes with transplants of bone marrow, fetal liver, or fetal thymus from a donor.

Practice Examination

Match the condition with the immunologic mechanism.

_____ 1. Graves disease

_____ 2. serum sickness

_____ 3. allergic rhinitis

_____ 4. systemic lupus erythematosus

_____ 5. contact dermatitis

_____ 6. hemolytic anemia

_____ 7. tuberculin reaction

a. IgE-mediated

b. cytotoxic/tissue-specific

c. immune complex

d. cell-mediated

8. Immunologic response(s) recognized as disease is/are:
   a. immediate hypersensitivities.
   b. delayed hypersensitivities.
   c. Both a and b are correct.
   d. Neither a nor b is correct.

9. Which is *not* characteristic of hypersensitivity?
   a. specificity
   b. immunologic mechanisms
   c. inappropriate or injurious response
   d. prior contact unnecessary to elicit a response

10. When the body produces antibodies against its own tissue, it is a/an:
    a. hypersensitivity.
    b. antibody reaction.
    c. cell-mediated immunity.
    d. autoimmune disease.
    e. opsonization.

11. Which hypersensitivity is caused by poison ivy?
    a. Type I
    b. Type II
    c. Type III
    d. Type IV

12. The mechanism of hypersensitivity for drugs is:
    a. Type I.
    b. Type II.
    c. Type III.
    d. Type IV.
    e. a, b, and c are correct.

13. Which is *not* an autoimmune disease?
    a. multiple sclerosis
    b. pernicious anemia
    c. transfusion reaction
    d. ulcerative colitis
    e. Goodpasture disease

14. Damage in SLE is due to the formation of antigen/antibody complexes mediated by:
    a. IgE.
    b. mast cells.
    c. the cell-mediated immune system.
    d. the humoral immune system and complement.
    e. lymphokines.

15. The classical complement cascade begins with:
    a. antigen/antibody complexes binding to a component of the complement system.
    b. opsonization.
    c. chemotaxis.
    d. cytolysis.

16. An alloimmune disorder is:
    a. erythroblastosis fetalis.
    b. insulin-dependent diabetes.
    c. myxedema.
    d. All of the above are correct.
    e. None of the above is correct.

17. Immunodeficiencies occur because of impaired function of:
    a. B and T cells.
    b. phagocytic cells.
    c. complement.
    d. All of the above are correct.
    e. Both a and c are correct.

18. An X-linked recessive disorder of immunodeficiency involves a deficit of:
    a. IgA.
    b. IgD.
    c. IgE.
    d. IgG.
    e. IgM.

19. Deficiencies in B cell immune responses are suspected when unusual or recurrent severe infections are caused by:
    a. fungi.
    b. yeasts.
    c. encapsulated bacteria.
    d. Both a and b are correct.
    e. a, b, and c are correct.

20. DiGeorge syndrome is a primary immunodeficiency caused by:
    a. failure of B cells to mature.
    b. congenital lack of thymic tissue.
    c. failure of the formed elements of blood to develop.
    d. selective deficiency of IgG.
    e. selective deficiency of IgA.

21. Acquired or secondary immunodeficiencies:
    a. develop after birth.
    b. may be caused by viral infections.
    c. may develop following immunosuppressive therapy.
    d. Both a and c are correct.
    e. a, b, and c are correct.

22. Rejection of a kidney transplant occurred after 2 weeks. The reaction was because of:
    a. immune response against recipient HLA antigens.
    b. immune response against donor HLA antigens.
    c. a Type IV hypersensitivity.
    d. Both a and b are correct.
    e. Both b and c are correct.

23. Zinc and vitamin deficits can depress:
    a. only B cell function.
    b. only T cell function.
    c. only complement activity.
    d. both B and T cell function.

24. A positive HIV antibody test signifies that the:
    a. individual is infected with HIV and likely so for life.
    b. asymptomatic individual will absolutely progress to AIDS.
    c. individual is not viremic.
    d. sexually active individual was infected last weekend.

25. Which is *incorrect* regarding AIDS?
    a. The T_4/T_8 ratio will be less than 1:1.
    b. The patient will be anti-HIV.
    c. The patient will likely develop opportunistic infections and cancer.
    d. The patient will have increased numbers of CD4 cells or T-helper cells.

8

Stress and Disease

Foundational Objectives

a. **Define stress.**
   Review page 222.

MEMORY CHECK!

- Stress arises when a person interacts or transacts with situations in certain ways. People are not disturbed by situations as they exist but by the ways they individually appraise and react to situations. Stress is a condition in which a demand exceeds a person's coping abilities. Stress reactions may include disturbance of cognition, emotion, and behavior that can adversely affect well-being.

b. **Describe Selye's original general adaptation syndrome; cite its stages.**
   Review pages 222-223; refer to Figure 8-1.

MEMORY CHECK!

- While attempting to discover a new sex hormone, Selye injected crude ovarian extracts into rats. Repeatedly, he found the following triad of structural changes: (1) enlargement of the cortex of the adrenal gland, (2) atrophy of the thymus gland and other lymphoid structures, and (3) development of bleeding ulcers of the stomach and duodenal lining. Selye discovered that this triad of manifestations was not specific for his ovarian extracts but also occurred after he exposed the rats to other noxious stimuli such as cold, surgical injury, and restraint. Selye concluded that this triad or syndrome of manifestations represented a nonspecific response to noxious stimuli. Because many diverse agents caused the same syndrome, Selye suggested that it be called the general adaptation syndrome (GAS).

- Selye later defined three successive stages in the development of the GAS: (1) the alarm stage, (2) the stage of resistance or adaptation, and (3) the stage of exhaustion. The nonspecific physiologic response identified by Selye consists of interaction among the sympathetic branch of the autonomic nervous system and two glands, the pituitary gland and the adrenal gland. The alarm phase of the GAS begins when a stressor triggers the actions of the pituitary gland and the sympathetic nervous system. The resistance or adaptation phase begins with the actions of cortisol, norepinephrine, and epinephrine. Exhaustion occurs if stress continues and adaptation is not successful. The ultimate signs of exhaustion are impairment of the immune response, heart failure, and kidney failure leading to death.

c. **Identify current concepts that modify Selye's work; define homeostasis and cite an example.**
   Review pages 223 and 225.

MEMORY CHECK!

- Studies show that activation of the adrenal cortex occurs in humans in response to psychologic stressors. Several factors, including degrees of discomfort/unpleasantness or suddenness of the stress, may account for the presence or absence of the physiologic stress response. In experiments in which psychologic reactions were minimized, physical stressors did not appear to stimulate the pituitary or adrenal cortex in a nonspecific fashion. To support Selye's concept of nonspecificity, evidence is needed that increased adrenal cortical or medullary activity can promote adaptations to both cold and heat. In fact, no single hormone responds to all stressful stimuli in an absolutely nonspecific fashion.

- Selye considered homeostasis the sum of the processes by which the body maintains itself at a relatively constant composition. He expanded Cannon's definition to mean that the body's need determines body responses and that adaptive responses are necessary to maintain body stability. Research has since demonstrated that homeostasis does not mean "constant composition" but rather a dynamic steady state representing the net effect of all the turnover or synthesis and breakdown of all bodily substances.

- Stressors cause a series of reactions that alter the dynamic steady state. This alteration may be either short- or long-term. For example, the normal concentration of glucose in the blood is about 80 mg/100 ml. The concentration of glucose rises with acute stress and then slowly returns to normal as stress subsides. If blood glucose remains high in the absence of a known stressor, it is diagnosed as a sign of disease, probably diabetes mellitus.

d. Summarize the major interactions of the nervous, endocrine, and immune systems in the stress response.
  Review the Health Alert on page 225 and pages 227-231; refer to Figures 8-2 through 8-5, and Tables 8-2 through 8-4.

MEMORY CHECK!

- Corticotropin-releasing factor (CRF) integrates many stress-induced alterations. It activates the pituitary gland and the sympathetic nervous system. Also, direct suppressive effects of CRF occur on two immune cell types processing CRF receptors, namely the monocyte-macrophage and T helper lymphocyte.
- Stress-induced endorphins lead to pain relief and inhibit or delay blood pressure increases.
- Prolonged stress leads to suppression of growth hormone.
- Testosterone is immunosuppressive; whereas estrogen enhances resistance to infection but increases risk for autoimmune disease
- Oxytocin is associated with reduced hypothalamic-pituitary-adrenal (HPA) activation and reduced anxiety; so it has antistress properties.

The following flow chart summarizes interaction of the three systems by common usage of molecules and receptors in each system:

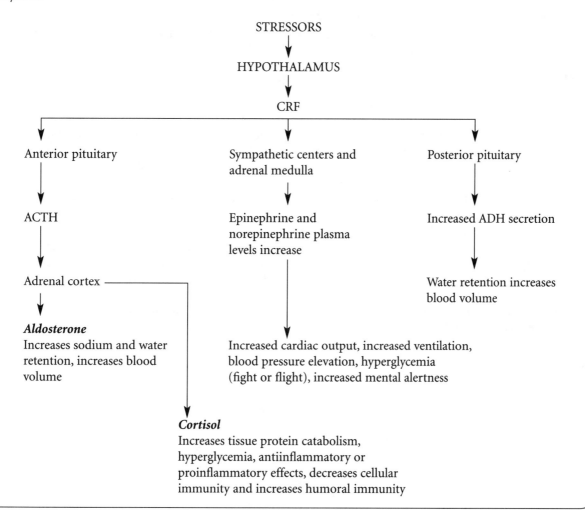

Objectives

After studying this chapter, the learner will be able to do the following:

1. **Cite examples of stress-related diseases.**
   Refer to Table 8-1.

Stress-Related Diseases or Conditions

System	Disease or Condition
Cardiovascular	Coronary artery disease, hypertension, stroke, arrhythmia
Musculoskeletal	Tension headaches, backache, rheumatoid arthritis, osteoporosis
Pulmonary	Asthma, hay fever, COPD
Immune	Immunosuppression, deficiency, autoimmunity
Digestive	Ulcer, irritable bowel syndrome, diarrhea, nausea and vomiting, ulcerative colitis, periodontal disease
Integumentary	Eczema, neurodermatitis, acne
Endocrine	Diabetes mellitus, amenorrhea
Central nervous system	Fatigue and lethargy, type A behavior, overeating, depression, insomnia, Alzheimer disease
Hematologic	Multiple myeloma, non-Hodgkin lymphoma, chronic lymphocytic leukemia

NOTE: The above is an abbreviated grouping of *tissues* and *systems* and their stress-related diseases or conditions.

2. **Describe stress and coping.**
   Study pages 231-232; refer to Figure 8-6.

Stress is not an independent entity but a system of interdependent processes that are moderated by the nature, intensity, and duration of the stressor. The perception, appraisal, and coping efficacy of the affected individual mediates the psychologic and physiologic responses to stress. Coping is managing stressful demands that exceed the individual's resources.

Periods of depression and emotional upheaval with ineffective coping place the affected individual at risk for immunologic deficits. Adverse life events that have the most negative effect on immunity have been characterized as those events that are uncontrollable, undesirable, and overtax the individual's ability to cope. Factors that may influence stress susceptibility or resilience include age, socioeconomic status, gender, social support status, personality, self-esteem, genetics, life events, past experiences, and current physical and mental status.

Problem-focused and social support coping processes have a beneficial influence during stressful experiences. An individual experiencing distress may draw upon internal and external resources to meet the demands. Social support groups can improve psychologic coping and immune function.

Practice Examination

Match the substance with its activity.

_____ 1. IL-1

_____ 2. oxytocin

_____ 3. somatotropin

_____ 4. testosterone

_____ 5. endorphin

a. secreted by the anterior pituitary

b. stimulates the perception of pain

c. produced by macrophages; stimulates release of CRF

d. suppressed by chronic stress

e. causes immunosuppression

f. antistress properties

g. relieves pain

h. released from mast cells, vasoactive

---

6. Which is *not* a characteristic of Selye's stress syndrome?
   a. adrenal atrophy
   b. shrinkage of the thymus
   c. bleeding gastrointestinal ulcers
   d. shrinkage of lymphatic organs

7. Which characterizes the alarm stage?
   a. increased lymphocytes
   b. increased sympathetic activity
   c. increased parasympathetic activity
   d. increased eosinophils

8. Glucocorticoids would be highest during the stage of:
   a. exhaustion.
   b. alarm.
   c. resistance.

9. Which is a correct sequence for Selye's hypothesis for stress?
   a. increased ACTH secretion, alarm
   b. increased ACTH in the blood, hypertrophy of the adrenal cortex
   c. stimulation of the sympathetic centers, alarm
   d. increased secretion of epinephrine, increased ACTH in the blood

10. CRF is released by the:
    a. adrenal medulla.
    b. adrenal cortex.
    c. anterior pituitary.
    d. hypothalamus.

11. Stress may be defined as any factor that:
    a. stimulates the posterior pituitary.
    b. stimulates the anterior pituitary.
    c. stimulates the hypothalamus to release CRF.
    d. stimulates the hypothalamus to release ADH.

12. Which statement is *not* true?
    a. Stressors are the same for all individuals.
    b. Stressors are extreme stimuli.
    c. The emotions of fear, anxiety, and grief can act as stressors.
    d. Stressors differ in different individuals and in one individual at different times.

13. What determines which stimuli are stressors for an individual?
    a. heredity
    b. past experience
    c. diet
    d. all of the above

14. Which statement is *not* true?
    a. Generally, psychologic stress is independent of physiologic stress.
    b. Physiologic stress is usually accompanied by some degree of psychologic stress.
    c. Identical psychologic stressors do not induce identical physiologic responses.
    d. For any one individual, adaptive responses are selective and counteract specific body changes.

15. The production of cortisol in response to stress can be initiated by:
    a. hypothalamus, anterior pituitary, adrenal cortex.
    b. hypothalamus, posterior pituitary, adrenal cortex.
    c. hypothalamus, sympathetic nerve fibers, adrenal cortex.
    d. hypothalamus, sympathetic nerve fibers, adrenal medulla.

16. Cortisol:
    a. increases protein catabolism.
    b. decreases blood sugar.
    c. increases immune response.
    d. increases allergic reactions.

17. Which would *not* occur in response to stress?
    a. increased systolic blood pressure
    b. increased epinephrine
    c. constriction of the pupils
    d. increased adrenocorticoids

18. Which would *not* be useful to assess stress?
    a. total blood cholesterol
    b. eosinophil count
    c. lymphocyte count
    d. adrenocorticoid levels

19. In response to stress, the adrenal cortex secretes:
    a. norepinephrine.
    b. norepinephrine and cortisol.
    c. cortisol and aldosterone.
    d. norepinephrine and aldosterone.

20. Severe stress results in all of the following *except:*
    a. an overactive immune system.
    b. increased heart rate.
    c. a rise in epinephrine levels.
    d. changes in breathing patterns.

Match the term with its definition or characteristic.

_____21. corticoids

_____22. stressors

_____23. stress response

_____24. exhaustion stage

_____25. alarm stage

a. sympathetic activity returns to normal

b. glucocorticoids return to normal

c. secreted by adrenal cortex in response to stress

d. Selye's changes seen in stress

e. stimulates the release of CRF

f. high resistance to stressor

g. bodily changes initiated by stress

h. impaired immune response

i. triggers sympathetic nervous system

Biology of Cancer

9

Foundational Objectives

a. **Describe the phases of cellular mitosis and cytokinesis and cell differentiation.**
   Review pages 19-20, 239, and 243; refer to Figures 9-4 and 9-5.

MEMORY CHECK!

- The reproduction or division of somatic cells involves two sequential phases: mitosis, or nuclear division, and cytokinesis, or cytoplasmic division. These phases occur in close succession, with cytokinesis beginning toward the end of mitosis. Before a cell can divide, it must double its mass and duplicate all of its contents. Most of the preparation for division occurs during the growth phase or interphase. The alternation between mitosis and interphase in all tissues having cellular turnover is known as the *cell cycle*.

- There are four designated phases of the cell cycle. They are (1) the S phase (synthesis), in which DNA is synthesized in the cell nucleus; (2) the G2 phase, in which RNA and protein synthesis occurs; (3) the M phase (mitosis), which includes both nuclear and cytoplasmic division; and (4) the G1 phase, which is the period between the M phase and the start of DNA synthesis. Interphase, consisting of the G1, S, and G2 phases, is the longest phase of the cell cycle.

- The M phase of the cell cycle, mitosis and cytokinesis, begins with prophase or the first appearance of chromosomes. Each chromosome has two identical halves called *chromatids* that lie side by side and are attached together at a site called a *centromere*. The nuclear membrane disappears in this phase. Spindle fibers are microtubules formed in the cytoplasm that radiate from two centrioles located at opposite poles of the cell.

- During metaphase, the next phase of mitosis and cytokinesis, the spindle fibers pull the centromeres until they are aligned in the middle of the spindle or at the equatorial plate.

- Anaphase begins when the centromeres separate and the genetically identical chromatids are pulled apart. The chromatids are pulled, centromeres first, toward opposite sides of the cell. When the identical chromatids are separated, each is considered to be a chromosome. Thus the cell has 92 chromosomes during this stage. By the end of anaphase, there are 46 chromosomes at each side of the identical cell. Each of the two groups of 46 chromosomes should be identical to the original 46 chromosomes present at the start of the cell cycle.

Continued

MEMORY CHECK!—cont'd

- During telophase, a new nuclear membrane is formed around each group of 46 chromosomes, the spindle fibers disappear, and the chromosomes begin to uncoil. Cytokinesis causes the cytoplasm to divide into roughly equal parts during this phase. At the end of telophase, two identical diploid cells, called daughter cells, have been formed from the original cell.

- The difference between slowly and rapidly dividing cells is the length of time spent in the G1 phase of the cell cycle. Some cells that divide very slowly can remain in the G1 phase for years. Once the S phase begins, progression through mitosis requires a relatively constant amount of time. Once a cell has progressed out of the G1 phase, it must complete the S, G2, and M phases.

b. Identify mechanisms that control cell division.
Review page 20; refer to Figure 1-19 and Table 1-4.

MEMORY CHECK!

- Protein growth factors govern the proliferation of different cell types in conjunction with genes involved in the social control or relationship of cells within tissues. It is likely that some genes code for growth factors, some for growth factor receptors, some for intracellular regulatory proteins involved in cell adhesion, and some for proteins that help relay signals for cell division to the cell nucleus.

- Cells require highly specific proteins to stimulate cell division. These growth factors are present in the serum in very low concentrations. For example, platelet-derived growth factor stimulates the production of connective tissue cells. Another important growth factor is interleukin, which stimulates proliferation of T cells. Cells responding to a particular growth factor have specific receptors for the specific growth factor in their plasma membrane. Some growth factors also are regulators of cellular differentiation.

Objectives

After studying this chapter, the learner will be able to do the following:

1. Define neoplasia or cancer.
Study page 238; refer to Figures 9-1 through 9-3.

Cancerous cells are defined by two heritable properties, autonomy and anaplasia. **Autonomy** is the cancer cell's independence from normal cellular controls. **Anaplasia** is the loss of differentiation or specialization. The cancer cell has lost its ability to function normally and to control its growth and division.

Cancer is considered a disorder of growth and differentiation because neoplasms resemble undifferentiated tissue. The less the tumor resembles normal tissue, the more undifferentiated or anaplastic it becomes. As malignant cells grow and divide, they lose their mature characteristics and no longer resemble their tissue of origin.

The word *tumor* originally referred to any swelling, for example, swelling caused by inflammation, but now the term is generally reserved for a new growth, or *neoplasm.* Not all tumors or neoplasms, however, are cancer. The term *cancer* refers to any malignant tumor, or neoplasm, and is not used to refer to benign growths such as lipomas or hypertrophy of an organ.

2. Cite the method for naming and classifying tumors; provide examples.
Refer to Tables 9-1 through 9-3.

Tumors are named according to the tissue of origin with the suffix "oma" added. Cancers having an epithelial tissue origin are identified as carcinomas, whereas those with a connective tissue origin are sarcomas. Lymphomas arise from lymphatic tissue, gliomas arise from glial cells of the central nervous system, and leukemias arise from the bone marrow. *Carcinoma in situ* (often abbreviated CIS) refers to pre-invasive epithelial tumors of glandular or squamous cell origin. These early stage tumors have not broken through basement membranes of the epithelium. (See first box on this page.)

3. **Contrast the properties of benign versus malignant tumors.**
   Refer to Table 9-1. (See box at bottom of this page.)

4. **Identify the stages of cancer spread.**
   Study page 239.

   Staging the tumor is an important component of cancer diagnosis. In general, a four stage system is used, with carci-

Common Benign and Malignant Tumors

Tissue	Benign Tumor	Malignant Tumor
Connective tissue		
Adult fibrous	Fibroma	Fibrosarcoma
Cartilage	Chondroma	Chondrosarcoma
Bone	Osteoma	Osteosarcoma
Fat	Lipoma	Liposarcoma
Muscle		
Smooth muscle	Leiomyoma	Leiomyosarcoma
Striated muscle	Rhabdomyoma	Rhabdomyosarcoma
Blood tissue		
Lymph vessels	Lymphangioma	Lymphangiosarcoma
Blood vessels	Hemangioma	Hemangiosarcoma
Lymphoid tissue	Infectious mononucleosis	Lymphosarcoma (lymphoma)
Bone marrow	Infectious mononucleosis	Leukemia
Neural tissue		
Nerve sheath	Neurilemmoma	Neurogenic sarcoma
Glial tissue	Gliosis	Glioma
Epithelium		
Squamous epithelium	Papilloma	Squamous carcinoma
Glandular epithelium	Adenoma	Adenocarcinoma

Properties of Benign/Malignant Tumors

Characteristic	Benign	Malignant
Differentiation	Yes, resemble tissue of origin	No, little resemblance to tissue of origin
Mitotic figures	Normal	Abnormal
Endocrine hormone secretion	Yes	No
Growth rate	Slow	Rapid
Growth mode	Expansive	Infiltrative
Capsulation	Yes	No
Cellular cohesiveness	Yes	No
Metastasis	No	Yes
Fatality rate	Low	High, if not treated

Examples of Tumor Markers

Marker	Name	Type of Cancer Suggested
AFP	α-fetoprotein	Hepatic, germ cell
CEA	Carcinoembryonic antigen	GI, pancreas, lung, breast
β-HCG	Human chorionic gonadotropin	Germ cell
PSA	Prostate-specific antigen	Prostate
Catecholamines (epinephrine)		Pheochromocytoma (adrenal medulla)
Urinary Bence-Jones protein		Multiple myeloma
ACTH	Adrenocorticotropic hormone	Pituitary adenomas

noma in situ regarded as a special case. Cancer confined to the site of origin is stage 1, cancer that is locally invasive is stage 2 or B, cancer that has spread to regional structures such as lymph nodes is stage 3 or C, and cancer that has spread to distant sites is stage 4, or D. In general, the lower the stage, the more amenable the cancer is to treatment.

5. Characterize tumor markers, cite some examples.
Study pages 243-244; refer to Table 9-4.

Tumor markers (biologic markers) are substances produced by cancer cells that are found on tumor plasma membranes or in the blood, spinal fluid, or urine. For diseases associated with a tumor marker, there is a "blood test for cancer." Tumor markers include hormones, enzymes, genes, antigens, and antibodies (see box above).

6. Postulate a model for the causes of neoplasia or cancer.
Study pages 244-253; refer to Figures 9-6 through 9-18 and 9-22 and Tables 9-5 through 9-7 and 9-9.

Why does a normal cell lose control and become abnormal? Genetic events are the primary cause of carcinogenesis. When sufficient "hits" or mutations over time have occurred, cancer develops. Mutations in germ-line cells (gametes) result in cancer-causing genes that can be inherited from generation to generation. Mutations in somatic cells are not transmitted to future generations. A chemical or other environmental agent can increase the frequency of mutations in somatic cells.

Viruses are another cause of cancer. These tiny packages of nucleic acids, either DNA or RNA, are capable of infecting cells and converting them to transformed cells. The bacterium, *H. pylori*, is responsible for the majority of gastric lymphomas and carcinomas. **Oncogenes** are genes that can transform a normal cell into a cancerous cell when inherited or activated by oncogenic viruses. Oncogenes can develop from normal genes (**proto-oncogenes**) that regulate growth and development by encoding for growth factors and growth factor receptors. These genes may undergo some change that either causes them to produce an abnormal product or disrupts their control so that they are expressed inappropriately and accelerate proliferation.

Some cancers are not caused by oncogenes but rather by genes called **tumor suppressor genes** that have mutated. These genes produce proteins that normally oppose the action of an oncogene or inhibit cell division. Carcinogenesis inactivates tumor suppressor genes by loss of **heterozygosity** (loss of one gene copy), which unmasks mutations in recessive genes, or by **silencing** (in which methylation of DNA shuts off genes without mutation) and activates oncogenes.

Cells have a self-destruct mechanism, known as **apoptosis,** triggered by normal development and excessive growth. The most common mutations causing resistance to apoptosis occur in the *p53* gene.

Other than germ cell, cells in the body can divide only a limited number of times. **Telomeres** are at the ends of each chromosome and block unlimited cell division. Telomerase maintains telomeres. Cancer cells activate telomerase to restore and maintain telomeres so cells can divide over and over again.

Whenever normal DNA integrity is disrupted during mitosis or by external mutagens, multiple mechanisms have evolved to protect and repair the genome. These repair mechanisms are directed by **caretaker genes.** These genes encode proteins that repair damaged DNA, and loss of caretaker genes leads to increased mutation rates.

Tumors appear to be derived from a single stem cell. Tumor development requires several independent mutational accidents to occur together in one cell. If a single mutation were responsible, the chance of developing cancer in any given year would be independent of age. However, the cancerous change increases at a rapid rate with increasing age.

In most cancers, the cells of the initial mutant clone undergo further mutation that enables them to divide more rapidly before they terminally differentiate. These cells acquire characteristics of cancer including increased growth rate, decreased apoptosis, or decreased death rate. Because of rapid division, the cancer cells begin to outnumber the normal cells as well as those having the primary mutation, leading to **clonal proliferation** or **clonal expansion** (see flow chart on p. 55).

Causes and Sequence of Carcinogenesis

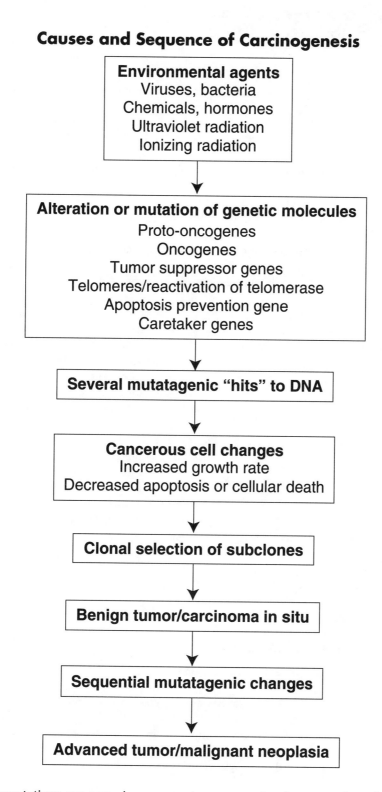

NOTE: Genetic mutations can occur in response to exposure to a large number of environmental agents. See Table 9-9 for agent exposures related to cancer.

Practice Examination

Match the term with its definition.

_____ 1. neoplasia

_____ 2. anaplasia

_____ 3. autonomy

a. variation in size, shape, and arrangement of cells

b. differentiation of dividing cells into cellular types not ordinarily found in a given area

c. abnormal, proliferating cells possessing a higher degree of autonomy than normal cells

d. increase in absolute number of cells

e. lack of cellular differentiation or specialization, primitive cells

f. cancer cells' independence from normal cellular controls

---

4. Which characterize(s) cancer cells?
    a. poorly differentiated
    b. metastasis
    c. infiltrative growth mode
    d. poor cellular cohesiveness
    e. All of the above are correct.

5. Which is *not* a malignant tumor?
    a. glioma
    b. adenocarcinoma
    c. rhabdomyoma
    d. leukemia

6. Endocrine hormone secretion is increased in:
    a. benign tumors.
    b. nonencapsulated tumors.
    c. tumors having little resemblance to tissue of origin.
    d. tumors having a high fatality rate.

7. Metastasis is:
    a. an alteration in normal cellular growth.
    b. growth of benign or malignant neoplastic cells.
    c. mutational.
    d. the ability to establish a secondary neoplasm at a new site.

8. Carcinoma in situ is:
    a. preinvasive.
    b. a glandular or epithelial lesion.
    c. a teratoma.
    d. a carcinoma that has broken through the basement membrane.
    e. Both a and b are correct.

Match the term with its definition/characteristic.

_____ 9. stage 3 or C

_____ 10. tumor markers

_____ 11. loss of heterozygosity

_____ 12. silencing

a. increased metabolite transport

b. cancer has spread to regional structures

c. unmasks mutations in recessive genes

d. methylation of DNA shuts off genes

e. "rounded-up" cells

f. substances produced by cancer cells

g. increased extracellular proteolysis

13. Which are carcinogens?
    a. viruses
    b. chemicals
    c. radiation
    d. Both b and c are correct.
    e. a, b, and c are correct.

14. Tumor suppressor genes are:
    a. genes having the ability to transform a normal cell into a cancerous cell.
    b. normal genes that regulate growth and development.
    c. genes that produce proteins that inhibit cellular division.
    d. Both b and c are correct.

15. In the current theory of carcinogenesis:
    a. the sequence is initiation-promotion-progression.
    b. several mutagenic "hits" are required.
    c. mutations in somatic cells are transmitted to future generations.
    d. sequential genetic changes occur.
    e. Both b and d are correct.

16. Proto-oncogenes:
    a. induce end-stage differentiation.
    b. encode for growth factors.
    c. inhibit growth factor stimulation.
    d. stimulate cell death.
    e. All of the above are correct.

17. Oncogenic viruses are:
    a. DNA viruses.
    b. RNA viruses.
    c. capable of incorporation into host genes.
    d. capable of transforming a normal cell into a cancerous cell.
    e. All of the above are correct.

18. The *p53* gene:
    a. enables cells to cope with DNA damage.
    b. blocks the proliferation of cells that have suffered carcinogenic mutations.
    c. mutations are the most common genetic lesion in human cancer.
    d. mutations disable an emergency brake on cell proliferation.
    e. All of the above are correct.

19. Chemical carcinogens:
    a. cause changes in the nucleotide sequence.
    b. cause chromosomal breaks.
    c. introduce foreign DNA into the cell.
    d. involve epigenetic changes.

20. Tumor suppressor genes are
    a. genes having the ability to transform a normal cell into a cancerous cell.
    b. normal genes that restrict differentiation.
    c. genes that produce proteins that inhibit cellular division.
    d. converted to oncogenes.

21. An adenoma is
    a. benign.
    b. a glandular epithelial neoplasm.
    c. a teratoma.
    d. a malignant epithelial tumor.
    e. a and b

Match the tumor markers with their expressing neoplastic cells.

_____22. AFP

_____23. CEA

_____24. urinary Bence-Jones protein

_____25. PSA

a. multiple myeloma

b. retinoblastomas

c. hepatic, germ cells

d. GI, pancreas

e. Wilms tumor

f. prostate gland

10

Tumor Spread and Treatment

Foundational Objective

a. **Describe mechanisms that confine cells and tissues to a specific anatomic site.**
   Review pages 20-24.

MEMORY CHECK!

- All cells are within a network of extracellular macromolecules known as the *extracellular matrix*. The extracellular matrix holds cells and tissues together and provides an organized framework in which cells can interact with one another.

- To confine themselves and form tissues, cells must have intercellular recognition and adhesion. Specialized cells likely form a tissue in one of two ways. The first way is mitosis of one or more founder cells. Founder cells, basic precursor cells, are prevented from "wandering away" by macromolecules in the extracellular matrix and by adherence to one another at specialized junctions on their plasma membranes. The second way specialized cells form tissues involves their migration to subsequent accumulation at the site of tissue formation. Migrant cells are thought to arrive at the specific site of tissue formation through chemotaxis or contact guidance. Cells at the migrant cells' destination secrete a chemical known as *chemotactic factor*, which attracts specific migrant cells. Contact guidance is movement along a pathway or "pavement" within the extracellular matrix. In order to stay together in groups, cells must recognize each other and remain distinct from the cells of surrounding tissues.

- Cells in direct physical contact with neighboring cells are often linked together at specialized regions of their plasma membranes. These regions are known as cell junctions. Cell junctions hold cells together and allow small molecules to pass from cell to cell. This coordinates the activities of cells that form tissues. There are three main types of cell junctions: (1) desmosomes, (2) tight junctions, and (3) gap junctions. Desmosomes hold cells together by forming either continuous bands of epithelial sheets or button-like points of contact. Desmosomes also provide a system of braces to maintain structural stability. Tight junctions act as a barrier to diffusion, prevent movement of substances through transport proteins of the plasma membrane, and prevent the leakage of small molecules between the plasma membranes of adjacent cells. Gap junctions are clusters of protein channels that allow small ions and molecules to pass directly from the inside of one cell to the inside of another. Cells connected by gap junctions are considered ionically and metabolically joined. Gap junctions coordinate the activities of adjacent cells. For example, these junctions synchronize contractions of heart muscle cells through ionic coupling. The junctions permit action potentials to spread rapidly from cell to cell in neural tissues.

Objectives

After studying this chapter, the learner will be able to do the following:

1. **Describe prerequisites for metastasis to occur.**
   Study pages 270-271; refer to Figures 10-1 through 10-3.

   Invasion or **local spread** is a prerequisite for metastasis and is the first step in the metastatic process. In early stages, **local invasion** may occur by direct tumor extension. Eventually, cells or clumps of cells become detached from the primary tumor and invade the surrounding interstitial spaces. Possible important factors in local invasion include (1) cellular multiplication, (2) mechanical pressure, (3) release of lytic enzymes, (4) decreased cell-to-cell adhesion, and (5) increased motility of individual tumor cells. These mechanisms are not mutually exclusive, and it is likely that in a given neoplasm any combination of the five may be involved.

   The rate of **cellular multiplication** depends on the cell generation time, the number of cells that are dividing, and the cell loss from the tumor. Malignant cells can divide rapidly, but the tumor may not grow because cells are rapidly dying.

   Mechanical pressure generates pressure that forces cellular sheets or finger-like projections along the lines of least mechanical resistance; spread is enhanced. The growing mass blocks local blood vessels and leads to local tissue death. This reduces mechanical resistance and further aids the spread.

   Many tumors have higher levels of protease and collagenases, plasminogen activators, and lysosomal enzymes than corresponding normal tissue. These **lytic enzymes** destroy normal tissue, which increases tumor invasion. At the leading edge of tumors, the balance between proteases and antiproteases favor proteases. Three classes of proteases aid invasion and metastasis: serine, cysteine, and metalloid proteinases (MMPs).

   Cancer cells do not adhere to one another as well as normal cells. This **decreased cell adhesion** has been attributed partially to fibronectin. Cancer cells may either produce a defective type of fibronectin or break down fibronectin as they produce it. Low levels or loss of this anchoring molecule may help cancer cells "slip" between normal cells and allow more invasion.

   Increased motility is essential for tumor cells to invade and travel. The neoplastic cell must detach and infiltrate into adjacent tissue, migrate through the vascular wall into the circulation, and then migrate out of the vascular wall into a secondary site. Tumor cells may actually move by means of their own chemotactic factors known as "autocrine motility factors"; the tumor cell secretes a factor that binds to a specific receptor on the cell surface to stimulate motility. Autotoxin (ATX) is one tumor-secreted autocrine motility factor. Thus the neoplastic cell acquires independent and continuous stimulation for its motile and invasive behavior.

2. **Describe the proposed sequence of events during tumor cell invasion of extracellular matrix.**
   Study pages 271-272; refer to Figures 10-4 and 10-5.

   A three-step theory likely describes the events during tumor cell invasion of the extracellular matrix. These steps involve tumor cell attachment to the basement membrane of vascular matrix, degradation or dissolution of the matrix, and locomotion or movement into the interstitial matrix. **Laminin** is a complex glycoprotein and a major constituent of all basement membranes and forms a bridge between laminin receptor and type IV collagen. Because membrane vesicles of tumor cells are rich in **laminin receptors,** the *first* step is complete when binding occurs between the vascular basement membrane laminin and its receptors. Once anchored, the tumor cell either secretes type II **collagenase** or induces host cells to produce proteolytic enzymes. Degradation of the matrix constitutes the *second* step. Such enzymes may degrade both the attachment proteins and the structural collagenous proteins of the vascular basement membrane matrix. The *third* step is tumor cell locomotion. Finger-like projections, called *pseudopodia,* extend from the tumor cell and attach to blood vessel walls that cross the basement membrane. Thus the tumor cells leave the vasculature and enter the interstitial stroma. The direction of locomotion site is likely influenced by chemotactic factors.

3. **Describe the avenues for metastatic spread.**
   Study pages 272-273; refer to Figure 10-6.

   Three routes for metastasis exist: direct or continuous extension, lymphatic spread, and bloodstream dissemination. These routes are not mutually exclusive. Tumor dissemination through one route often facilitates metastasis through others because tumor cells move through numerous microscopic anatomic connections.

   Direct tumor extension is thought to be initiated by a complex sequence of events. These events are initiated by loss of intracellular adhesion, enabling cells to "slip" past one another. Movement of cells through tissue barriers is further influenced by protease and autocrine motility factors.

   The process of metastasis involves invasion and penetration of tumor cells into and from blood vessels or via lymphatics or both. The most common route for distant metastases is **lymphatic spread.** Tumors generally lack a well-formed lymphatic network; rather, lymphatic channels occur at the periphery of the tumor and not within the tumor mass. Tumor cells entering the lymphatic vessels from interstitial sites are carried to regional lymph nodes that initially may prevent the further spread of tumor cells into the lymphatics. A cancer cell that becomes lodged in lymph nodes may die as a result of local inflammatory reaction or, because of an incompatible local environment, grow into a discernable lump, remain dormant for unknown reasons, or detach and enter the efferent lymphatics. If tumor cell emboli are released into efferent lymphatic vessels, lymphatic metastasis occurs. The shedding of emboli may be caused by changes in vessel pressure, by turbulent alterations in lymphatic flow, or by manipulation of the tumor during diagnostic tests or surgery. Tumor cells eventually move into the venous drainage because of numerous venolymphatic communications.

Hematogenous spread requires tumor cells to penetrate and detach from blood vessels and spread to distant organs. To establish a metastatic site, tumor cells must "escape" host defenses, survive mechanical trauma in the bloodstream, and lodge in the vascular bed of the target organ. Tumor cells circulate and attach directly to the endothelial surface of the basement membrane. The formation of a leukocyte-fibrin-platelet complex around tumor cells is thought to protect tumor cells within these complexes from host defenses and to assist successful attachment to the vascular epithelium. After invading the vascular wall, these neoplastic cells leave the vascular bed, enter the interstitial stroma, and invade the parenchyma of the target organ.

See the flow chart on p. 61 to complement objectives 3 and 4.

4. **Describe angiogenesis; identify factors that may determine sites of distant metastases.**
    Study pages 273-275; refer to Table 10-1.

Tumors likely cannot grow more than a few millimeters in diameter without developing new blood vessels. This new vascular network development is called **angiogenesis.** Development of blood vessels is the result of diffusible substances secreted by the tumor. These secreted substances are known as **tumor-angiogenesis factors (TAF)** and include several growth factors. Also, production of **thrombospondin**—a protein that inhibits growth of new blood vessels—drops suddenly in cancer cells.

The ability of metastatic cells to grow and develop requires not only the development of a vascular network but also evasion of host defenses and a compatible new environment. The metastatic potential of many common carcinomas is related to the size of the primary tumor. Larger tumors may overwhelm host defenses, thus favoring survival of disseminated malignant cells. Also, the "stresses" endured by cancer cells may promote the emergence of stronger, more aggressive tumors.

Distant metastatic sites may not be the first capillary bed encountered by the circulating cells. Instead, preferential growth in specific organs may be observed. This feature is called "organ tropism." This tropism may result from local growth factors or hormones present in the target organ, preferential adherence by tumor receptors to the surface of certain target organs, or the presence of chemotactic factors diffusing from the target organ, which cause circulating tumor cells to extravasate from the vessels and accumulate in the target organ. Evidence exists that organ tropism is genetically determined, as different proteolytic enzymes are expressed in different sites.

5. **Describe the clinical manifestations of cancer.**
    Study pages 276-278; refer to Figure 10-8 and Table 10-2.

Usually little or no **pain** is associated with the early stages of malignant disease, but pain will affect 60% to 80% of individuals terminally ill with cancer. The pain may be directly related to the malignancy but also may be the result of inflammation and infection. A very common cause of pain is bone metastasis; it is caused by periosteal irritation, medullary pressure, or pathologic fractures. Abdominal pain is often caused by stretching, obstructions, or surgical adhesions of the hollow visceral organs. An enlarged liver from hepatic malignancies results in a dull pain or fullness over the right upper quadrant of the abdomen. Any tumor having very little space to grow without compressing blood vessels and nerve endings against bone will elicit pain. Tissue destruction from infection and necrosis can cause pain.

Fatigue is the most frequently reported symptom of cancer and cancer treatment. Likely causes of fatigue include sleep disturbance, biochemical changes, psychologic factors, altered nutritional status, and level of activity.

Decreased muscle contractibility and function are observed in individuals with cancer. Muscle loss may result from cancer treatment or from circulating tumor necrosis factor and interleukin-1.

Cachexia is a severe wasting, emaciation, and decreased quality of life seen in those with malignancy. Anorexia, or loss of appetite, contributes to the syndrome of cachexia. Reductions in sensitivities to sweet, sour, and salty tastes make ordinarily seasoned foods seem bland. Also, aversions to food likely develop because of poor use

Metastatic Sequence

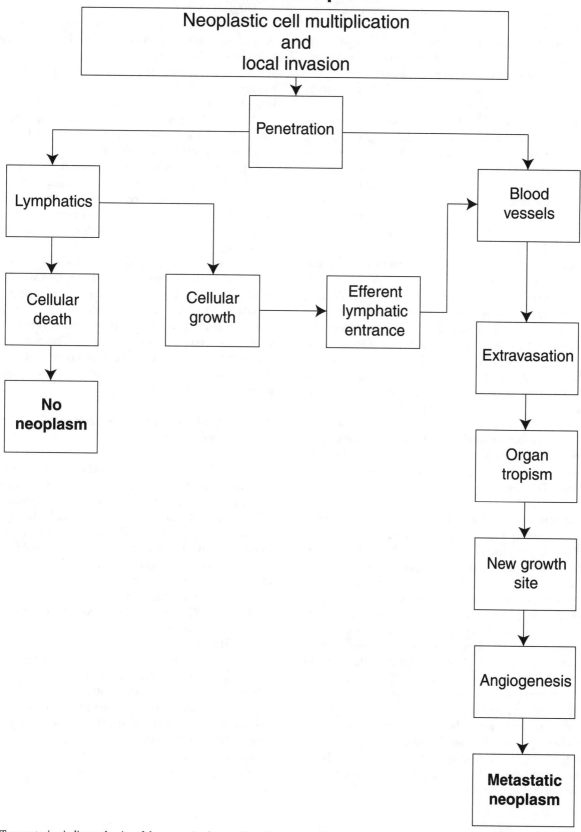

NOTE: Tumor staging indicates the size of the tumor, its degree of local invasion, and its extent of spread. Prognosis declines with increasing tumor size, lymph node involvement, and metastasis.

of glucose and increased mobilization of protein, or increased degradation resulting from an increased function of the ubiquitin-protease protein degradation pathway. Elevated glucose and amino acid levels in the blood stimulate the satiety center, resulting in reduced appetite.

Anemia is commonly associated with malignancy. The majority of individuals with cancer usually have a mild anemia, although 20% may have hemoglobin concentrations that are depressed to below 9 g/dl. Chronic bleeding, severe malnutrition, medical therapies, or malignancy in blood-forming organs may cause anemia.

Direct tumor invasion into the bone marrow causes decreased leukocyte counts and decreased numbers of platelets. Chemotherapy and radiotherapy of areas of the bone marrow cause **leukopenia** and **thrombocytopenia.**

Infection is the most significant cause of complications and death in individuals with malignant disease. Individuals with cancer are very susceptible to infection because of reductions in immunologic functions, debility from advanced disease, and immunosuppression from radiotherapy and chemotherapy. Surgery can create favorable residual sites for infection. The incidence of hospital-related or nosocomial infections for cancer patients is increased because of indwelling medical devices, compromised wound care, and the introduction of microorganisms from visitors and other patients.

6. **Compare the modalities for the treatment of neoplasms; identify the advantages of immune therapy.**
   Study pages 278-279 and 281-282; refer to Figure 10-9 and Tables 10-3 through 10-5.

Cancer is treated by chemotherapy, radiotherapy, surgery, immunotherapy, and combinations of these modalities. The mechanism by which **chemotherapy** acts to eradicate tumor cells depends largely on its effect on the cell cycle. To be effective, chemotherapy must eliminate enough neoplastic cells so that the body's own defenses can eradicate the remaining cells. Combination chemotherapy is the synergistic use of severed agents. This approach helps decrease single agent drug resistance and reduce harmful effects on normal cells. Neoadjuvant chemotherapy enables early use of agents to decrease initial tumor size before radiation therapy or surgical therapy.

To eradicate neoplastic cells without producing excessive toxicity and to avoid damage to normal structures is the challenge of **radiation therapy.** Ionizing radiation damages important macromolecules, especially DNA. Rapidly renewing and dividing cells are generally more radiosensitive than other cells.

Surgical therapy is useful for nonmetastatic disease when the neoplasm is accessible and has not yet spread beyond the limits of surgical excision. Palliative surgery, alleviation without cure, may be used to relieve or avoid symptoms of malignancy. Debulking surgery in which the majority of the tumor is removed can allow more success with adjuvant chemotherapy or irradiation.

Immunotherapy is a promising modality for the treatment of cancer. A specific method, such as immunotherapy, may eliminate transformed cells without damaging normal tissues. Also, immune memory cells are long-lived and capable of providing extended protection against the emergence of recurrent primary tumor cells and metastatic cancer cells. Development of tumor-specific vaccines has been notable with malignant melanoma.

Immunotherapies for the treatment of cancer are known as **biologic response modifiers (BRMs).** These BRMs can have a direct cytotoxic effect on cancer cells, initiate or augment the host's tumor-immune rejection response, or modify cancer cells' susceptibility to the lytic or tumor-arresting effects of the immune system. The BRMs include immunomodulating agents, interferons, thymosins, antigens, effector cells, lymphokines, cytokines, and monoclonal antibodies.

7. **Identify side effects of cancer treatment.**
   Study pages 282-283.

Most side effects accompanying cancer treatment are directly related to the targeting of rapidly growing cells. In the gastrointestinal tract, both chemotherapy and irradiation may cause decreased cell turnover leading to oral ulcers, malabsorption, and diarrhea. Disruption of barrier defenses increases the risk of gastrointestinal tract infection. Nausea may occur because of the agent's direct action on the vomiting center.

Chemotherapy can cause bone marrow suppression of RBCs, WBCs, and platelets. Decreased numbers of these formed elements lead to anemia, increased infections, and bleeding.

Hair loss (alopecia) results from chemotherapy effects on hair follicles. Alopecia is usually temporary and is not caused by all chemotherapeutic agents.

The reproductive tract may be affected by irradiation and chemotherapy causing decreased fertility and premature menopause. Prepubertal gonads seem more resistant to damage. In craniospinal irradiation, the hypothalamus or pituitary gland may be affected and result in gonadal failure.

Practice Examination

1. Tumor spread depends on:
   a. growth rate of the tumor and its degree of differentiation.
   b. unknown factors.
   c. the presence or absence of anatomic barriers.
   d. Both a and c are correct.
   e. a, b, and c are correct.

2. Which is the correct sequence during the process of metastasis?
   a. vascularization, adherence of neoplastic cells, invasion into lymph and vascular systems
   b. transport, vascularization, adherence of neoplastic cells
   c. local invasion, invasion into lymph and vascular systems, transport
   d. vascularization, extravasation, transport

3. In order for metastasis to occur, local invasive factors must include all of the following *except:*
   a. cellular multiplication.
   b. mechanical pressure.
   c. lytic enzyme release.
   d. increased cellular adhesion.
   e. increased individual tumor cells.

4. Known routes for metastasis of malignant cells include:
   a. continuous extension.
   b. lymphatic spread.
   c. bloodstream dissemination.
   d. Both b and c are correct.
   e. a, b, and c are correct.

5. Common sites for metastatic cells include all of the following *except:*
   a. lung.
   b. liver.
   c. brain.
   d. bone.
   e. heart.

6. A malignant cell that becomes lodged in a lymph node may:
   a. die.
   b. divide.
   c. become dormant.
   d. enter efferent lymphatics.
   e. All of the above are correct.

7. The process by which tumors develop new vascular networks is:
   a. heparinization.
   b. angiogenesis.
   c. anaplasia.
   d. autonomy.
   e. differentiation.

8. Organ tropism involves:
   a. local growth factors.
   b. chemotactic factors.
   c. tumor receptors.
   d. genetic determinants.
   e. All of the above are correct.

9. Likely causes for the fatigue observed in individuals with cancer include:
   a. biochemical changes because of treatment.
   b. muscle loss.
   c. psychologic factors.
   d. All of the above are correct.
   e. Both a and c are correct.

10. Neoplasms may cause all of the following *except:*
    a. obstruction of passageways.
    b. hormonal imbalances.
    c. viral infections.
    d. nutrient depletion.

11. Metastatic behavior may be caused by:
    a. altered cytoplasm.
    b. altered ribosomes.
    c. altered genetic code.
    d. chromosomal breakage.

12. The pain experienced with cancer:
    a. affects the individual in the early stages of malignancy.
    b. occurs in bone metastasis.
    c. results from tissue necrosis.
    d. Both b and c are correct.
    e. a, b, and c are correct.

13. The anorexia or loss of appetite seen in the syndrome of cancer cachexia may occur because of:
    a. altered blood serum levels of glucose and amino acids.
    b. hyperinsulinism.
    c. late satiety.
    d. hypoproteinemia.

14. The anemia associated with malignancy can be:
    a. due to depletion of hemoglobin building blocks.
    b. severe in the majority of cases.
    c. caused by destruction of bone marrow.
    d. All of the above are correct.
    e. Both a and c are correct.

15. Chemotherapy for cancer:
    a. prevents transcription.
    b. damages cells undergoing mitosis.
    c. Both a and b are correct.
    d. Neither a nor b is correct.

16. Immunotherapy for cancer:
    a. is a nonspecific treatment.
    b. injures both transformed and normal cells.
    c. suppresses tumor-immune response.
    d. is augmented by memory cells.
    e. None of the above is correct.

17. BRMs:
    a. directly kill cancer cells.
    b. augment the tumor-immune rejection response.
    c. modify the cancer cell's susceptibility to lysis.
    d. All of the above are correct.
    e. None of the above is correct.

18. Which is *not* involved in metastasis?
    a. initial establishment
    b. interference
    c. invasion
    d. dissemination
    e. proliferation

Match the term with its characteristic.

_____19. metalloproteinase

_____20. locomotion

a. chronic bleeding

b. taste alterations

c. aids invasion and metastasis

d. inflammation

e. exits vasculature and enters the interstitial stroma

Match the cancer treatment with its characteristic.

_____21. radiation

_____22. monoclonal antibodies

_____23. immunomodulating agents

_____24. debulking surgery

_____25. neoadjuvant chemotherapy

a. decreases initial tumor size

b. T cell transfer

c. specific antibodies for tumor antigen

d. cancerous cells attacked in cell cycle

e. stimulation of immune system

f. facilitates adjuvant chemotherapy or irradiation

g. direct ionization

Cancer in Children

11

Foundational Objective

a. Describe mechanisms that confine cells and tissues to a specific anatomic site.
   Review Foundational Objective **a** in Chapter 10.

Objectives

After studying this chapter, the learner will be able to do the following:

1. Compare childhood neoplasms to adult neoplasms. Refer to Table 11-1.

COMPARISON OF CHILDHOOD AND ADULT CANCERS

Characteristic	Childhood Cancers	Adult Cancers
Incidence	<1% of all cancers	>99% of all cancers
Environmental causation	Weak relationship to environmental exposures and life-style	Strong relationship to environmental exposures and life-style
Latency (from initiation to diagnosis)	Short	Long
Sites involved	Tissue	Organs
Cells involved	Nonepithelial (connective tissue): sarcomas, embryonal, leukemia, lymphoma	Epithelial: carcinomas
Prevention	Few strategies to prevent	80% may be preventable
Early detection	Generally accidental	Possible by early detection screening tests/exams
Stage at diagnosis	80% have metastasized	Local or regional spread
Treatment/side effects	Less difficulty with acute toxicity but more significant long-term consequences	More difficulty with acute toxicity but fewer long-term consequences
Response to treatment	Very responsive to chemotherapy	Less responsive to chemotherapy
Prognosis	>60% cure	<60% cure

2. Describe the incidence and types of childhood cancers.
Study page 288; refer to Tables 11-2 and 11-3.

Approximately 9000 children up to the age of 15 years are diagnosed with cancer each year. The incidence of cancer in children between birth and the age of 15 years is estimated to be 128 children per million per year. Projections reveal that 1 in every 250 individuals between the ages of 15 and 45 years will be a survivor of childhood cancer in the year 2010.

Cancer is 10% to 25% more common in white than in black children due to the lower incidence of acute lymphocytic leukemia, lymphomas, and Ewing sarcoma in black children. In the United States, childhood cancer is slightly more common in boys than in girls; the male to female ratio is 1.2:1.

Most childhood cancers originate from the mesodermal germ layer that gives rise to connective tissue, bone, cartilage, muscle, blood and blood vessels, gonads, kidney, and the lymphatic system. Thus the more common childhood cancers are leukemias, sarcomas, and embryonic tumors. Embryonic tumors originate during intrauterine life and contain immature tissue unable to mature or differentiate into functional cells. Embryonic tumors are diagnosed early, usually by 5 years of age.

Carcinomas almost never occur in children because these cancers usually result from environmental carcinogens and require a long time from exposure to the appearance of the lesion. However, epithelial tumors begin to increase between the ages of 15 and 19 years and become the most common cancer type after adolescence.

The most common malignancy in children is **leukemia,** accounting for more than one-third of childhood cancers. The second most common group is cancers of the nervous system, primarily brain lesions. All other pediatric malignancies occur much less often. **Neuroblastoma** is a tumor of the sympathetic nervous system. **Wilms tumor** is a malignancy of the kidney; its histologic name is nephroblastoma. **Rhabdomyosarcoma** is a soft tissue sarcoma of striated muscle. Two major bone tumors, **osteosarcoma** and **Ewing sarcoma,** occur in children.

Childhood cancers usually are diagnosed during peak times of growth and maturation. In general, they are extremely fast-growing cancers. Many childhood cancers have a peak incidence before the child is 5 years of age. Among these are the leukemias, neuroblastoma, Wilms tumor, and **retinoblastoma.** Central nervous system tumors are more common in children less than 15 years of age. Bone tumors, soft tissue sarcomas, and **lymphomas** are more likely to occur between 15 and 19 years of age.

3. Describe the etiologic factors for childhood cancers.
Study pages 289-292; refer to Tables 11-4 and 11-5.

Some environmental and host factors predispose a child to cancer, but causal factors have not been established for most childhood cancers. Many host factors are genetic risk factors or congenital conditions. Childhood cancer most likely can be attributed to the complex interaction of both genetic and environmental factors.

Genetic factors may involve chromosome aberrations, single-gene defects, or chromosome abnormalities including aneuploidy, deletions, translocations, and fragility. Some congenital malformations and syndromes herald the onset of pediatric malignancies. One of the more recognized syndromes is the association of Down syndrome with an increased susceptibility to acute leukemia. For children with this syndrome, the risk of developing leukemia is 10 to 20 times greater during the first 10 years of life than the risk is in healthy children.

Wilms tumor is particularly recognized for its association with a number of malformations, including horseshoe kidney, undescended testicles, collecting system defects, congenital absence of the iris of the eye, and muscular overgrowth of one half of the body or face. Approximately 10% of children diagnosed with Wilms tumor demonstrate one of these congenital abnormalities. Wilms tumor genes—*WT1* gene, *WT2*, and *WT3*—have been found. Retinoblastoma, a malignant embryonic tumor of the eye, occurs as an inherited defect or as an acquired mutation of the retinoblastoma gene, *RB1* gene. Single-gene defects have been associated with the subsequent development of childhood tumors. Two autosomal recessive diseases involving increased chromosomal fragility, Fanconi anemia and Bloom syndrome, are risk factors predisposing the child to acute nonlymphocytic leukemia.

The relative ineffectiveness of the immune surveillance system during intrauterine life may explain the occurrence of embryonic tumors. During rapid proliferation and differentiation of cells in the developing fetus, cell mutation could result in embryonic tumors.

Children with immunodeficiencies have a striking risk of subsequent cancer over healthy children. These conditions may be either congenital, generally involving X-linked recessive inheritance, or acquired. Therapeutic immunosuppression after organ transplantation or treatment for aplastic anemia may cause cancer.

A few malignancies seem to demonstrate a familial tendency because these specific cancers cluster in particular families. A child who has a sibling with leukemia has a risk for the development of leukemia that is 2 to 4 times greater than a child with a normal sibling.

Few childhood tumors share a strong association with environmental agents. This is because of the lengthy latency period required between exposure and development of cancer; early exposure to carcinogens does not usually result in a tumor until the child is an adult.

Prenatal exposure to some drugs and to ionizing radiation have been linked to subsequent cancers. Perhaps the most well-known such drug is diethylstilbestrol (DES), a drug taken to avert early abortion. DES is a transplacental chemical carcinogen. Adenocarcinoma of the vagina has developed in a small percentage of the daughters of mothers who took DES while pregnant.

An area of study is the role of parental occupational exposures and subsequent cancers in offspring. The exposure could lead to genetic changes of the ova or sperm or to transplacental transfer of the carcinogen. Several associations have been found for parental occupations involving hydrocarbon, petroleum, chemical, and paint exposure. Intrauterine exposure to radiation during pregnancy likely causes an increased risk for all types of childhood cancer.

Childhood exposures to drugs, ionizing radiation, and viruses have been implicated as risk factors for specific cancers. Drugs implicated include (1) anabolic androgenic steroids, which are used in the treatment of aplastic anemia or used illegally by teenage athletes for body development and have been associated with subsequent hepatocellular carcinoma; (2) cytotoxic agents used in the treatment of pediatric cancers, which may predispose a child to leukemia in later years; and (3) immunosuppressive agents, particularly those used for transplants, which have been shown to increase the risk for lymphoma. In children, the strongest viral carcinogenic relationship is the Epstein-Barr virus and Burkitt lymphoma.

4. Indicate the prognosis for childhood cancers.
Study page 292.

More than 77% of children diagnosed with cancer can now be expected to survive for 5 years or more. Estimates indicate that these individuals are at increased risk for a second cancer because of their previous exposure to cancer therapy and, possibly, their genetic constitution. The risk of a secondary cancer 20 years after childhood cancer is approximately 3%. Overall, children have a more favorable prognosis than do adults. Children appear to be more responsive to available treatments and are better able to tolerate the immediate side effects of therapies.

Even those cancers that cannot be cured can be treated, resulting in significant quality time. Cured children do face residual and late effects of treatment. These late effects are more significant in children than in adults because childhood treatment occurs in a physically immature, growing individual.

Practice Examination

True/False

Childhood cancers:

_____ 1. are more common than adult cancers.

_____ 2. have a strong relationship to environmental agents.

_____ 3. possess a short latency period.

_____ 4. involve tissues more than organs.

_____ 5. involve epithelial cells more often than connective tissue cells.

_____ 6. are generally detected accidentally.

_____ 7. often have metastasized at the time of diagnosis.

_____ 8. are less responsive to chemotherapy than are adult cancers.

_____ 9. have more long-term consequences than adult cancers.

_____10. have a better prognosis than adult cancers.

Match the syndrome/disorder with the risk factor.

_____11. Down syndrome

_____12. Wilms tumor

_____13. retinoblastoma

_____14. Fanconi anemia

_____15. vaginal adenocarcinoma

_____16. Ataxia-telangiectasia

a. *RB1* gene

b. DES

c. lymphoma

d. nonlymphocytic leukemia

e. acute leukemia

f. congenital absence of iris of the eye

True/False

_____17. Most childhood cancers originate from the mesoderm.

_____18. Embryonic tumors are diagnosed during teenage years.

_____19. Carcinomas are prevalent before the age of adolescence.

_____20. The most common malignancy in children involves the nervous system.

_____21. Cancer is more common in white than in black children.

_____22. The male-to-female ratio for childhood cancer in the United States is 1.2:1.

_____23. Children with immunodeficiencies have a low risk of subsequent cancers.

_____24. Fewer than 50% of children diagnosed with cancer can expect to survive for 5 years.

_____25. Cured children face few residual and late effects from their therapy.

12

Structure and Function of the Neurologic System

Objectives

After reviewing this chapter, the learner will be able to do the following:

1. Identify the structural and functional subdivisions of the nervous system.
   Review page 296.

2. Compare the functions of neurons with those of neuroglia; identify the parts of neurons.
   Review pages 296-297; refer to Figures 12-1 through 12-3 and Table 12-1.

3. Describe the circumstances under which nervous tissue can regenerate.
   Review page 297; refer to Figure 12-4.

4. Describe transmission of impulses by neurotransmitters.
   Review pages 299 and 320-321; refer to Tables 12-2 and 12-7.

5. Identify the three main divisions of the brain; characterize their associated structures and functions.
   Review pages 301, 303, and 305-306; refer to Figures 12-5 through 12-7 and Table 12-3.

6. Identify the significance of decussation of motor fibers.
   Review page 306; refer to Figure 12-8.

7. Describe the location and structure of the spinal cord; define a reflex arc.
   Review pages 306-309; refer to Figures 12-9 through 12-13.

8. Identify the structures responsible for maintaining and protecting the central nervous system.
   Review pages 309-311; refer to Figures 12-14 through 12-16 and Table 12-4.

9. Identify the route of blood circulation within the central nervous system; note the significance of the circle of Willis.
   Review pages 312 and 314-315; refer to Figures 12-17 through 12-21 and Table 12-5.

10. Describe the structure of cranial and spinal nerves; locate plexuses.
    Review page 315; refer to Figure 12-22.

11. Name the cranial nerves and state functions of each.
    Refer to Table 12-6.

12. Identify the subdivisions of the autonomic nervous system, their origins, and general functions.
    Review pages 318-320, 322 and 324; refer to Figures 12-24, 12-25, and 12-27.

13. **Identify the type of neurotransmitter secreted by preganglionic and postganglionic fibers in the autonomic nervous system.**
    Review page 320; refer to Figures 12-23 and 12-26 and Table 12-7.

14. **Identify the structural, cellular, vascular, and functional changes that occur with aging.**
    Review page 324.

Practice Examination

1. One function of the somatic nervous system that is *not* performed by the autonomic nervous system is:
   a. conduction of impulses to involuntary muscles and glands.
   b. conduction of impulses to the central nervous system.
   c. conduction of impulses to skeletal muscles.
   d. conduction of impulses between the brain and spinal cord.

2. A neuron with a single dendrite at one end of the cell body and a single axon at the other end of the cell body would be classified as:
   a. unipolar.
   b. multipolar.
   c. monopolar.
   d. bipolar.

3. Neurons that carry impulses away from the CNS are called:
   a. afferent neurons.
   b. sensory neurons.
   c. efferent neurons.
   d. association neurons.

Match the structure with its function or description.

_____ 4. Schwann cell

_____ 5. dendrite

a. is the outer, nucleated layer of a certain cell type

b. produces myelin sheath

c. carries impulses away from perikaryon

d. covers neuron fibers

e. conducts impulses to cell body

6. Neurons are specialized for the conduction of impulses, whereas neuroglia:
   a. support nerve tissue.
   b. serve as motor end plates.
   c. synthesize acetylcholine and cholinesterase.
   d. All of the above are correct.

7. There is one-way conduction at a synapse because:
   a. only postsynaptic neurons contain synaptic vesicles.
   b. acetylcholine prevents nerve impulses from traveling in both directions.
   c. only the presynaptic neuron contains neurotransmitters.
   d. only dendrites release neurotransmitters.

8. Which contains the thalamus and hypothalamus?
   a. diencephalon
   b. cerebrum
   c. medulla oblongata
   d. brain stem

9. The reticular activating system:
   a. programs for fine repetitive motor movements.
   b. maintains wakefulness.
   c. maintains constant internal environments.
   d. affects the positioning of the head to improve hearing.

10. Which phrases best describe the spinal cord? (More than one answer may be correct.)
    a. descends inferior to the lumbar vertebrae
    b. conducts motor impulses from the brain
    c. descends to the fourth lumbar vertebra
    d. conducts sensory impulses to the brain

Match the component of a reflex arc with its descriptor.

_____11. sensory neuron

_____12. effector

a. carries impulses to the CNS

b. carries impulses to a responding organ

c. responds to motor impulse

d. is stimulated by one neuron and passes impulse on to another neuron

e. responds directly to changes in environment

13. Which is *not* a protective covering of the CNS?
    a. cauda equine
    b. dura mater
    c. arachnoid
    d. cranial bone

14. The composition of cerebrospinal fluid is:
    a. the same as blood.
    b. distilled H_2O with dissolved salts.
    c. a plasma-like liquid with glucose, salts, and proteins.
    d. a heavy mucous solution with dissolved salts, glucose, and urea.

Match the function with the cranial nerve.

_____15. tasting   a. facial

_____16. balance maintenance   b. olfactory

                                         c. vestibulocochlear

                                         d. hypoglossal

                                         e. optic

17. An autonomic ganglion can be described as:
    a. the site of synapses between visceral efferent
       neurons.
    b. a site where spinal reflexes occur.
    c. a point of synapse between parasympathetic and
       sympathetic neurons.
    d. the place where unconscious sensations occur.

18. The sympathetic division of the autonomic nervous
    system:
    a. mobilizes energy in times of need.
    b. is innervated by cell bodies from T1 through L2.
    c. is innervated by cell bodies located in the cranial
       nerve nuclei.
    d. Both a and b are correct.
    e. Both a and c are correct.

19. The parasympathetic division of the autonomic
    nervous system:
    a. conserves and stores energy.
    b. has relatively short postganglionic neurons.
    c. Both a and b are correct.
    d. has paravertebral ganglia.

Match the characteristic with the related division of the autonomic nervous system.

_____20. more extensive use of norepinephrine as   a. sympathetic
           a transmitter substance
                                                         b. parasympathetic
_____21. more widespread and generalized effects

_____22. elicits rest-response

Classify the effect of sympathetic nerve stimulation on the structure.

_____23. breathing passageways   a. increases diameter

_____24. intestines   b. decreases diameter

_____25. liver   c. increases activity

                                         d. decreases activity

13

Pain, Temperature, Sleep, and Sensory Function

a. **Identify receptors, pathways, and perceptors for pain.**
   Review pages 330-331; refer to Figure 13-1.

MEMORY CHECK!

- Pain receptors, also known as *nociceptors,* are small unmyelinated and lightly myelinated nerve endings of afferent neurons found in nearly every tissue in the body. These neurons respond to chemical, thermal, and mechanical stimuli. Sensory nerves transmit the stimuli from pain receptors into the dorsal horn of the spinal cord. The impulses ascend by either the neospinothalamic tract or the paleospinothalamic tract. The paleospinothalamic tract carries information to the reticular formation, the pons, the limbic system, and the midbrain. The neospinothalamic tract carries information to the midbrain, the postcentral gyrus where pain is perceived, and the cortex where precision and discrimination occur.

b. **Describe thermoregulation.**
   Review pages 335-337; refer to Table 13-5.

MEMORY CHECK!

- The control of body temperature is a function of centers located in the hypothalamus. Thermoreceptors provide the hypothalamus with information about peripheral and core temperatures. If the temperature is low, the body initiates heat conservation measures by a series of hormonal mechanisms. Heat production begins with hypothalamic release of TSH-RH, which stimulates release of TSH from the anterior pituitary. The TSH causes release of thyroxine from the thyroid gland. This hormone causes release of epinephrine from the adrenal medulla. Epinephrine causes vasoconstriction, glycolysis, and increased metabolic rates, which increase heat production. Warmer peripheral and core temperatures reverse the process. Decreasing the sympathetic pathway produces vasodilation, decreased muscle tone, and increased perspiration.

c. **Identify the normal sleep stages; describe nervous system control of sleep.**
   Review pages 338-340.

MEMORY CHECK!

- Normal sleep has two phases that can be documented by electroencephalography (EEG): rapid eye movement (REM) sleep and non-REM, or slow wave, sleep. Non-REM sleep is initiated by the withdrawal of neurotransmitters from the reticular formation and by the inhibition of arousal mechanisms. During non-REM sleep, respiration is controlled by metabolic processes. The basal metabolic rate, temperature, heart rate, blood pressure, and muscle tone all decrease. Knee-jerk reflexes are absent. Pupils are constricted. During various stages, cerebral blood flow to the brain decreases, growth hormone is released, and levels of corticosteroids and catecholamines are depressed.

- REM sleep occurs about every 90 minutes beginning after 1 or 2 hours of non-REM sleep. The EEG pattern of REM sleep is similar to the normal awake pattern. Alternating periods of REM and non-REM sleep occur throughout the night, with lengthening intervals of REM sleep and fewer intervals of the deeper stages of non-REM sleep toward morning. REM sleep is characterized by rapid eye movement; loss of tone of antigravity muscles; loss of temperature regulation; alteration in heart rate, blood pressure, and respiration; penile erection in men and clitoral engorgement in women; and a high rate of memorable dreams. Steroids are released in short bursts and cerebral blood flow is increased. The reticular formation is primarily responsible for generating REM sleep. Projections from the reticular formation and other areas of the mesencephalon and brain stem produce non-REM sleep.

d. **Describe the eye and its structure.**
   Review pages 340-342; refer to Figures 13-6 through 13-8.

MEMORY CHECK!

- The wall of the eye is formed of three layers: sclera, choroid, and retina. It becomes transparent at the cornea in the central anterior region, which allows light to enter the eye. The choroid is the pigmented middle layer that prevents light from scattering inside the eye. The iris, part of the choroid, has a round opening, the pupil, through which light passes.

- The innermost layer of the eye, the retina, contains the rods and cones. These photoreceptors convert light energy into nerve impulses.

- Nerve impulses pass through the optic nerves to the optic chiasm. Nerves from the nasal halves of the retinas cross and join fibers from the temporal halves of the retinas to form the optic tracts. The optic tracts connect to the primary visual cortex in the occipital lobe of the brain. Light entering the eye is focused on the retina by the lens, which is a flexible, biconvex, crystal-like structure. The lens separates the anterior cavity from the vitreous chamber. The aqueous humor of the anterior cavity helps maintain pressure inside the eye and provides nutrients to the lens and the cornea. The vitreous chamber is filled with a gel-like vitreous humor that prevents the eyeball from collapsing inward.

- Six extrinsic eye muscles allow gross eye movements and permit eyes to follow a moving object. The external structures protecting the eye include the eyelids, conjunctiva, and lacrimal apparatus.

e. **Describe the parts of the ear.**
   Review pages 344-346; refer to Figures 13-11 and 13-12.

- The ear is divided into three areas: the external ear, involved only with hearing; the middle ear, involved only with hearing; and the inner ear, involved with hearing and equilibrium.

- The external ear is composed of the pinna, which is visible, and the external auditory canal that leads to the middle ear. Sound waves entering the external auditory canal cause the tympanic membrane to vibrate. This membrane separates the external ear from the middle ear.

- The middle ear is composed of the tympanic cavity within the temporal bone. Three ossicles transmit the vibration of the tympanic membrane to the inner ear and set the fluids of the inner ear in motion.

- The inner ear is a system of osseous labyrinths filled with perilymph. The bony labyrinth is divided into the cochlea, the vestibule, and the semicircular canals.

- Sound waves that reach the cochlea through vibrations of the tympanic membrane, ossicles, and oval window set the cochlear fluids in motion. Receptor cells on the basilar membrane are stimulated and transmit impulses along the cochlear nerve, a division of the vestibulocochlear nerve, to the auditory cortex of the temporal lobe for sound interpretation.

- The semicircular canals and vestibule of the inner ear contain equilibrium receptors. In the semicircular canals, the dynamic equilibrium receptors respond to changes in direction of movement. The vestibule in the inner ear contains receptors essential to the body's sense of static equilibrium. Both of these impulses are transmitted through the vestibular nerve, a division of the vestibulocochlear nerve, to the cerebellum.

Objectives

After studying this chapter, the learner will be able to do the following:

1. **Describe pain modulation and note stimuli that activate nociceptors.**
   Study pages 331-332; refer to Figures 13-2 and 13-3 and Table 13-1.

According to the **gate control theory,** nociceptive impulses are transmitted from specialized skin receptors to the spinal cord through large A and small C fibers. These fibers terminate in the dorsal horn of the spinal cord. Cells in the substantia gelatinosa of the dorsal horn function as a gate and permit some impulses to reach the central nervous system for interpretation. Stimulation of larger, faster-transmitting fibers causes the cells in the substantia gelatinosa to "close the gate," which diminishes pain perception. Slower-transmitting small-fiber input inhibits cells in the substantia gelatinosa and "opens the gate," and enhances pain perception. In addition to gate control through large- and small-fiber stimulation, the central nervous system through efferent pathways may close, partially close, or open the gate. This theory does not explain chronic pain problems such as phantom limb pain.

Tissue injury and chronic inflammation result in the release of prostaglandins and lymphokines that trigger release of neuromodulators that mediate information about painful stimuli. These neuromodulators include **substance P, calcitonin-gene-related peptide, norepinephrine,** and **5-hydroxytryptamine.**

Endorphins (endogenous morphines) are neuropeptides that inhibit transmission of pain impulses in the spinal cord and brain. All endorphins attach to opiate receptors on the plasma membrane of the afferent neuron. The combination of the opiate receptor and endorphin inhibits the release of excitatory neurotransmitters, thereby blocking the transmission of the painful stimulus. Stress, excessive physical exertion, acupuncture, and intercourse are factors that increase the level of circulating endorphins, serotonin, norepinephrine, and other neurotransmitters, thus raising the pain threshold.

2. **Differentiate among categories of pain.**
   Study pages 332-335; refer to Figure 13-4 and Tables 13-2 and 13-3.

   Somatogenic pain is pain with an identifiable cause. **Psychogenic pain** is pain without a known physical cause.

   Acute pain may be somatic, visceral, or referred. **Somatic pain** comes from the skin or close to the surface of the body and is well localized. Visceral pain occurs in internal organs, the abdomen, or skeleton. It is poorly localized. It is associated with nausea and vomiting, hypotension, restlessness, and possible shock. **Visceral pain** often radiates or is referred. **Referred pain** is present in an area removed or distant from its point of origin. The area of referred pain is supplied by the same spinal segment as the actual site of injury. Impulses from many cutaneous and visceral neurons converge on the same ascending neuron, and the brain cannot distinguish between the origins of the two.

   Chronic pain is prolonged; it may last longer than 6 months and may either persist or be intermittent. Causes of chronic pain include decreased levels of endorphins or a predominance of C neuron stimulation. Physiologic responses to chronic pain depend on the persistent or intermittent nature of the pain. **Intermittent pain** produces physiologic response similar to acute pain, whereas **persistent pain** permits physiologic adaptation. Individuals with chronic pain often are depressed, have difficulty sleeping and eating, and may become preoccupied with their pain.

   Neuropathic pain results from abnormal processing of sensory information by the peripheral and central nervous systems. *Central pain* is caused by a lesion or dysfunction in the brain or spinal cord, such as phantom pain or reflex sympathetic dystrophy. *Peripheral pain* is the result of trauma or disease that affects peripheral nerves, such as nerve entrapment or diabetic neuropathy.

3. **Describe the alterations occurring in fever, hyperthermia, and hypothermia.**
   Study pages 337-338; refer to Figure 13-5.

   Fever is not the failure of the normal thermoregulatory mechanism. Instead, it is considered "a resetting of the hypothalamic thermostat" to a higher level. The normal thermoregulatory mechanisms are raised so that the thermoregulatory center adjusts heat production, conservation, and loss to maintain the core temperature at a new, higher set-point temperature.

   The pathophysiology of fever begins with exogenous pyrogens or endotoxins stimulating the release of interleukin-1, tumor necrosis factor, interleukin-6, and interferon, which raise the set-point. As the set-point is raised, the hypothalamus signals an increase in heat production and conservation to raise body temperature to the new level.

   As fever breaks, the set-point is returned to normal. The hypothalamus signals a decrease in heat production and an increase in heat reduction.

   Fever can be beneficial. Elevated body temperature kills many microorganisms and has adverse effects on the growth and replication of others. Increased temperature causes lysosomal breakdown with autodestruction of cells; this prevents viral replication in infected cells. Heat increases lymphocytic transformation and motility of polymorphonuclear neutrophils, which facilitate the immune response.

   Hyperthermia can produce nerve damage, coagulation of cell proteins, and death. At 41° C (106° F), nerve damage produces convulsions in the adult. At 43° C (109° F), death follows. In hyperthermia, there is no resetting of the hypothalamic set-point. Forms of accidental hyperthermia are heat cramps, heat exhaustion, and heatstroke.

   Heat cramps are severe, spasmodic cramps in the abdomen and extremities subsequent to prolonged sweating and associated sodium loss. Heat cramps usually appear in individuals who are unaccustomed to heat or who perform strenuous work in very warm climates. Fever, rapid pulse, and increased blood pressure often accompany the cramps.

   Heat exhaustion or collapse results from prolonged high body core or environmental temperatures. These high temperatures cause profound vasodilation and profuse sweating. Over a prolonged period of elevated temperatures, the hypothalamic responses produce dehydration, decreased plasma volumes, hypotension, decreased cardiac output, and tachycardia.

   Heatstroke is a potentially lethal consequence of a breakdown in control of an overstressed thermoregulatory center. In cases of very high core temperatures (>40° C), the regulatory center may cease to function appropriately.

   High core temperatures and vascular collapse produce cerebral edema, degeneration of the central nervous system, and renal tubular necrosis. Death results unless immediate, effective treatment is initiated.

   Malignant hyperthermia is a potentially lethal complication of an inherited muscle disorder. Malignant hyperthermia causes intracellular calcium levels to rise, producing sustained, uncoordinated muscle contractions. As a result of these contractions, acidosis develops. Cardiac dysrhythmias, hypotension, decreased cardiac output, or cardiac arrest may follow.

Hypothermia (marked cooling of core temperature) produces depression of the central nervous and respiratory systems. In severe hypothermia, ice crystals form on the inside of the cell, causing cells to rupture and die. Tissue hypothermia slows cell metabolism, increases the blood viscosity, slows microcirculatory blood flow, facilitates blood coagulation, and stimulates profound vasoconstriction. Hypothermia may be accidental or therapeutic.

4. **Describe sleep disorders; cite examples.**
   Study page 340.

Sleep disorders are classified by signs and symptoms rather than by their etiologies. Sleep disorders can be classified as (1) disorders of initiating sleep, (2) disorders of excessive somnolence, (3) disorders of the sleep-wake schedule, and (4) dysfunctions of sleep, sleep stages, or partial arousals.

Disorders of initiating sleep are classified as **insomnia,** the inability to fall or stay asleep. Insomnia may be transient and related to travel across time zones, or it may be due to acute stress. Long-term insomnia is associated with drug or alcohol abuse, chronic pain disorders, or chronic depression.

Two disorders of excessive daytime sleepiness are **obstructive sleep apnea syndrome** and **hypersomnia sleep apnea (HSA) syndrome.** Both are associated with periodic breathing and episodes of apnea.

In obstructive sleep apnea syndrome, the apneic periods are generally due to obesity, decreased chemosensitivity to carbon dioxide and oxygen tensions, or upper airway obstruction occurring while sleeping. HSA syndrome is primarily a result of upper airway obstruction occurring during sleep. The sleep apnea reduces oxygen saturation and eventually produces polycythemia, pulmonary hypertension, right-sided congestive heart failure, liver congestion, cyanosis, and peripheral edema.

Common **disorders of the sleep-wake schedule** include rapid time-zone change or "jet-lag syndrome," an altered sleep schedule with an advance or a delay of 3 hours or more in sleep time, or a change in total sleep time from day to day. Vigilance of psychomotor performance and arousal are markedly depressed after alterations in the sleep-wake schedule.

Dysfunctions of sleep, sleep stages, or **partial arousals** are common in children. They are somnambulism, night terrors, and enuresis. **Somnambulism,** or sleepwalking, appears to resolve itself within several years after the onset of the sleepwalking episodes. During the sleepwalking episode, the child functions at a very low level of arousal and has no memory of the event upon awakening.

Night terrors are characterized by "sudden apparent arousals in which the child expresses intense fear or emotion." However, the child is not awake and is very difficult to arouse. Once awakened, the child has no memory of the night terror event. Neither somnambulism nor night terrors are associated with dreams.

Enuresis, or bedwetting, is disturbing because of social pressure. It is not associated with dreaming. Children eventually "outgrow" the enuretic episodes.

5. **Identify common diseases that are associated with the special senses and describe their etiologies and manifestations.**
   Study pages 341-349; refer to Figures 13-9 and 13-10 and Tables 13-6 and 13-7.

Vision

Blepharitis is an inflammation of the eyelids caused by staphylococcal infections or seborrheic dermatitis.

Conjunctivitis is an inflammation of the conjunctiva, or the mucous membrane covering the front part of the eyeball. It may be caused by bacteria, viruses, allergies, or chemical irritations.

Keratitis is an infection of the cornea usually caused by bacteria or viruses. Bacterial infections often cause corneal ulceration and require extensive antibiotic treatment. Type I herpes virus usually infects the cornea and conjunctiva.

Strabismus is the deviation of one eye from the other when the person is looking directly at an object. It is due to a weak or hypertonic muscle in one of the eyes. The deviation may be upward, downward, inward, or outward.

Amblyopia is a vision reduction or dimness for unknown reasons. Amblyopia is associated with diabetes mellitus, renal failure, malaria, and toxic substances such as alcohol and tobacco.

A **scotoma** is a circumscribed defect of the central field of vision. It is most often a sequel to an inflammatory lesion of the optic nerve and is often associated with multiple sclerosis.

A **cataract** is a cloudy or opaque ocular lens. The most common form of cataract is degenerative.

Papilledema is edema and inflammation of the optic nerve at its point of entrance into the eyeball. Generally, papilledema is caused by obstruction to the venous return from the retina.

Dark adaptation affects visual acuity. Changes in rhodopsin, a substance found in the rods and responsible for low-light vision, are likely responsible for reduced dark adaptation in older adults. Vitamin A deficiencies can cause the same disorder in individuals of any age.

Glaucoma is characterized by intraocular pressures above the normal range of 12 to 20 mm Hg maintained by the aqueous fluid in homeostasis. Intraocular fluid accumulation blocks the flow of nutrients to optic nerve fibers, leading to their death.

Loss of accommodation associated with aging is termed **presbyopia,** a condition in which the ocular lens becomes larger, firmer, and less elastic. The major symptom is reduced near vision, causing reading material to be held at arm's length.

In **myopia,** or nearsightedness, light rays are focused in front of the retina when the person is looking at a distant object. In **hyperopia,** or farsightedness, light rays are focused behind the retina when the person is looking at a near object. **Astigmatism** is caused by an unequal curvature of the cornea; light rays are bent unevenly and do not come to a single focus on the retina.

Hearing

A **conductive hearing loss** occurs when a change in the outer and/or middle ear impairs sound conduction from the outer to the inner ear. Conditions that commonly cause a conductive hearing loss include impacted cerumen, foreign bodies lodged in the ear canal, neoplasms of the external auditory canal and/or middle ear, eustachian tube dysfunction, otitis media, cholesteatoma, and otosclerosis. Symptoms of conductive hearing loss include diminished hearing and soft speaking voice. The voice is soft because the individual may hear his or her voice conducted by bone ossicles.

A **sensorineural hearing loss** is due to impairment of the organ of Corti and its hearing receptors or its central connections. Conditions that commonly cause sensorineural hearing loss include congenital and hereditary factors, noise exposure, aging, ototoxicity, and systemic diseases. Congenital and neonatal sensorineural hearing loss may be caused by maternal rubella, infant prematurity, traumatic delivery, or erythroblastosis fetalis.

Otitis externa is an infection of the outer ear associated with prolonged exposure to moisture.

Otitis media is an infection of the middle ear common in children.

Olfaction

Hyposmia is an impaired sense of smell; anosmia is the complete loss of smell. **Olfactory** hallucinations arise from hyperactivity in cortical neurons and involve the smelling of odors that actually are not present. **Parosmia** is an abnormal or perverted sense of smell.

Taste

Hypogeusia is decreased taste sensation; **ageusia** is the absence of taste. These disorders are the result of cranial nerve injuries and can be specific to the area of tongue innervated.

Parageusia is a perversion of taste in which substances that are usually palatable instead illicit an unpleasant flavor. Parageusia is common in individuals receiving chemotherapy for cancer. Parageusia often leads to anorexia.

Touch

Any impairment of reception, transmission, perception, or interpretation of touch alters tactile sensation. Trauma, tumor, infection, metabolic changes, vascular changes, and degenerative disease may cause tactile dysfunction.

Proprioception

Proprioception is the perception and awareness of the position of the body and its parts. It depends on impulses from the inner ear and from receptors in joints and ligaments. **Proprioceptive dysfunction** may be caused by alterations at any level of the nervous system, similar to that observed in tactile dysfunction.

Vestibular nystagmus is the constant, involuntary movement of the eyeball caused when the semicircular canal system is overstimulated.

Vertigo is the sensation of spinning that occurs with inflammation of the semicircular canals in the ear.

Ménière disease is a vestibular disorder that can cause proprioceptive dysfunction. The individual with acute Ménière disease may experience loss of proprioception and become unable to stand or walk.

Peripheral neuropathies are probably associated with renal disease and diabetes mellitus. The result is a diminished or absent sense of body position or position of body parts. Gait changes often occur.

Practice Examination

Match the pain characteristic with the nervous system component.

_____ 1. basic perception of pain

_____ 2. initiation of pain stimulus

_____ 3. discrimination and precision given to painful stimulus

a. nociceptive receptors

b. postcentral gyrus

c. brain stem

d. A fibers

e. cortex

4. Endorphins:
   a. increase pain sensations.
   b. decrease pain sensations.
   c. may increase or decrease pain sensations.
   d. have no effect on pain sensations.

5. Referred pain from upper abdominal diseases involves:
   a. the sacral region.
   b. L2 to L4.
   c. T8, L1, and L2.
   d. the gluteal regions, posterior thighs, and calves.

6. In the gate control theory of pain:
   a. a "closed gate" increases pain perception.
   b. stimulation of large A fibers "closes the gate."
   c. Both a and b are correct.
   d. Neither a nor b is correct.

7. Which is *not* a neuromodulator of pain?
   a. prostaglandins
   b. 5-hydroxytryptamine
   c. norepinephrine
   d. lymphokines
   e. heparin

8. Interleukin-1:
   a. raises the hypothalamic set-point.
   b. is an endogenous pyrogen.
   c. is stimulated by exogenous pyrogens.
   d. None of the above is correct.
   e. a, b, and c are correct.

9. Increased serum levels of epinephrine increase body temperature by:
   a. increasing shivering.
   b. increasing muscle tone.
   c. increasing heat production.
   d. decreasing basal metabolic rate.

10. In heatstroke:
    a. core temperature usually doesn't exceed 101° F.
    b. sodium loss follows sweating.
    c. core temperature increases as the regulatory center fails.
    d. Both b and c are correct.

11. Which is involved in fever?
    a. tumor necrosis factor
    b. endotoxins
    c. elevation of the set-point in the hypothalamus
    d. Both a and b are correct.
    e. a, b, and c are correct.

12. In hypothermia:
    a. the viscosity of blood is decreased.
    b. acidosis can develop.
    c. the hypothalamic center prevents shivering.
    d. All of the above are correct.

13. Although non-REM and REM sleep are defined by electrical recordings, they are characterized by physiologic events. Which does *not* occur?
    a. During non-REM sleep, muscle tone decreases.
    b. Non-REM is initiated by withdrawal of neurotransmitters from the reticular formation.
    c. During non-REM, cerebral blood flow to the cortex is decreased.
    d. During non-REM, levels of corticosteroids are increased.

14. Ménière disease:
    a. affects the outer ear.
    b. disrupts both vestibular and hearing functions.
    c. is the common cause of sensorineural hearing loss.
    d. is caused by impacted cerumen.

15. Acute otitis media (AOM):
    a. has no genetic determinants.
    b. displays a tympanic membrane progressing from erythema to opaqueness with bulging.
    c. has breast-feeding as a risk factor.
    d. is commonly caused by *Staphylococcus aureus*.

16. Age-related macular degeneration (AMD):
    a. has a higher incidence in hypotensive individuals.
    b. occurs in individuals before the age of 60 years.
    c. exhibits retinal detachment and loss of photoreceptors.
    d. exhibits loss of accommodation.

17. Vestibular nystagmus:
    a. is the constant, involuntary movement of the eyeball caused by ear disturbances.
    b. is the sensation of spinning.
    c. may be caused by alterations in nervous system from receptor to the cerebral cortex.
    d. causes a diminished sense of the position of body parts.

18. Sleep apnea:
    a. is lack of breathing during sleep.
    b. results from airway obstruction during sleep.
    c. is associated with "jet-lag syndrome."
    d. All of the above are correct.
    e. Both a and b are correct.

19. Individuals affected by sleep apnea may experience:
    a. polycythemia.
    b. cyanosis.
    c. pulmonary hypertension.
    d. All of the above are correct

Match the term with its defining characteristic.

_____20. blepharitis

_____21. strabismus

_____22. anosmia

_____23. hypogeusia

_____24. vertigo

_____25. glaucoma

a. inflammation of mucous membrane covering the eyeball

b. infection of the cornea

c. weak muscle in one of the eyes

d. reduction or dimness of vision

e. inflammation of the eyelids

f. high intraocular pressures

g. elevated intraocular pressure

h. inflammation of the semicircular canals

i. decreased taste sensation

j. complete loss of smell

Case Study

Mrs. D. is a 45-year-old female who sought care for chronic insomnia of 15 months' duration. She stated that she awakes 15 to 20 times a night and rarely sleeps more than 4 hours. Various hypnotics had been unsuccessful in relieving her symptoms.

Her history revealed that about 18 months earlier some important stressful life changes occurred. Her only child, a daughter, left for an out-of-state university. A lifelong friend, who was a confidante, moved to another community. Her husband, a successful dentist, had become more involved in various men's organizations than in the past.

A sedating antidepressant was prescribed and a second appointment was made for 10 days later. At the second appointment, which lasted 1 hour, she noted her sleep patterns had improved. She was able to articulate that she felt unneeded, incompetent, and old.

As a caregiver, how would you assess Mrs. D.'s case?

Concepts of Neurologic Dysfunction

14

Foundational Objectives

a. Describe the RAS as a modulator of consciousness.
   Review page 301; refer to Figure 12-5.

MEMORY CHECK!

- The reticular activating system (RAS) maintains wakefulness. It ascends from the lower brain stem and projects throughout the cerebral cortex. The ability to respond to stimuli or arousal depends on an intact RAS in the brain stem and the ability to respond to the environment. Cognition relies on an intact cerebral cortex. Therefore, consciousness or responsiveness requires functioning along the reticular formation in the brain stem to the cerebral cortex.

b. Identify the structural and functional components of the brain.
   Review pages 301, 303, and 305-306; refer to Figures 12-3 through 12-7 and Table 12-3.

MEMORY CHECK!

- The central nervous system (CNS) consists of the brain and spinal cord encased within the meninges and bathed in cerebrospinal fluid (CSF). The brain is divided into several areas, including the cerebrum, midbrain, cerebellum, pons, and medulla oblongata. The midbrain, the medulla, and the pons comprise the brain stem.

- The outer covering of the cerebrum is the cortex. The entire cerebrum is divided into two halves, or hemispheres, connected by a neural bridge, the corpus callosum, that coordinates activities between hemispheres. The cortex is concerned with thinking and sensory perception. Emotional responses and control of body temperature, water and food intake, and sex drive have their origin in the midbrain area. The cerebellum primarily integrates muscular movements to produce coordination in walking, talking, and other complex muscular activities. The medulla oblongata controls vital functions such as respiration, heart rate, and blood pressure, although these are modified by higher brain centers.

- Within the cerebral hemispheres are subdivisions, or lobes. The frontal lobe is located in the anterior portion of each hemisphere. The temporal lobe is located in the lower middle region of each hemisphere. The parietal lobe is the upper, rear portion. The occipital lobe is the lower, rear portion of each hemisphere.

- The basal ganglia are a collection of cell bodies in several areas of the brain's gray matter including the caudate nucleus, globus pallidus, putamen, and substantia nigra. The function of the basal ganglia is thought to involve the planning and programming of movement.

c. **Identify the parts of the CNS that control voluntary muscle movement.**
   Review pages 303 and 305-306; refer to Figures 12-6 through 12-8, and 12-11.

MEMORY CHECK!

- The cerebral cortex plays a major role in controlling precise, voluntary muscular movements. Motor output to skeletal muscles travels down the spinal cord in two types of descending tracts, the pyramidal tracts and the extrapyramidal tracts. The pyramidal tracts originate in the motor cortex and terminate in the brain stem. They cross to the opposite side at the medulla-spinal cord junction. The pyramidal tracts convey impulses causing precise, voluntary movements of skeletal muscles. The extrapyramidal tracts arise from the cortex and project to innervate the motor neurons; they do not cross to the opposite side. Extrapyramidal tracts convey nerve impulses that program fine repetitive motor movements.

Objectives

After studying this chapter, the learner will be able to do the following:

1. **Define terms describing levels of consciousness.**
   Refer to Table 14-3.

   Consciousness is alertness with orientation to person, place, and time. **Confusion** is an inability to think. First there is **disorientation** to time, then to place, and eventually to person. The attention span is shortened. A state of **lethargy** may exhibit orientation to person, place, and time; however, slow vocalization and decreased motor skills are present. **Obtundation** is awakening in response to stimulation. Continuous stimulation is needed for arousal. **Stupor** is vocalization only in response to vigorous stimuli. Markedly decreased spontaneous movement is seen. **Coma** displays no vocalization and no arousal to any stimulus.

2. **Identify sites and causes for alterations in arousal.**
   Study page 356; refer to Tables 14-1 and 14-2.

   Possible causes of an **altered level of arousal** may be separated into three major groups: structural, metabolic, and psychogenic. **Structural causes** are divided according to whether the original pathologic condition is above (**supratentorial**) or below (**infratentorial**) the tentorial plate.
   Supratentorial processes produce a decreased level of consciousness because of compression or displacement of the diencephalon or brain stem. **Infratentorial processes** produce a reduction in arousal by diseases that destroy the brain stem.
   Disorders outside the brain, such as neoplasms, bleeding from trauma, and pus, can produce arousal dys-

function. Bleeding, infarcts, emboli, and neoplasms within the brain also can contribute to altered levels of arousal.
   A wide spectrum of disorders or agents may produce a **metabolically** induced alteration in arousal. Hypoxia, electrolyte disturbances, hypoglycemia, drugs, and toxins alter arousal.
   Psychogenic unresponsiveness may develop in general psychiatric disorders. Despite apparent unconsciousness, the person is actually physiologically awake.

3. **Summarize the changes in levels of consciousness, pupillary response, muscle tone, and respiratory activity as the diencephalon through the medulla is affected.**
   Study pages 356-357 and 359-361; refer to Figures 14-1 through 14-6 and Tables 14-4 and 14-5. (See box on page 84 of *Workbook*.)

4. **Distinguish between cerebral death and brain death.**
   Study pages 362-363 and Box 14-1.
   Cerebral death, or irreversible coma, is death of the cerebral hemispheres, exclusive of the brain stem and cerebellum. The individual is permanently unable to respond in any significant way to the environment. The brain may continue to maintain internal homeostasis.
   Brain death occurs when irreversible brain damage is so extensive that the brain can no longer maintain the body's internal respiratory and cerebral vascular functions. There is destruction of the brain stem and cerebellum.

ROSTRAL-CAUDAL PROGRESSION OF NONRESPONSIVENESS

Area Involved	Level of Consciousness	Pupils	Muscle Tone	Breathing Pattern
Diencephalon (thalamus/ hypothalamus)	Decreased concentration, agitation, dullness, lethargy, obtundation	Respond to light briskly; full-range eye movements only on "doll's eyes"—none in direction of rotation or after injection of hot or cold water in ear canal (caloric posturing)	Some purposeful movement in response to pain, combative movement Decorticate—flexion in upper extremities and extension in lower extremities	Yawning and sighing to Cheyne-Stokes
Midbrain	Stupor to coma	Midposition fixed (MPF)	Decerebrate—arms rigid, palms turned away from body	Neurogenic hyperventilation
Pons	Coma	MPF	Decerebrate	Apneustic—prolonged inspiration and expiration
Medulla	Coma	MPF	Flaccid	Ataxic—uncoordinated and irregular

5. **Define seizure and cite conditions associated with seizure disorders.**
Study pages 363-366; refer to Tables 14-6 through 14-8.

A **seizure** is a sudden, explosive disorderly discharge of cerebral neurons and is characterized by a sudden, transient alteration in brain function, usually involving motor, sensory, autonomic, or psychic clinical manifestations and an alteration in level of arousal. The alteration in level of arousal is temporary. Among the causes of seizure activity are:

metabolic defects	motor syndromes
congenital malformations	infections
genetic predisposition	brain tumors
perinatal injury	vascular diseases
postnatal trauma	fever

Epilepsy, seizure activity recurring in absence of treatment, is now believed to be caused by genetic mutations that cause brain wiring abnormalities and/or chemical imbalances in brain signals or abnormal nerve connections made while attempting repair after injury.

An **epileptogenic focus** may be a group of neurons that have lost their afferent stimulation. The plasma membranes of these neuronal cells appear to be hypersensitive. This makes them more easily activated by hyperthermia, hypoxia, hypoglycemia, hyponatremia, repeated sensory stimulation, and certain sleep phases. The neural excitation spreads to the subcortical, thalamic, and brain stem areas to initiate the tonic phase of muscle contraction, which is followed by increased muscle tone and loss of consciousness.

The clonic phase of alternating contraction and relaxation of muscles begins as inhibitory neurons in the cortex, anterior thalamus, and basal ganglia begin to inhibit the cortical excitation. This inhibition interrupts seizure discharge and produces an intermittent pattern of muscle contractions; the contractions gradually decrease and then finally cease.

6. **Differentiate between partial and generalized seizures.**
Refer to Table 14-7.

COMMON EPILEPTIC SEIZURE TYPES

Disorder	Areas Involved	Changes in Consciousness	Impaired Capacities/Symptoms
Partial			
Jacksonian	Simple unilateral	No change in consciousness generally	Disturbance in motor capacity
Psychomotor	Complex unilateral	Loss of consciousness, automatism	Dyscognitive states, loss of awareness
Generalized			
Generalized tonic-clonic movement (grand mal)	Bilateral	Loss of consciousness with postictal sleeping	Major tonic-clonic movement; muscular contraction followed by relaxation or a longer phase of contraction
Absence (petit mal)	Bilateral	Transient losses of consciousness	Blank spells, akinetic seizures, myoclonic jerks

7. **Define general descriptive terms of cognitive deficits.**
   Study pages 366-368; refer to Table 14-9.

Selective attention deficit refers to the inability to select appropriately from available, competing environmental stimuli for conscious processing.
Anterograde amnesia is an inability to form new memories.
Retrograde amnesia is loss of past memories.
Executive function deficit prevents programming, verification, and correction.
   Generally, the primary pathophysiologic mechanism that operates in cognitive system disorders is due directly to ischemia and hypoxia or indirectly to compression, toxins, and chemicals.

8. **Identify terms used to describe specific cognition disorders.**
   Study pages 368 and 370-372; refer to Figure 14-7 and Tables 14-10 through 14-13.

Agnosia is a defect of recognition of the form and nature of objects. Although it most commonly is associated with cerebrovascular accidents, it may arise from any pathologic process that injures specific areas of the brain.
Dysphasia is impairment of comprehension or production of language. Comprehension or use of symbols, in either written or verbal language, is disturbed or lost. Dysphasias usually are associated with cerebrovascular

accidents involving the middle cerebral artery or one of its many branches. Dysphasia results from dysfunction in the left cerebral hemisphere and usually involves the frontotemporal region. Dysphagia may be nonfluent; the individual cannot find words to express thoughts and exhibits difficulty in writing. Dysphasia also may be fluent; uttered verbal language is meaningless; inappropriate words are used.

Acute confusional states result from cerebral dysfunction secondary to drug intoxication or nervous system disease. These states may begin either suddenly or gradually depending on the amount of toxin exposure. The predominant feature of an acute confusional state is impaired or lost vigilance. The individual is unable to concentrate on incoming sensory information or on any one particular mental or motor task.

The **dementias** are characterized by the loss of more than one cognitive or intellectual function. There may be a decrease in orientation, general knowledge and information, vigilance, recent memory, remote memory, concept formation, abstraction, reasoning, and language. Causes of dementia include degeneration, cerebrovascular accidents, compression, toxins, metabolic disorders, biochemical imbalance, demyelinization, and infections. Symptoms of dementia may be categorized as cortical, subcortical, or both. Cortical dementia manifests as amnesic dementia (loss of recent memory), or cognitive dementia (loss of remote memory). Subcortical dementia exhibits slowed thought processes, personality changes, and loss of motor function.

9. Characterize the stages of increased intracranial pressure; describe herniation syndrome and cerebral edema.

Study pages 372-375; refer to Figures 14-8 through 14-10 and Box 14-2.

Increased intracranial pressure may result from an increase in intracranial content, which occurs with tumor growth, edema, excess cerebrospinal fluid, or hemorrhage. A rise in intracranial pressure from one component requires an equal reduction in volume of other components. The most readily displaced content of the cranial vault is cerebrospinal fluid (CSF).

In Stage 1 of intracranial hypertension, vasoconstriction and external compression of the venous system occur in an attempt to decrease further the intracranial pressure following CSF displacement from the cranial vault.

With continued expansion of the intracranial content, the resulting increase in intracranial pressure may exceed the brain's compensatory capacity to adjust to the increasing pressure (stage 2). The pressure begins to compromise neurotissues (stage 3), and eventually herniates brain tissue (stage 4) from one brain compartment to another.

The four types of cerebral edema are (1) vasogenic edema, (2) cytotoxic (metabolic) edema, (3) ischemic edema, and (4) interstitial edema.

Vasogenic edema is clinically the most important type. It is caused by the increased permeability of the capillary endothelium of the brain after injury to the vascular structure. Plasma proteins leak into the extracellular spaces, drawing water to them, so the water content of the brain parenchyma increases. Vasogenic edema starts in the area of injury and spreads with preferential accumulation in the white matter of the ipsilateral side because the parallel myelinated fibers separate more easily.

In **cytotoxic (metabolic) edema,** toxic factors directly affect the neuronal, glial, and endothelial cells, causing failure of the active transport systems. The cells lose their potassium and gain larger amounts of sodium. Water follows by osmosis into the cells, causing the cells to swell. Cytotoxic edema principally occurs in the gray matter.

Ischemic edema follows cerebral infarction. The initial edema is confined to the intracellular compartment. Later in the process, brain cells begin to undergo necrosis and die. The released lysosomes increase the blood-brain barrier's permeability by lysing it.

Interstitial edema is caused by movement of cerebrospinal fluid from the ventricles into the extracellular spaces of the brain tissues. The brain fluid volume is mostly increased around the ventricles; increased pressure is within the white matter.

10. Describe hydrocephalus.

Study pages 375-376; refer to Table 14-14.

Hydrocephalus refers to various conditions characterized by excess fluid in the cranial vault, subarachnoid space, or both. It occurs because of interference with cerebrospinal fluid flow caused by increased fluid production, obstruction within the ventricular system, or defective reabsorption of the fluid.

Hydrocephalus may develop from infancy through adulthood. Congenital hydrocephalus is rare. **Noncommunicating,** or internal, hydrocephalus in which the flow from the ventricles is obstructed is seen more often in children, and the **communicating** type without obstruction is seen more often in adults.

Obstructed cerebrospinal fluid is under pressure and causes atrophy of the cerebral cortex and degeneration of the white matter tracts. There is selective preservation of gray matter.

Acute hydrocephalus manifests signs of rapidly developing increased intracranial pressure. If not promptly treated, the individual quickly becomes comatose. Normal pressure hydrocephalus develops slowly, showing declining memory and cognitive function. In infancy, head enlargement is predominant before cranial suture closure.

The diagnosis is based on physical examination, CT scan, and MRI. Hydrocephalus can be treated by surgery to resect cysts, neoplasms, or hematomas. Ventricular bypass into the normal intracranial channel or into an extracranial compartment by a shunt is also used therapeutically.

11. Define terms that describe alterations in motor functions.

Study pages 376, 378, and 380-386; refer to Figures 14-11 through 14-18, and Tables 14-15 through 14-19.

Movements are influenced by the cerebral cortex, the pyramidal system, the extrapyramidal system, and the motor units. Dysfunction in any of these areas may cause motor dysfunction.

Hypotonia is decreased muscle tone shown by passive movement of a muscle against resistance. It likely is due to decreased muscle spindle activity secondary to decreased excitability of neurons. Hypotonia is caused by cerebellar damage or, in rare cases, by pyramidal tract damage.

Hypertonia is increased muscle tone shown by passive movement of a muscle with resistance. **Spasticity,** a type of hypertonia, results from hyperexcitability of the stretch reflexes and is associated with damage to the motor, premotor, and supplementary motor areas and lateral corticospinal tracts. **Rigidity,** another hypertonia, is produced by tonic reflex activity. The involved muscles are firm and tense; the increase in muscle movement is even and uniform throughout the range of passive movement.

Hyperkinesia is excessive movement, whereas **dyskinesias** are abnormal, involuntary movements. **Hypokinesia,** or decreased movement, is a loss of voluntary movement despite consciousness and normal peripheral nerve and muscle function. Types of hypokinesia include paresis/paralysis, akinesia, bradykinesia, and loss of associated movement.

Hemiparesis/hemiplegia is paresis/paralysis of the upper and lower extremity on one side. **Diplegia** is the paralysis of both upper or both lower extremities due to cerebral hemisphere injuries. **Paraparesis/paraplegia** refers to weakness/paralysis of the lower extremities. **Quadriparesis/quadriplegia** refers to paresis/paralysis of all four extremities. Both paraparesis/paraplegia and quadriparesis/quadriplegia may be caused by dysfunction of the spinal cord.

When the pyramidal system is destroyed below the level of the pons, **spinal shock** occurs. This is the complete cessation of spinal cord functions below the lesion. Spinal shock is characterized by complete flaccid paralysis, absence of reflexes, and marked disturbances in bowel and bladder function.

Lower motor syndrome originating in the anterior horn cells or the motor nuclei of the cranial nerves are called **amyotrophies.** Paralytic poliomyelitis is the prototype of these disorders. In the amyotrophies, muscle strength, muscle tone, and muscle bulk are affected in the muscles innervated by the involved motor neurons.

Several brain stem syndromes involve damage to one or more of the cranial nerve nuclei. These are called **nuclear palsies** and may be caused by vascular occlusion, tumor, aneurysm, tuberculosis, or hemorrhage.

Akinesia is a decrease in associated and voluntary movements. It is related to dysfunction of the extrapyramidal system. Pathogenesis is related to either a deficiency of dopamine or a defect of the postsynaptic dopamine receptors. **Bradykinesia** is slowness of voluntary movements. In **hypokinesia,** the normal, habitually associated movements that provide skill, grace, and balance to voluntary movements are lost. An expressionless face, a statuesque posture, absence of speech inflection, and absence of spontaneous gestures are exhibited as well.

Dystonia is the maintenance of abnormal posture through muscular contractions. **Decorticate posture** is characterized by upper extremities that are flexed at the elbows and held close to the body and lower extremities that are externally rotated and extended. Decorticate posture is thought to occur when the brain stem is not inhibited by the motor function of the cerebral cortex. **Decerebrate posture** refers to a position of extended and internally rotated arms with the legs extended and feet in plantar flexion. The decerebrate posture is caused by severe injury to the brain and brain stem. **Basal ganglion posture** refers to a stooped, hyperflexed posture with a narrow-based, short-stepped gait. **Senile posture** is characterized by an increasingly flexed posture similar to a basal ganglion posture. The posture is associated with frontal lobe dysfunction.

A **spastic gait** is associated with unilateral, pyramidal injury and is manifested by a shuffling gait with the leg extended and held stiff. This gait causes a scraping over the walking surface. A **scissors gait** is associated with bilateral pyramidal injury and spasticity. The legs are abducted, so the legs touch each other. A **cerebellar gait** manifests as a wide-based gait with the feet apart and often turned outward and inward for greater stability. Cerebellar dysfunction accounts for this particular gait. A **basal ganglion gait** is a broad-based gait. Small steps are taken, and there is a decreased arm swing during walking. The individual's head and body are flexed and the arms are semiflexed and abducted, whereas the legs are flexed and rigid in more advanced states. Basal ganglion and frontal lobe dysfunction, respectively, account for these two gaits.

Hypermimesis, a disorder of expression, is most commonly manifested as pathologic laughter or crying. Pathologic laughter is associated with right hemisphere injury, whereas pathologic crying is associated with left hemisphere injury. **Hypomimesis** is manifested as aprosodias, or the loss of emotional language. **Aprosodias** involve an inability to understand emotion in speech and facial expression. Aprosodias are associated with right hemisphere damage.

Dyspraxia/apraxia is the inability to perform purposeful or skilled motor acts in the absence of paralysis, sensory loss, abnormal posture and tone, abnormal involuntary movement, incoordination, or inattentiveness. Dyspraxias arise when the connecting pathways between the left and right cortical areas are interrupted; conceptualization and execution of complex motor acts are impaired.

12. **Show the relationships between pyramidal and extrapyramidal motor syndromes and between upper motor neuron and lower motor neuron syndromes.**
    Study pages 378, 380, and 386; refer to Figures 14-15 through 14-17 and Tables 14-17 and 14-19.

Disturbances in motor function are classified along upper and lower motor neuron structures. Amyotrophic lateral sclerosis can involve both upper and lower neuron structures. Upper motor neuron disorders include cerebral palsies, cerebrovascular accidents, multiple sclerosis, and Parkinson disease. Lower motor neuron disorders include poliomyelitis, muscular dystrophies, myasthenia gravis, and polymyositis.

Motor Syndrome Types

Cerebral cortex

Pyramidal tract   Extrapyramidal tract

Upper motor neuron (UMN)   Lower motor neuron (LMN)

Brain stem
Cranial nerve nuclei
Medulla pyramids

Spinal cord
Associated neurons
Anterior horn

UMN injury features
• Spastic paralysis
• Increased tendon reflexes
• Disuse atrophy

LMN injury features
• Flaccid paralysis; possible rigidity
• Weak or absent tendon reflexes
• Pronounced muscle atrophy
• Visible, uncoordinated twitching

Examples of UMN are:
• Childhood cerebral palsies, CVAs, MS, and Parkinson disease

Common pathway

Examples of LMN are:
• Polymyelitis, myasthenia gravis, and polymyositis

Skeletal muscles

Practice Examination

Match the level of consciousness with its characteristic.

_____ 1. confusion

_____ 2. coma

a. orientation to person, time, and place

b. slow vocalization, decreased oculomotor activity

c. inability to think clearly

d. vocalization in response to pain stimuli

e. no arousal

3. Supratentorial processes reduce arousal by:
   a. developing the reticular activating system.
   b. encephalitis.
   c. destroying the brain stem.
   d. Both a and c are correct.
   e. None of the above is correct.

4. An individual shows flexion in upper extremities and extension in lower extremities. This is:
   a. decorticate posturing.
   b. decerebrate posturing.
   c. excitation posturing.
   d. caloric posturing.

5. Cerebral death:
   a. is death of the cerebellum.
   b. permits normal internal homeostasis.
   c. no longer maintains respiratory and cardiovascular functions.
   d. is death of the brain stem.

6. Precipitating causes of seizure include all of the following *except*:
   a. meningitis.
   b. stroke.
   c. hyperglycemia.
   d. hyperthermia.
   e. All of the above are correct.

7. Which epileptic seizure is characterized by temporal lobe spikes in the EEG?
   a. autonomic
   b. status epilepticus
   c. absence
   d. Jacksonian
   e. psychomotor

8. Postictal sleeping can be seen in _____ seizures.
   a. partial
   b. unilateral
   c. absence
   d. grand mal
   e. psychomotor

Match the term with its definition.

_____ 9. cortical dementia

_____10. agnosia

_____11. subcortical dementia

a. inability to understand relationships

b. inability to verify and correct input

c. inability to control motor function

d. inability to recognize sound

e. inability to remember

12. Hypotonia is:
    a. spasticity.
    b. caused by cerebellar damage.
    c. rigidity.
    d. abnormal, involuntary movement.
    e. All of the above are correct.

13. Dystonia is:
    a. abnormal posture maintained by muscular contractions.
    b. flexed posture.
    c. stooped, hyperflexed posture.
    d. a spastic gait.

14. An individual with increased intracranial pressure from a head injury shows dilated and sluggish pupils, widened pulse pressure, and bradycardia. Which stage of ICP exists?
    a. Stage 1
    b. Stage 2
    c. Stage 3
    d. Stage 4

15. Infratentorial herniation occurs with:
    a. shifting of the mesencephalon.
    b. shifting of the diencephalon.
    c. shifting of the cerebellum.
    d. Both a and b are correct.
    e. None of the above is correct.

16. In cerebral vasogenic edema:
    a. active transport fails.
    b. there is autodigestion.
    c. plasma proteins leak into extracellular spaces.
    d. cerebrospinal fluid leaves the ventricles.

17. Which statement is *not* true regarding increasing intracranial pressures?
    a. Accumulating CO_2 causes vasoconstriction.
    b. The brain volume increases.
    c. The blood volume in the vessels increases.
    d. Brain tissue shifts from the compartment of greater pressure to one of lesser pressure.
    e. Both b and c are correct.

18. Intellectual function is impaired in the dementing process. Which intellectual function is *not* impaired?
    a. anterograde memory
    b. retrograde memory
    c. abstraction
    d. language deficits
    e. All of the above functions are impaired.

Match the term with its characteristic.

_____19. hypertonia

_____20. rigidity

_____21. hemiparesis

_____22. akinesia

_____23. senile posture

_____24. dyspraxia

_____25. lower motor neuron syndrome

a. paralysis of both upper and lower extremities

b. difficult initiation of spontaneous and voluntary movements

c. absence of spontaneous gestures

d. abnormal posture maintained through muscular contractions

e. frontal lobe dysfunction

f. impaired conceptualization and execution of complex acts

g. individual muscles affected

h. involuntary writing movements

i. organically caused impairment of intellectual functions

j. increased muscle tone

k. tonic reflex activity

l. upper and lower extremity paralysis on same side

Case Study

A 12-year-old male complained of strange odors before loss of consciousness and a major tonic-clonic seizure. During the seizure, his parents rushed him to the emergency room of a local hospital. On arrival at the hospital, he appeared to be asleep.

Studies at the hospital showed routine laboratory work within normal limits (WNL), lumbar puncture (CSF) was WNL, no evidence of skull fracture on x-ray study was revealed, and an electroencephalograph (EEG) showed no abnormalities.

How would you interpret the episode and findings?

Alterations of Neurologic Function

Foundational Objectives

a. **Identify the protective structures of the central nervous system.**
   Review pages 309-311; refer to Figures 12-14 through 12-16 and Table 12-4.

MEMORY CHECK!

- The cranium is composed of eight bones that fuse early in childhood. The cranial vault encloses and protects the brain and its associated structures. The floor of the cranial vault is irregular and contains many foramina or openings for cranial nerves, blood vessels, and the spinal cord to exit. The foramen magnum is large enough for the spinal cord to exit. Surrounding the brain and spinal cord are three protective membranes called the *meninges:* the dura mater, the arachnoid membrane, and the pia mater.

- The dura mater is composed of two layers and has venous sinuses between the layers. The outermost dural layer forms the periosteum of the skull. The inner dural meningeal layer forms the rigid plates that support and separate various brain structures.

- One of these membranous plates, the falx cerebri, transverses between the two cerebral hemispheres and anchors the base of the brain to the ethmoid bone. The tentorium cerebelli is a membrane that surrounds the brain stem and separates the cerebellum from the cerebral structures.

- Below the dura mater lies the arachnoid membrane, which is characterized by its spongy, weblike structure. The space between the dura and arachnoid membrane is the subdural space. Many small bridging veins traverse the subdural space. The subarachnoid space between the arachnoid membrane and the pia mater contains cerebrospinal fluid. The delicate pia mater provides support for blood vessels serving the brain tissue. The choroid plexuses, structures that produce cerebrospinal fluid, arise from the pial membrane. The spinal cord is anchored to the vertebrae by extension of the meninges. Between the dura mater and skull is a potential space, the epidural space.

- Cerebrospinal fluid (CSF) is a clear, colorless fluid similar to blood plasma and interstitial fluid. The CNS's soft tissues are cushioned from traumatic jolts and blows because of the CSF's buoyant properties. The choroid plexuses in the lateral, third, and fourth ventricles produce the major portion of the CSF.

b. Describe the blood supply to the brain.
Review page 312; refer to Figures 12-17 through 12-20 and Table 12-5.

MEMORY CHECK!

- The brain receives approximately 20% of the cardiac output, or 800 to 1000 ml of blood flow per minute. Carbon dioxide is a potent vasodilator in the CNS and ensures an adequate cerebral blood supply. The brain derives its arterial supply from two systems: the internal carotid arteries and the vertebral arteries.

- The internal carotid arteries originate from the common carotid arteries, enter the cranium through the base of the skull, and pass through the cavernous sinus. After giving off some small branches, they divide into the anterior and middle cerebral arteries. The vertebral arteries originate at the subclavian arteries and pass through the transverse foramina of the cervical vertebrae and enter the cranium through the foramen magnum. They join to form the basilar artery. The basilar artery divides at the level of the midbrain to form paired posterior cerebral arteries. Superficial arteries supply small branches that project into the brain. The circle of Willis is a structure having the ability to provide collateral blood flow. It is formed by many communicating arteries that extend to various brain structures.

- The venous drainage of the brain stem and cerebellum parallels the arterial supply; the venous drainage of the cerebrum does not. The cerebral veins are classified as superficial and deep. The veins drain into venous plexuses and dural sinuses and eventually drain into the internal jugular veins at the base of the skull. The blood-brain barrier selectively inhibits certain substances in the blood from entering the interstitial spaces of the brain or CSF. It is believed that the supporting cells and tight junctions between endothelial cells are involved in the formation of the blood-brain barrier and are responsible for its impermeability.

c. State the functions of the parts and associated structures of the brain.
Review pages 301, 303, and 305-306; refer to Figures 12-5 through 12-7 and Table 12-3.

MEMORY CHECK!

STRUCTURAL FUNCTIONS OF THE BRAIN

Structure	Function
Brain stem	Performs sensory, motor, and reflex functions; controls cardiac, vasomotor, and respiratory centers; cranial nerve reflex
Cerebellum	Coordinates the activities of groups of muscles, maintains equilibrium, controls posture
Diencephalon	
Thalamus	Conscious recognition of crude pain, temperature, and touch; relays sensory impulses except smell to cerebrum; emotions; arousal mechanism; complex reflex movements
Hypothalamus	Links nervous system to endocrine system; coordinates ANS; controls body temperature, hunger, thirst, and sleep
Cerebrum	
Cerebral cortex lobes	
Frontal	Voluntary control of skeletal muscles, unconscious skeletal muscle movement, speaking and writing
Temporal	Interpretation of odor and sound
Parietal	General body sensations
Occipital	Interpretation of sight
All lobes	Memory, emotions, reasoning, and intelligence
Left hemisphere	Language, numerical skills, motor control of right side of body
Right hemisphere	Musical and artistic awareness, space and pattern perception, insight, motor control of left side of body

d. Cite some examples of neurotransmitters and neuroreceptors.
   Review pages 299 and 320-321; refer to Figures 12-23 and 12-26 and Tables 12-2 and 12-7.

MEMORY CHECK!

RESPONSES OF SELECTED EFFECTOR ORGANS TO AUTOMATIC NERVE IMPULSES

Effector	Receptor Type	Adrenergic Response	Cholinergic Response
Eye			
Radial muscle, iris	∂	Contraction	—
Sphincter muscle, iris	β_1	—	Contraction
Heart			
SA node	β_1	Increases heart rate	Decreases heart rate
Ventricles	β_1	Increases contractility	—
Arterioles			
Pulmonary	∂, β_2	Dilation predominates	—
Skeletal muscle	∂, β_2	Dilation predominates	—
Cerebral	∂	Constriction	—
Lung			
Bronchial muscle	β_2	Relaxation	Contraction
Adrenal medulla	—	—	Secretion of epinephrine and norepinephrine

- Sympathetic preganglionic fibers, parasympathetic preganglionic fibers, and postganglionic fibers release acetylcholine. These fibers are characterized by cholinergic transmission. Most postganglionic sympathetic fibers release norepinephrine (adrenaline) and are considered to function by adrenergic transmission.

- Two types of adrenergic receptors exist, ∂ and β. Cells of effector organs may have only one or both types of these adrenergic receptors. ∂_1 receptors are associated with excitation, whereas ∂_2 receptors are associated with inhibition. β_1 receptors stimulate cardiac muscle and cause release of renin from the kidney, whereas β_2 receptors facilitate all other effects attributed to receptors.

Objectives

After studying this chapter, the learner will be able to do the following:

1. **Differentiate between focal and diffuse brain trauma.**
   Study pages 392-396; refer to Figures 15-1 through 15-3 and Tables 15-1 through 15-3.

Traumatic brain injuries are broadly categorized into blunt or closed trauma and open or penetrating trauma. In blunt trauma, the head strikes a hard surface or a rapidly moving object strikes the head. The dura remains intact and brain tissues are not exposed to the environment. Blunt trauma may result in both focal brain injuries and diffuse axonal injuries. When a break in the dura exposes the cranial contents to the environment, open trauma has occurred. Open trauma results in focal brain injuries.

Focal brain injury involves specific, grossly observable brain lesions seen in cortical contusions, epidural hemorrhage, subdural hematoma, and intracerebral hematoma. The force of impact typically produces **contusions,** or bruises, on the brain. The contusion, in turn, produces epidural hemorrhage, subdural hematomas, and intracerebral hematomas. Contusion and bleeding occur because of small tears in blood vessels resulting from these forces. The smaller the area of impact, the greater the severity of injury because the force is concentrated into a smaller area. The focal injury may be coup or contrecoup. **Coup** is the direct impact area. **Contrecoup** lies opposite the line of force; the lesions occur where the brain strikes hard tissue on the opposite side.

The clinical manifestations of a contusion may include immediate loss of consciousness, loss of reflexes, transient cessation of respiration, a brief period of brady-cardia, and a fall in blood pressure. Vital signs may stabilize in a few seconds. Reflexes return next and the person begins to regain consciousness. Returning to full alertness takes variable periods of time from minutes to days.

Large contusions and lacerations with hemorrhage may be surgically excised. Otherwise treatment is directed at controlling intracranial pressure and managing symptoms.

Extradural hematomas, also called *epidural hematomas* or *epidural hemorrhages,* most often have an artery as the source of bleeding. Extradural hemorrhages may result in herniation through the foramen magnum.

Tearing of the bridging veins is the major cause of rapidly developing and subacutely developing **subdural hematomas.** However, torn cortical veins or venous sinuses and contused tissue may be the source of the bleeding. The subdural space gradually fills with blood, and herniation can result.

In **intracerebral hematomas,** small blood vessels are traumatized by shearing forces. The intracerebral hematoma expands and increases intracranial pressure with compression of brain tissues.

Individuals with classic temporal extradural hematomas lose consciousness at the time of injury; some lucid periods follow. As the hematoma mass accumulates, a headache of increasing severity, vomiting, drowsiness, confusion, seizure, and hemiparesis may develop. Level of consciousness declines rapidly as the temporal lobe herniation begins. Clinical manifestations of temporal lobe herniation also include ipsilateral pupillary dilation and contralateral hemiparesis. Surgical therapy evacuates the hematoma through burr holes followed by ligation of the bleeding vessel(s).

An acute subdural hematoma classically begins with headache, drowsiness, restlessness or agitation, slowed cognition, and confusion. These symptoms worsen over time and progress to loss of consciousness, respiratory pattern changes, and pupillary dilation. Most persons with chronic subdural hematomas appear to have a progressive dementia accompanied by generalized rigidity. Chronic subdural hematomas require a craniotomy to evacuate the gelatinous blood.

In intracerebral hematomas, as the intracranial pressure rises, clinical manifestations of temporal lobe herniation may appear. Delayed intracerebral hematoma results in the following: sudden, rapidly progressive decreased levels of consciousness with pupillary dilation, breathing pattern changes, hemiplegia, and bilateral positive Babinski reflexes. Evacuation of a singular intracerebral hematoma is occasionally helpful for subcortical white matter hematomas. Otherwise treatment is directed at reducing the intracranial pressure and allowing the hematoma to reabsorb slowly.

Diffuse brain injury or **diffuse axonal injury (DAI)** results from the inertial force to the head; it is associated with high levels of acceleration and deceleration. Severity of the diffuse injury correlates with how much shearing force is applied to the brain stem. In DAI, increased intravascular blood within the brain, vasodilation, and increased cerebral blood volume are often seen. Several categories of diffuse brain injury exist: mild concussion, classical concussion, mild DAI, moderate DAI, and severe DAI.

Mild concussion involves temporary axonal disturbances. Cerebral cortical dysfunction related to attentional and memory systems results, and consciousness is not lost.

Classical cerebral concussion causes reflexes to fail transiently. Confusional states last for hours or days. Loss of consciousness lasts more than 6 hours.

In **mild DAI,** individuals display decerebrate or decorticate posturing. They may experience prolonged stupor or restlessness; 78% recover in 3 months.

In **moderate DAI,** widespread physiologic impairment exists throughout the cerebral cortex and diencephalon. Actual tearing of some axons in both hemispheres occurs. Basal skull fracture is commonly associated with moderate DAI. Prolonged coma lasting more than 24 hours is present, and recovery is often incomplete in surviving individuals. Of these, 38% recover in 3 months.

Severe DAI, formerly called *primary brain stem injury* or *brain stem contusion,* involves severe mechanical disruption of many axons in both cerebral hemispheres and those extending to the diencephalon and brain stem. Of patients with severe DAI, 15% recover in 3 months.

DAI is associated with physical, cognitive, psychologic/behavioral, and social consequences. Spastic paralysis, peripheral nerve injury, swallowing disorders, dysarthria, visual and hearing impairments, and taste and smell deficits are some of the physical consequences. Common cognitive deficits include disorientation and confusion, short attention span, memory deficits, learning difficulties, dysphasia, poor judgment, and perceptual deficits. Behavioral disorders that emerge include agitation, impulsivity, blunted affect, social withdrawal, and depression.

2. **Discuss pathogenesis and manifestations of spinal cord injuries.**
   Study pages 396-401; refer to Figures 15-4 through 15-8 and Tables 15-4 through 15-6.

Spinal cord injuries occur most often as a result of vertebral injuries. Traumatic forces injure the vertebral and/or neural tissues by compressing the tissue, pulling or exerting a traction on the tissue, or shearing tissues so that they slide into one another.

Vertebral injuries occur most often at the first to second cervical, fourth to seventh cervical, and twelfth thoracic to second lumbar vertebrae. These are the most mobile portions of the vertebral column. The cord occupies most of the vertebral canal in these areas, and its size makes it more easily injured. Within a few minutes after injury, microscopic hemorrhages appear in the central gray matter and pia-arachnoid. Edema progresses into the white matter, impairing the microcirculation of the cord with reduced vascular perfusion and development of metabolic changes in spinal cord tissues, including lactate and increasing concentrations of norepinephrine. The elevated norepinephrine levels may produce further ischemia, vascular damage, and necrosis of tissue. Cord swelling increases the individual's degree of dysfunction. In the cervical region cord, swelling may be life-threatening because of impairment of diaphragm function. The traumatized cord is replaced by acellular collagenous tissue usually in 3 to 4 weeks. Meninges thicken as part of the scarring process.

Normal activity of the spinal cord cells at and below the level of injury ceases because of the lack of continuous tonic discharges from the brain or brain stem and inhibition of suprasegmental impulses immediately after cord injury. This causes **spinal shock,** which is characterized by a complete loss of reflex function in all segments below the level of the lesion. This condition involves all skeletal muscles; bladder, bowel, and sexual function; and autonomic control.

Spinal shock may last for 7 to 20 days following onset; it may persist as long as 3 months. Indications that spinal shock is terminating include the reappearance of reflex activity, hyperreflexia, spasticity, and reflex emptying of the bladder. Loss of motor function and sensory function depends upon the level and degree of injury. Paraplegia or quadriplegia can result. Return of spinal neuron excitability occurs slowly. Either motor, sensory, reflex, and autonomic functions return to normal, or autonomic neural activity in the isolated segment develops.

Autonomic hyperreflexia is a syndrome that may occur at any time after spinal shock resolves. The syndrome is associated with a massive, uncompensated cardiovascular response to stimulation of the sympathetic nervous system. Individuals most likely to be affected have lesions at the T6 level or above. Hyperreflexia involves the stimulation of sensory receptors below the level of the cord injury. The intact autonomic nervous system reflexively responds with an arteriolar spasm that increases blood

pressure. Baroreceptors in the cerebral vessels, the carotid sinus, and the aorta sense the hypertension and stimulate the parasympathetic system. The heart rate decreases, but the visceral and peripheral vessels do not dilate because efferent impulses cannot pass through the cord and cardiovascular compensation is incomplete. The most common precipitating cause is a distended bladder or rectum, but any sensory stimulation can elicit autonomic hyperreflexia.

For a suspected or confirmed vertebral fracture or dislocation, the immediate intervention is immobilization of the spine to prevent further injury. Decompression and surgical fixation may be necessary. Corticosteroids are given to decrease secondary cord injury. In cases of autonomic hyperreflexia, intervention must be prompt because a cerebrovascular accident is possible. The head of the bed should be elevated, and the injurious stimulus should be found and removed. Medications may be used if these measures do not effectively reduce blood pressure.

3. **Describe degenerative disorders of the spine.**
   Study pages 401-403; refer to Figures 15-9 and 15-10.

The local processes involved in **low back pain** include tension caused by tumors or disk prolapse, bursitis, synovitis, degenerative joint disease, abnormal bone pressures, spinal immobility, and inflammation caused by osteomyelitis, bony fractures, or ligamentous strains. Pain may be referred from viscera or the posterior peritoneum. General processes resulting in low back pain include bone diseases such as osteoporosis or osteomalacia seen in hyperparathyroidism.

The etiology for **degenerative disk disease** includes biochemical and biomechanical alterations of tissue comprising the intervertebral disk. Fibrocartilage replaces the gelatinous mucoid material of the nucleus pulposus as the disk changes with aging; the narrowing disk results in variable segmental instability. The process seems to stabilize when segmental fibrosis results; often, the incidence of back pain decreases also.

Spondylolysis is a structural defect involving the lamina or neural arch of the vertebra. The most common site is the lumbar spine. Heredity plays a significant role, and spondylolysis is associated with other congenital spinal defects. As a result of torsional and rotational stress, microfractures occur at the affected site and eventually cause dissolution of the pars interarticularis. **Spondylolisthesis** is caused when a vertebra slides forward in relation to an inferior vertebra. Spinal stenosis may represent several conditions ranging from entrapment of a single nerve root in the lateral recess to diffuse central stenosis involving many roots.

Most individuals having acute low back pain benefit from bed rest, analgesic medications, exercises, physical therapy, and education. Surgical treatments include diskectomy and spinal fusions. Individuals with chronic low back pain can be treated with antiinflammatory and muscle relaxant medications and exercise programs. Spinal surgery has a limited role in curing chronic low back pain.

Herniation of an intervertebral disk is a protrusion of part of the nucleus pulposus through a tear in the fibrous capsule enclosing the gelatinous center of the disk. Rupture of intervertebral disks is usually caused by trauma, degenerative disease, or both. Lifting with the trunk flexed and sudden straining when the back is in an unstable position are the most common causes; males are more affected than females. Most commonly affected are the lumbosacral disks; disk herniation occasionally occurs in the cervical area. The symptoms may be immediate or occur within a few hours, or they may take months to years to develop. The pain of a herniated disk in the lumbosacral area radiates along the sciatic nerve over the buttock and into the calf or ankle. With the herniation of a lower cervical disk, paresthesia and pain are present in the upper arm, forearm, and hand according to the affected nerve root distribution.

The conservative therapeutic approach comprises traction, bed rest, heat and ice to the affected areas, and an effective analgesic regimen. The surgical approach is indicated if there is weakness and decreased deep tendon reflexes and bladder/bowel reflexes or if the conservative approach is unsuccessful.

4. **Compare and contrast cerebrovascular accidents.**
   Study pages 403-408; refer to Figures 15-11 and 15-12 and Table 15-7.

Cerebrovascular accidents are classified as thrombotic, embolic, or hemorrhagic. The accidents are vascular in origin but are manifested neurologically. **Thrombotic strokes** arise from arterial occlusions caused by thrombi formed in the intracranial vessels or the arteries supplying the brain.

The risk factors for cerebrovascular occlusive disease are:
   hypertension
   cigarette smoking
   elevated blood cholesterol
   elevated triglyceride levels
   diabetes mellitus
   sedentary life-style
   hypothyroidism
   use of oral contraceptives
   sickle cell disease
   coagulation disorders
   polycythemia vera
   arteritis
   subclavian steal syndrome
   chronic hypoxia
   dehydration

The development of a cerebral thrombosis is most often attributed to atherosclerosis and inflammatory disease processes that damage arterial walls. Atheromatous plaques tend to form at branchings and curves in the cerebral circulation. Degeneration or bleeding into the vessel wall may cause endothelial damage. Platelets and fibrin adhere to the damaged wall and delicate thrombi form. Small thrombi collect over time; gradual occlusion of the artery occurs. Once the artery is occluded, the thrombus may enlarge lengthwise in the vessel.

Thrombotic strokes may be further subdivided on the basis of clinical manifestations into transient ischemic attacks, strokes-in-evolution, and completed strokes. **Transient ischemic attacks (TIAs)** represent thrombotic particles that cause an intermittent or temporary blockage of circulation. In a true transient ischemic attack, all neurologic deficits must completely clear within 24 hours and leave no residual dysfunction. The typical development of thrombotic stroke causes the clinical syndrome

CEREBROVASCULAR ACCIDENTS (STROKE SYNDROMES)

	Thrombotic	Embolic	Hemorrhagic
History of earlier transient ischemia attacks (TIAs)	Frequent	Occasional	Infrequent
Onset	Acute, hours to days	Acute	Acute, progressive, worsening
Associated headache	Occasional, not severe	Often moderately severe	Frequent, severe
Stiff neck	Rare	Rare	Frequent
Loss of consciousness	Occasional, not at onset	Occasional, brief	Frequent
Blood in CSF	Rare	Rare	Frequent

known as a **stroke-in-evolution.** An intermittent progression of a neurologic deficit over hours to days is characteristic of thrombotic stroke or slow intracranial hemorrhage. The **completed stroke** has reached its maximum destructiveness in producing deficits, although cerebral edema may not have reached its maximum.

An **embolic stroke** involves fragments that break from a thrombus formed outside the brain. Common origin sites are in the heart, aorta, common carotid, or thorax. The embolus usually involves small vessels and obstructs a bifurcation or other narrowing to cause ischemia. Conditions associated with an embolic stroke include atrial fibrillation, myocardial infarction, endocarditis, rheumatic heart disease, valvular prostheses, atrial-septal defects, and disorders of the aorta, carotids, or vertebral-basilar circulation. In persons who experience an embolic stroke, usually a second stroke follows at some point because the source of emboli continues to exist. Emboli usually lodge in the distribution of the middle cerebral artery.

Hemorrhagic stroke or intracranial hemorrhage is a common cause of cerebrovascular accidents. The most common causes of hemorrhagic stroke are hypertension, ruptured aneurysms or arteriovenous malformation, and hemorrhage associated with bleeding disorders.

Hypertensive hemorrhage is associated with a significant increase in systolic-diastolic pressure over several years and usually occurs within the brain tissue. A mass of blood forms as its volume increases; adjacent brain tissue is displaced and compressed. Rupture or seepage into the ventricular system occurs in many of the cases. The most common sites for hypertensive hemorrhages are in the putamen of the basal ganglia.

Lacunar strokes, or lacunar infarcts, are very small and involve the small arteries predominantly in the basal ganglia, internal capsules, and brain stem. Because of the subcortical location and small area of infarction, these strokes may have limited motor and sensory deficits.

Cerebral infarction results when an area of the brain loses blood supply due to vascular occlusion. In ischemic infarcts, neuronal cell bodies change, myelin sheaths and axis cylinders are interrupted and disintegrate, and there is loss of function.

The symptoms depend on the blood vessel involved. Essentially, if the internal carotid artery branches are involved, there is confusion, inability to plan, aphasia, perception disorders, paralysis, or blindness. If the vertebral artery branches are involved, there is diplopia, ataxia, vertigo, dysphagia, and dysphonia. If a TIA is the cause of the thrombotic lesion, the neurologic deficit will usually clear within 24 hours. Other CVAs usually have permanent neurologic deficits.

In thrombotic strokes, treatment is directed at supportive management to control cerebral edema and increased intracranial pressure. Intervention to restore blood supply may be indicated. Arresting the disease process by controlling risk factors is critical. In embolic strokes, treatment is directed at preventing further embolization by instituting anticoagulation therapy and correcting the primary problem. Rehabilitation is indicated in both thrombotic and embolic stroke. Treatment of an intracranial stroke, regardless of cause, is focused on stopping or reducing the bleeding, controlling the increased intracranial pressures, preventing another hemorrhagic episode, and preventing vasospasm. At times, an attempt is made to evacuate or aspirate the blood.

MENINGITIS AND ENCEPHALITIS

	Bacterial Meningitis	Aseptic Meningitis	Encephalitis
Site	Pia mater, arachnoid, subarachnoid space, CSF, ventricles	Meninges	Meninges, white and gray matter
Infectious agents	*Neisseria meningitidis, Streptococcus pneumoniae, Haemophilus influenzae*	Enteroviral viruses, herpes simplex 1, mumps, adenoviruses	Arthropod-borne viruses, herpes simplex 1, complications of systemic viral infection
Lesion	Meningeal vessels become hyperemic and permeable	Similar to bacterial	Nerve cell degeneration
Manifestations	Throbbing headache, flexion of legs and thighs, stiff neck, projectile vomiting, confusion	Mild but similar symptoms compared to bacterial meningitis	Fever, delirium, confusion, coma, seizure, cranial nerve palsies, paresis and paralysis
CSF	Increased pressure, bacteria, elevated protein levels, decreased glucose levels, neutrophils and monocytes	Increased pressure, normal glucose levels, lymphocytes	Same as aseptic meningitis
Treatment	Antibiotics	Antiviral agents and steroids	Herpes infections—antiviral agents, control of intracranial pressure

NOTE: Fungal meningitis is a chronic, much less common infection than bacterial or viral meningitis.

5. **Compare meningitis with encephalitis.**
   Study pages 408-409 and 411; refer to Table 15-8.

6. **Characterize CNS abscesses.**
   Study pages 409-410; refer to Figure 15-13.

Abscesses are localized collections of pus within the parenchyma or functioning cells of the brain and spinal cord. Abscesses occur following open trauma and during neurosurgery; from foci of infection such as the middle ear, mastoid cells, nasal cavity, and nasal sinuses; and through metastatic or hematogenous spread from distant foci. Streptococci, staphylococci, and *Bacteroides* in combination with anaerobes are the most common bacteria that cause abscesses. However, yeast and fungi have also been found in CNS abscesses.

Initially, a localized inflammatory process leads to edema, hyperemia, softening, and petechial hemorrhage. After a few days, fibroblasts from capillaries deposit collagen fibers that contain and encapsulate the purulent focus. The infection becomes limited with a center of pus and a wall of granular tissue.

Clinical manifestations of **brain abscesses** include fever, headache, nausea, vomiting, decreasing cognitive abilities, paresis, and seizures. These signs and symptoms develop because of the infection and expanding mass.

Clinical manifestations of **spinal cord abscesses** are spinal discomfort, root pain accompanied by spasms of the back muscles and limited vertebral movement due to pain and spasm, weakness due to progressive cord compression, and paralysis.

Aspiration or excision accompanied by antibiotic therapy is the recommended but somewhat controversial treatment for brain abscesses. Intracranial pressure must be managed. Spinal cord abscesses are treated with surgical excision or aspiration because decompression is necessary. Antibiotic and supportive therapy is also required.

7. **Identify the neurologic complications of AIDS.**
   Study pages 411-412.

Approximately 40% to 60% of all persons with AIDS develop neurologic complications. The most common neurologic disorder is HIV encephalopathy. Other common neurologic disorders are peripheral neuropathies, vacuolar myelopathy, opportunistic infection of the CNS, and neoplasms.

HIV encephalopathy is characterized by progressive cognitive dysfunction in conjunction with motor and behavioral alterations. HIV encephalopathy is likely the result of direct brain tissue infection by the virus. HIV is mostly found in white matter subcortical areas.

HIV myelopathy involving diffuse degeneration of the spinal cord may occur in persons with AIDS. A progressive spastic paraparesis with ataxia is the predominant clinical manifestation. Leg weakness, upper motor neuron signs, incontinence, and posterior column sensory loss may be present.

Peripheral neuropathy (HIV neuropathy) is a sensory neuropathy. Individuals experience painful dysesthesias and paresthesias in the extremities. Weakness and decreased or absent distal reflexes may be present.

Some individuals develop an acute **aseptic meningitis** at approximately the time of positive seroconversion. Headache, fever, and meningismus with cranial nerve involvement, especially V and VII, may appear.

Opportunistic infections may be bacterial, fungal, or viral and may produce central nervous system disease. Meningitis, encephalitis, or brain abscesses also may develop.

Opportunistic nonviral infections are the most common CNS disorders associated with AIDS. Clinical manifestations of CNS toxoplasmosis, a common AIDS disorder, are highly variable and include clumsiness to hemiplegia, aphasia, seizures, ataxia, and cognitive changes.

CNS neoplasms associated with AIDS include CNS lymphoma, systemic non-Hodgkin lymphoma, and metastatic Kaposi sarcoma.

8. Describe Alzheimer disease.

Study pages 413-414; refer to Figures 15-14 and 15-15.

Alzheimer disease (AD) is one of the most common causes of severe cognitive dysfunction in older persons. The exact cause of Alzheimer disease is unknown. Several possible theories are notable, including loss of neurotransmitter stimulation by choline acetyltransferase, mutation for encoding amyloid precursor protein, and alteration in apolipoprotein E (apo *E*), which binds beta amyloid. Early- and late-onset familial Alzheimer disease (FAD) are linked to genetic defects. Early-onset FAD has been linked to mutations on chromosomes 1, 14, and 21, whereas late-onset FAD and sporadic AD are associated with chromosome 19 and involved with its apolipoprotein E (Apo E-IV) gene. The more prevalent forms are late-onset FAD and nonhereditary, or sporadic, late-onset AD. Aggregation and precipitation of insoluble amyloid occur with these disorders.

Alzheimer disease also has been linked to a lysosomal pathway that yields a neurotoxic substance. An autoimmune etiology is also being investigated, as well as aging and injury effects.

Microscopically, the protein in the neurons becomes distorted and twisted, forming a tangle called a **neurofibrillary tangle.** These abnormal protein fibers accumulate within the neurons. Groups of nerve cells, especially terminal axons, degenerate and coalesce around an amyloid core. These areas appear like plaques and are called **senile plaques.** These plaques disrupt nerve impulse transmission. Senile plaques and neurofibrillary tangles are more concentrated in the cerebral cortex and hippocampus. The greater the number of senile plaques and neurofibrillary tangles, the greater the dysfunction.

Dyspraxias, or the inability to perform coordinated acts, may appear. Motor changes may occur if the posterior frontal lobes are involved. The individual may exhibit rigidity with flexion posturing, propulsion, and retropulsion. There is great variability in age of onset, intensity, and sequence of symptoms and in the location and extent of brain pathology among individuals with the disease.

DEGENERATIVE CNS DISEASES

	Parkinson	Huntington	Multiple Sclerosis	ALS
Lesion site	Basal ganglia, degeneration of dopaminergic receptors	Basal ganglia frontal cortex, depletion of GABA	CNS demyelination	Scarring of corticospinal tract in lateral column of spinal cord—upper and lower motor neurons
Etiology	Dopamine insufficiency, trauma, infection, neoplasms, drugs, toxins	Autosomal dominant, chromosome 4	Immunogenetic-viral, genetic/environmental, T cells become autoreactive to myelin protein	Genetics, defective free radical destruction gene
Onset	> age 40, peak 60s	30s and 50s	Between 20 and 40 years of age	40s, peaks in early 50s
Manifestations	Resting tremor, muscle stiffness, poverty of movement or akinesia, flexed or forward leaning, possible late-stage dementia	Dementia, delusions, and depression; chorea-type movements beginning in face and arms and finally progressing to the entire body	Remissions and exacerbations but progressive paresthesia, diplopia, cerebellar incoordination, urinary dysfunction	Muscle weakness and atrophy, progress to paralysis, normal intellectual and sensory function until death
Treatment	Symptomatic, dopaminergic drugs, possible fetal cell transplants	No known treatment, possible recombinant genetic techniques	Antiinflammatory agents for exacerbations, immunosuppression to slow or stop progression	No known treatment to alter overall course, drug extends time before ventilatory assistance

9. **Distinguish among the degenerative diseases of Parkinson, Huntington, multiple sclerosis, and amyotrophic lateral sclerosis (ALS).**
   Study pages 414-418; refer to Figures 15-16 through 15-18.

10. **Describe peripheral nervous system disorders; characterize myasthenia gravis.**
    Study pages 418-420; refer to Table 15-9.

Radiculopathies and **radiculitis** are disorders of the spinal nerve roots. As spinal roots emerge from or enter into the vertebral canal, they may be injured or damaged by compression, inflammation, or direct trauma that stretches or tears the roots.

Plexus injuries involve the nerve plexus distal to the spinal roots but proximal to the peripheral nerves. Such injuries may be caused by trauma, compression, or infiltration or iatrogenically by positioning during surgery or by intramuscular injections. Clinical manifestations include motor weakness, muscle atrophy, and sensory loss in affected areas. Paralysis can occur with complete plexus lesions.

Where the peripheral nerves themselves are affected, **neuropathy** develops. Sensory neuropathies are mostly caused by leprosy, some industrial solvents, chloramphenicol, and heredity. Motor neuropathies are predominantly caused by Guillain-Barré syndrome, infectious mononucleosis, viral hepatitis, acute porphyria, lead, mercury, and triorthocresylphosphates (TCP).

Sensory alterations are seen in sensory neuropathy. These include paresthesia and dysesthesia, as well as decreased or absent primary sensations.

The neurologic dysfunctions observed in **Guillain-Barré syndrome** are associated with earlier respiratory or gastrointestinal infections. The individual may have a symmetrical weakness or paralysis involving the legs, the trunk, and possibly the neck and face. Any paresthesia ascends upward. Individuals then may experience respiratory arrest or cardiovascular collapse.

Myasthenia gravis is a disorder of voluntary or striated muscles characterized by muscle weakness and fatigability because of a defect in nerve impulse transmission at the neuromuscular junction. Between 70% and 80% of persons with myasthenia gravis have pathologic changes in the thymus; this disorder is an autoimmune disease. Different types of myasthenia gravis exist. **Ocular myasthenia,** which is more common in males, involves muscle weakness confined to the eye muscles. **Generalized autoimmune myasthenia** involves the proximal musculature throughout the body and exhibits varying rates of progression with possible remissions.

In myasthenia gravis, postsynaptic acetylcholine receptors on the muscle cell's plasma membrane are no longer recognized as "self." Therefore, IgG antibody is secreted against the acetylcholine receptors. These antibodies fix onto the receptor sites and block the binding of acetylcholine. Eventually, the antibody action causes the destruction of receptor sites and the diminished transmission of the nerve impulse across the neuromuscular junction.

The muscles of the eyes, face, mouth, throat, and neck are usually affected first. Manifestations include diplopia, ptosis, and ocular palsies; facial droop and an expressionless face; difficulty chewing and swallowing; drooling, episodes of choking, and aspirations; and a nasal, low-volume but high-pitched monotonous speech pattern. The muscles of the neck, shoulder girdle, and hip flexor are less often affected.

Myasthenic crisis occurs when severe muscle weakness causes extreme quadriparesis or quadriplegia, respiratory insufficiency that can lead to respiratory arrest, and extreme difficulty in swallowing. **Cholinergic crisis** is caused by the muscle hyperactivity secondary to excessive accumulation of acetylcholine at the neuromuscular junctions and excessive parasympathetic activity. As in myasthenic crisis, the individual is in danger of respiratory arrest.

Anticholinesterase drugs, steroids, and immunosuppressant drugs are used to treat myasthenia gravis and myasthenic crisis. Treatment of individuals with cholinergic crisis involves withholding anticholinergic drugs until blood levels fall out of the toxic range while providing ventilatory support.

Myopathies are primary muscle disorders. Primary muscle disease is associated with marked weakness that is usually symmetric and proximal; occasionally, it is distal as in myotonic dystrophy. No denervation nor sensory changes are found.

11. **Describe the pathophysiology, manifestations, and treatment of CNS tumors; classify common CNS tumors.**
    Study pages 420-421 and 423-425; refer to Figures 15-19 and 15-20 and Tables 15-10 and 15-11.

Cranial tumors can be either primary or metastatic. **Primary intracerebral tumors** originate from brain substance, neuroglia, neurons, cells of the blood vessels, and connective tissue. **Primary extracerebral tumors** originate outside the substance of the brain and include meningiomas, acoustic nerve tumors, and tumors of the pituitary and pineal glands. **Metastatic tumors** can be found inside and/or outside the brain substance.

Cranial tumors cause local and generalized clinical manifestations. The local effects are due to the destructive action of a particular site in the brain and to compression that reduces cerebral blood flow. The effects are varied and include seizures, visual disturbances, unstable gait, and cranial nerve dysfunction. The generalized effects result from increased ICP.

Intracranial brain tumors do not metastasize as readily as tumors in other organs because there are no lymphatic channels within the brain substance. If metastasis does occur, it is usually through seeding of cerebral blood or cerebrospinal fluid, during cranial surgery, or through artificial shunts.

CLASSIFICATION OF COMMON PRIMARY CNS TUMORS

Type	Frequency	Age Group	Feature
Astrocytoma	50% (brain/spinal cord)	Adults	Slow-growing, invasive
Oligodendroglioma	10%-15% (brain)	Adults	Slow-growing
Ependymoma	6%-10% (brain ventricles)	All ages	Variable growth rate; invasive
Meningioma	15%-20% (brain)	All ages	Slow-growing, encapsulated

The principal treatment for cerebral neoplasms is surgical or radiosurgical excision or surgical decompression if total excision is not possible. Chemotherapy and radiotherapy also may be used. Supportive treatment is directed at reducing edema.

An estimated 25% of persons with cancer develop metastasis to the brain. One-third of metastatic brain tumors arise from the lung, approximately one-sixth from the breast, and a lesser number from the gastrointestinal tract and kidney. Other tumors metastasize less often. Carcinomas are disseminated to the brain by the circulation. Metastatic brain tumors carry a poor prognosis. If a solitary tumor is found, surgery and/or radiation therapy is used; but if multiple tumors exist, symptomatic relief only is pursued.

Spinal cord tumors are classified as **intramedullary tumors,** those originating within the neural tissues, or **extramedullary tumors,** those originating from tissues outside the spinal cord. Intramedullary tumors have the same cellular origins as brain tumors. Extramedullary tumors arise from the meninges, epidural tissue, or vertebral structure. The most common primary extramedullary spinal cord tumors are neurofibromas and meningiomas. Metastatic spinal cord tumors are usually carcinomas, lymphomas, or myelomas. Their location is often extradural.

The acute onset of clinical manifestations suggests a vascular insult caused by thrombosis of vessels supplying the spinal cord. Clinical manifestations fall into three major categories: a compressive syndrome, an irritative syndrome, or, rarely, a syringomyelic syndrome. In the **compressive syndrome,** the motor dysfunction is paresis and spasticity depending on the level of involvement. The sensory manifestations of tingling paresthesias have a similar pattern to that of the motor signs. Pain and temperature dysfunctions are more commonly found than touch, vibration, and proprioceptive changes. Bladder and bowel deficits usually appear when paresis develops in the legs.

The **irritative syndrome** combines the clinical manifestations of a cord compression with radicular pain. This pain is in the sensory root distribution and indicates root irritation. Sensory changes include paresthesia and impaired pain and touch perception; motor disturbances include cramps, atrophy, fasciculation, and decreased or absent deep tendon reflexes.

Intradural-extramedullary tumors are surgically removed or decompressed by excision of the posterior vertebral arch or laminectomy. Laminectomy with decompression and excision is used for gliomas and is followed by radiotherapy. Extradural metastatic tumors are often managed by radiotherapy, chemotherapy, hormonal therapy, or pain management protocols.

Practice Examination

1. In blunt head trauma:
   a. brain tissues are exposed.
   b. only focal injury occurs.
   c. the dura is severed.
   d. the dura remains intact.

2. In an automobile accident, an individual's forehead struck the windshield. The coup/contrecoup injury would be in the:
   a. frontal/parietal region.
   b. frontal/occipital region.
   c. parietal/occipital region.
   d. occipital/frontal region.

3. In moderate diffuse axonal injury:
   a. coma lasts more than 24 hours.
   b. coma lasts less than 24 hours.
   c. disruption of axons occurs in cerebral hemispheres and those extending into the diencephalon and brain stem.
   d. tearing of axons in the cerebral hemisphere occurs.
   e. Both a and d are correct.

Match the injury with its characteristic.

_____ 4. concussion

_____ 5. contusion

_____ 6. extradural hematoma

_____ 7. subdural hematoma

_____ 8. intracerebral hematoma

a. bleeding into the brain's parenchyma

b. bruising of part of the brain

c. violent displacement of brain tissue due to acceleration or deceleration

d. arterial bleeding

e. venous bleeding

9. Most spinal cord injuries occur in the:
   a. cervical and thoracic regions.
   b. cervical and lumbar regions.
   c. thoracic and lumbar regions.
   d. lumbar and sacral regions.

10. Injury of the cervical cord may be life-threatening because of:
    a. increased intracranial pressure.
    b. disrupted reflexes.
    c. spinal shock.
    d. loss of bladder and rectal control.
    e. diaphragmatic impairment.

11. Autonomic hyperreflexia is characterized by all of the following *except:*
    a. hypotension.
    b. slower heart rate.
    c. stimulation of sensory receptors below the level of the cord lesion.
    d. precipitation because of a distended bladder or rectum.

12. Intervertebral disk herniation:
    a. usually occurs at the thoracic level.
    b. in the lumbosacral area causes pain over the gluteal region and into the calf or ankle.
    c. is infrequent in the lumbosacral disks.
    d. Both b and c are correct.
    e. a, b, and c are correct.

13. Transient ischemic attacks (TIAs) are:
    a. unilateral neurologic deficits that slowly resolve.
    b. generalized neurologic deficits that occur a few seconds every hour.
    c. focal neurologic deficits that develop suddenly, last for several minutes, and clear in 24 hours.
    d. neurologic deficits that slowly evolve or develop.

14. Which is a risk factor for the development of CVAs?
    a. polycythemia vera
    b. hypertension
    c. diabetes mellitus
    d. elevated blood cholesterol
    e. All of the above are risk factors.

15. Which most typically characterizes the victims of a cerebral embolic stroke?
    a. individuals older than 65 years of age with a history of hypertension
    b. individuals with a long history of TIAs
    c. middle-aged individuals with a history of heart disease
    d. individuals with gradually occurring symptoms that then rapidly disappear

16. Ruptured aneurysms are most likely in _____ cerebrovascular accidents.
    a. TIA
    b. thrombotic
    c. embolic
    d. hemorrhagic

17. Which is *not* a primary intracerebral neoplasm?
    a. astrocytoma
    b. meningioma
    c. oligodendroglioma
    d. ependymoma

18. In bacterial meningitis, the CSF has:
    a. normal glucose levels.
    b. an elevated number of lymphocytes.
    c. neutrophilic infiltration.
    d. None of the above is correct.
    e. a, b, and c are correct.

19. Chorea-type movements are present in:
    a. Parkinson disease.
    b. Huntington disease.
    c. multiple sclerosis.
    d. ALS.

20. Manifestations of Parkinson disease include which of the following? (More than one answer may be correct.)
    a. resting tremor
    b. muscle flaccidity
    c. akinesia
    d. early-stage dementia

Match the disease with its site of dysfunction.

_____21. Parkinson disease

_____22. myasthenia gravis

_____23. multiple sclerosis

_____24. Guillain-Barré syndrome

_____25. amyotrophic lateral sclerosis

a. cerebral cortex

b. basal ganglia

c. peripheral nerve myelin

d. neuromuscular junction

e. ventricular system of brain

f. corticospinal tracts and anterior roots

g. CNS myelin

h. muscles

Case Study 1

Mrs. B. is an overweight 71-year-old white female. Upon hospital admission, she exhibited slurred speech and some severe right-handed numbness with a weak hand grip on the left. Her smile was asymmetric with right-sided facial weakness that had persisted for 48 hours. Mrs. B. has a history of smoking moderately for 50 years. Her mother had adult-onset diabetes and died of breast cancer at age 62; one sister died of a subarachnoid hemorrhage at age 63; and another sister is hemiparetic because of a CVA. One brother is hypertensive, and three other younger siblings are apparently healthy.

Vital signs showed a normal temperature, elevated heart rate, and normal respirations but a severely elevated blood pressure. A lumbar puncture was negative for blood with normal protein and glucose levels. A normal electrocardiogram was found. EEG showed localized activity in the left hemisphere. A CT scan showed increased density on the left. Blood chemistry was normal except for elevated glucose.

How would you assess Mrs. B.'s history, her family history, and her symptoms and signs?

16

Alterations of Neurologic Function in Children

a. **Identify the normal infant neurologic reflexes.**
   Refer to Table 16-1.

MEMORY CHECK!

- Many reflex patterns are mediated by the brain stem and spinal cord at birth. As the infant matures, the neonatal reflexes disappear in a predictable order as voluntary motor functions replace them. If these reflexes persist, developmental delays or central motor lesions are likely.

b. **Identify the major differences between adult and infant neurologic functioning.**
   Review page 430.

MEMORY CHECK!

- Several differences between adults and children are notable. First, the head of a normal infant accounts for approximately one-fourth of the total height, whereas an adult's head is one-eighth of the total body height. Second, the bones of the infant's skull are separated at the suture line to form anterior and posterior fontanelles, or "soft spots." The posterior fontanelle may be open until 2 to 3 months of age, whereas the anterior fontanelle normally closes by 18 months. The adult's cranium is a closed cavity with sutures firmly holding the cranial bones together, whereas the infant's cranium has room for expansion through the fontanelles and increases in circumference during the first 5 years of life. An adult's head size cannot expand, regardless of trauma or increased production of cerebrospinal fluid. The head is the fastest-growing body part during infancy. In children, abnormal intracranial conditions characterized by increased intracranial pressure also may increase head circumference in excess of that expected with normal growth. Health care providers carefully monitor head growth during the first 5 years of life by measuring head circumference and comparing the results with a standardized growth chart.

Objectives

After studying this chapter, the learner will be able to do the following:

1. **Describe the major forms of central nervous system malformation.**

   Study pages 430-435; refer to Figures 16-2 through 16-5 and Tables 16-2 and 16-3.

   Neural tube defects are caused by an arrest in embryologic development and have an incidence of 0.7 to 1.0 per 1000 live births in the United States. A strong association with fetal death obscures the actual incidence somewhat. These can be subdivided into posterior defects or anencephaly, the myelodysplasias or defects of the vertebral column and spinal cord, and the less common anterior midline defects.

   Anencephaly is the absence of the skull and parts of the brain. It is a fatal disorder.

   Encephalocele is herniation of the brain and meninges through a defect in the skull. Most encephaloceles occur in the occipital area. Others are found in the frontal, parietal, or nasopharyngeal regions.

   Meningocele is the protrusion of meninges through a vertebral defect. The spinal cord is not involved. The meningocele is present at birth as a protruding sac at the level of the defect. Meningoceles occur with equal frequency in the cervical, thoracic, and lumbar areas.

   Myelomeningocele, or spina bifida, is a herniation of the meninges, spinal fluid, spinal cord, and nerves through a vertebral defect; 80% are located in the lumbosacral region. The covering membrane may leak cerebrospinal fluid (CSF), increasing the risks of infection and neural damage. Deficits will be distal to the defect and include weakness, paralysis, spasticity, and either bowel or bladder dysfunction. These deficits may worsen with age because of tethering of the cord with development. Hydrocephalus occurs in 85% of cases.

   Spina bifida occulta is a less serious form of myelomeningocele, with the defect occurring in the lumbar or sacral area of the spine because of incomplete fusion of the vertebral laminae. Spina bifida occulta is more common than myelomeningocele and usually causes no neurologic deficits; it may occur in 10% to 25% of infants. Physical findings may include abnormal hair growth along the spine, a midline sacral dimple with or without a sinus tract, angioma over the defect, or an overlying subcutaneous mass.

   Craniosynostosis is the premature closure of cranial sutures during the first 20 months of life. Asymmetry of the skull or interference with brain growth may result if multiple sutures are involved. Brain damage from compression may cause neurologic dysfunction.

   Microcephaly is a defect in brain growth as a whole. Primary microcephaly may be due to chromosomal abnormality, toxin exposure, radiation, or chemical exposure during periods of induction and major cell migration. Secondary microcephaly may be due to various insults during the third trimester.

   Congenital hydrocephalus is characterized by an increase in the volume of CSF that may be due to overproduction, a defect in reabsorption, or blockage of the ventricular drainage system. The incidence rate is approximately 2 of every 1000 live births. Before fusion of the sutures, the skull is able to accommodate the increased fluid, which preserves neuronal function.

2. **Compare and contrast the encephalopathic processes of cerebral palsy, phenylketonuria, and Reye syndrome.**

   Study pages 435-436; refer to Figure 16-6 and Table 16-4.

   Cerebral palsy (CP) is a static encephalopathy, meaning that the resulting damage does not change over time. Clinical manifestations, however, may change as the child continues to develop. CP can be classified according to the neurologic symptoms produced. These include spasticity, ataxia, dyskinesia, or a combination of all three. Many factors contribute to cerebral palsy, including birth asphyxia, low birth weight, vascular abnormalities, pre- or postnatal trauma, and a host of other insults not well understood.

   Phenylketonuria (PKU) is an encephalopathy caused by an inherited metabolic disorder and is progressive in nature. The disorder involves an inability to metabolize the amino acid phenylalanine and occurs once in every 10,000 births worldwide. A high level of phenylalanine causes insufficient amounts of other amino acids to enter the brain, which results in malformation, defective myelination, or cystic degeneration of the white and gray matter. Diagnosis is usually made by nonselective newborn screening. Treatment is to restrict phenylalanine in the diet, which generally results in normal growth and development.

   Reye syndrome is an acute encephalopathy caused by an interaction of salicylate, viruses, and liver dysfunction. Clinical manifestations begin with vomiting and lethargy (stage 1) and progress to disorientation, delirium, central neurologic hyperventilation, and stupor (stage 2). Obtundation, coma, and decorticate rigidity ensue (stage 3), followed by rapidly developing seizures, flaccidity, and respiratory arrest (stage 4). Avoiding aspirin administration during viral illnesses in children is the widely accepted preventive measure. Treatment depends on the stage of development.

3. Describe the seizure disorders of children, noting their manifestations.
Study pages 436-437; refer to Table 16-5.

Seizures during infancy and childhood may be the result of asphyxia, intracranial bleeding, CNS infection, electrolyte imbalance, or inborn errors of metabolism. Many seizure disorders are idiopathic, having no known cause. Seizure disorders in infancy and childhood include **infantile spasms, Lennox-Gastaut syndrome, juvenile myoclonic epilepsy,** and **febrile seizures.**

4. Identify the most common pathogens responsible for bacterial meningitis in infancy and childhood; characterize viral meningitis.
Study page 440.

Haemophilus influenzae type B, *Streptococcus pneumoniae,* and *Neisseria meningitidis* (60% of all pediatric cases) are responsible for bacterial meningitis in infants and children. *H. influenzae* type B is most common in children less than 5 years of age. *S. pneumoniae* is found in children older than 4 years of age. *E. coli* is most common in the newborn period.

The hallmark of **viral meningitis** is a mononuclear response in the CSF instead of a neutrophilic response as in bacterial meningitis and normal sugar levels instead of decreased sugar levels as in bacterial meningitis. The symptoms are similar but milder than those in bacterial meningitis. Malaise, fever, headache, stiff neck, nausea, and vomiting are common.

5. Identify the most common site of infection for human immunodeficiency virus (HIV) in children and identify the common effects of this infection.
Study pages 440-441.

The site most commonly affected by **HIV** in infants and children is the CNS. Manifestations include progressive encephalopathy, indicating a poor prognosis, failure to attain developmental milestones or loss of intellectual ability, impaired brain growth, and acquired symmetric motor deficits.

6. Describe the types of brain tumors in children and characterize their presentation.
Study pages 441 and 443-445; refer to Figures 16-8 through 16-10 and Tables 16-7 and 16-8.

Brain tumors are the most common solid tumor in childhood and the second most common neoplasm in children; leukemia is the most common neoplasm. Genetic, environmental, and immune factors are all implicated in causation. Parental employment also is a possible etiologic factor. Childhood brain tumors arise from any central nervous system cell, with two-thirds of tumors found in the posterior fossa or infratentorial area.

Brain tumors are unique in their presentation by virtue of their locations. **Supratentorial tumors** of the cerebral hemispheres are uncommon in children. **Infratentorial tumors** often present with localized neurologic findings such as truncal ataxia, impaired coordination, gait anomalies, and loss of balance. The most common brain tumors in childhood are **medulloblastoma, ependymoma, astrocytoma, brain stem glioma,** and **optic nerve glioma.** These tumors are generally amenable to a wide range of surgical, chemical, and radiation therapies. Prognosis is variable and specific to the individual process.

Practice Examination

True/False

_____ 1. An 11-month-old infant who displays a strong asymmetric tonic neck is probably just "slow" in development and should be assumed to have normal neurologic function.

_____ 2. Ninety percent of neural tube defects are anencephaly.

_____ 3. Anencephaly is the result of premature closure of the sutures of the skull.

_____ 4. Environmental influences play an important role in neural tube defects.

_____ 5. Encephalocele is the result of herniation of the brain and meninges through a defect of the lower vertebrae.

_____ 6. Neurologic function at birth is chiefly at the subcortical level.

_____ 7. The prognosis for an individual with meningomyelocele depends on the level and extent of the defect.

_____ 8. Hydrocephaly may be due to overproduction of CSF, blockage of CSF flow, or inhibition of reabsorption.

_____ 9. Hydrocephaly is almost never a neural tube defect, because such defects usually permit leakage of the CSF out of the defect.

_____10. Seizure disorders in children are usually static and resolve naturally because the neurons and the neuronal pathways are constantly maturing.

_____11. An obvious "sac" on the back of a newborn should be thoroughly probed and examined in order to determine where it is attached to underlying structures.

Fill-In-the-Blanks

12. Aspirin administration during a viral illness has been associated with _____ syndrome, which is considered to be a _____ encephalopathy.

13. Early morning vomiting without associated nausea may be indicative of a _____ fossa brain tumor.

14. Focal neurologic findings such as ataxia may be associated with an _____ fossa brain tumor.

15. A child becoming significantly more ill with symptoms of headache, lethargy, and stiff neck after several days of treatment for otitis media may be showing findings consistent with _____.

16. _____ is a disease associated with premature closure of the sutures of the skull.

Match the description with the alteration.

_____17. may restrict brain growth

_____18. may result from increased CSF

_____19. protrusion of the meninges through a vertebral defect

_____20. may require cesarean section for delivery

_____21. static disease that has changing findings over time

_____22. defect in metabolism of an amino acid with severe neurologic involvement

_____23. associated with ingestion of aspirin during upper respiratory infection

_____24. very small head

_____25. infectious process that may cause profound damage to cranial nerves

a. meningitis

b. microcephaly

c. Reye syndrome

d. PKU

e. cerebral palsy

f. hydrocephaly

g. meningocele

h. congenital hydrocephaly

i. craniosynostosis

Case Study

Allen S. is an 11-year-old white male who presents to the pediatric nurse practitioner's office for a school physical. His past medical history is unremarkable and the family history also is benign. After the examination has started, his mother requests that the practitioner pay particular attention to her son's lower back. He has an area "down there" that is extremely tender and that has been tender as long as she can remember. The problem worsened this year when Allen was hit from behind while playing sandlot football and was paralyzed and "numb" from the hips down for approximately 15 minutes. When asked about the findings when he was taken to the emergency room for the injury, his mother states that she never sought care for him because his symptoms subsided within a few minutes and he "seemed fine!"

As the physical examination continues, it is noted that he has an extremely tender area over the lower lumbar spine and palpation causes pain in both legs. This area feels and appears perfectly normal. He is noted to have a very deep, dime-sized sacral dimple and highly fissured skin over the lower sacral spine. Deep tendon reflexes, strength, and sensation are all within normal limits. Bowel and bladder function are normal as well. Spinal x-rays are ordered.

What would you expect the x-rays to reveal and what would be the next step(s)?

17

Mechanisms of Hormonal Regulation

Objectives

After reviewing this chapter, the learner will be able to do the following:

1. **Identify the functions of the endocrine system and describe the regulation of hormone secretion.**
   Review pages 450-453; refer to Figures 17-2 through 17-4.

2. **Classify the types of hormones, their receptors, and proposed mechanisms of action.**
   Review pages 453-455; refer to Figures 17-5 through 17-7 and Tables 17-1 through 17-3.

3. **State the relationship between the hypothalamus and the pituitary; identify the hormones of the anterior pituitary and posterior pituitary, their target organs, and their functions.**
   Review pages 456-458 and 460; refer to Figures 17-8 through 17-11 and Tables 17-4 and 17-5.

4. **Identify the thyroid hormones and state their functions.**
   Review pages 460-462; refer to Figures 17-12 and 17-13 and Table 17-6.

5. **Cite the physiologic effects of parathyroid hormone and the variables that affect its secretion.**
   Review page 462; refer to Figure 17-12.

6. **Identify the production sites of pancreatic somatostatin, insulin, and glucagon and state their roles in metabolism.**
   Review pages 463-464; refer to Figures 17-14 and 17-15.

7. **Describe the effects of the adrenal cortical glucocorticoids, mineralocorticoids, and gonadotropins; note the adrenal medullary secretions and their roles.**
   Review pages 465-468; refer to Figures 17-16 through 17-19.

Practice Examination

1. Organs that respond to a particular hormone are called the:
   a. target organs.
   b. integrated organs.
   c. responder organs.
   d. hormone attack organs.
   e. None of the above is correct.

2. A major feature of the "plasma membrane receptor" mechanism of hormonal action is:
   a. action of cyclic AMP.
   b. increased lysosomal activity.
   c. requirement of a "second messenger."
   d. All of the above are correct.
   e. Both a and c are correct.

110

3. A major feature of the "activation of genes" mechanism of hormonal action is:
   a. a "second messenger" is used.
   b. a hormone-Golgi complex is used.
   c. the hormone enters the cell.
   d. lysosomal activity increases.
   e. All of the above are correct.

4. A hormone having an antidiuretic effect similar to
   that of ADH is:
   a. insulin.
   b. oxytocin.
   c. hGH.
   d. aldosterone.
   e. ACTH.

5. The hypothalamus controls the adenohypophysis by
   direct involvement of:
   a. nerve impulses.
   b. prostaglandins.
   c. cerebrocortical controlling factors (CCCF).
   d. regulating hormones.
   e. None of the above is correct.

6. Hormones convey regulatory information by:
   a. endocrine signaling.
   b. paracrine signaling.
   c. autocrine signaling.
   d. synaptic signaling.
   e. All of the above are correct.

7. If calcium levels in the blood were too high, thyro-
   calcitonin (calcitonin) concentrations in the blood
   should:
   a. increase, thereby inhibiting osteoclasts.
   b. increase, thereby stimulating osteoclasts.
   c. increase, but this would not affect osteoclasts.
   d. decrease, thereby inhibiting osteoclasts.
   e. decrease, thereby stimulating osteoclasts.

8. In the negative feedback mechanism controlling
   thyroid hormone secretion, which is the nonregula-
   tory hormone?
   a. TRH
   b. TSH
   c. thyroxine
   d. All of the above are regulatory for thyroid hor-
      mone secretion.

9. The control of parathyroid hormone is most accurately described as:
   a. negative feedback controlled by the hypothala-
      mus.
   b. positive feedback controlled by the pituitary.
   c. negative feedback involving the pituitary.
   d. negative feedback *not* involving the pituitary.
   e. Both a and c are correct.

Match the group of adrenocortical hormones with their function.

_____10. mineralocorticoids   a. blood cell formation

_____11. glucocorticoids   b. antiinflammatory

                                      c. conserves sodium

                                      d. usually no function

                                      e. bone mineralization

12. The renin-angiotensin-aldosterone system begins to
    function when renin is secreted by the:
    a. adrenal cortex.
    b. adrenal medulla.
    c. pancreas.
    d. kidneys.
    e. None of the above is correct.

13. The effects of adrenal medullary hormones and the
    effects of sympathetic stimulation can be described as:
    a. opposites in all respects.
    b. overlapping in some respects.
    c. opposites in some respects.
    d. variable depending on the sex involved.
    e. overlapping in most respects.

14. Which best describes the respective effects of insulin and glucagon on blood sugar?
    a. Insulin raises blood sugar; glucagon lowers it.
    b. Both raise blood sugar.
    c. Insulin lowers blood sugar; glucagon raises it.
    d. Both lower blood sugar.
    e. None of the above is correct.

15. The releasing hormones produced in the hypothalamus travel to the anterior pituitary via the:
    a. stem neurons.
    b. infundibular stem.
    c. hypophyseal stalk.
    d. hypophyseal arteries.

16. Which is an anabolic protein hormone?
    a. T$_4$
    b. aldosterone
    c. FSH
    d. insulin

17. Aldosterone maintains electrolyte balance by:
    a. retention of potassium.
    b. elimination of sodium.
    c. retention of both Na and K.
    d. Both a and b are correct.
    e. None of the above is correct.

Match the hormone with its target organ.

_____18. ACTH

_____19. TSH

_____20. TRF

_____21. prolactin

a. mammary glands

b. adrenal cortex

c. adrenal medulla

d. thyroid gland

e. adenohypophysis

Match the hormone with its role.

_____22. epinephrine

_____23. glucocorticoids

_____24. mineralocorticoids

_____25. gonadocorticoids

a. influence(s) immunity

b. inhibit(s) growth

c. cause(s) fight-or-flight response

d. control(s) Na$^+$, H$^+$, and K$^+$ levels

e. effect(s) metabolism and resistance to stress

f. act(s) as minor sex hormones

18

Alterations of Hormonal Regulation

a. **Diagram the negative feedback system of hormone secretion.**
   Review page 450; refer to Figure 17-2.

MEMORY CHECK!

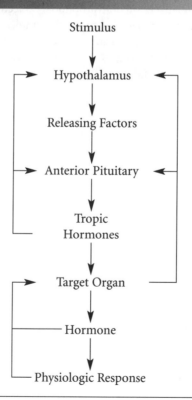

Stimulus
↓
Hypothalamus
↓
Releasing Factors
↓
Anterior Pituitary
↓
Tropic
Hormones
↓
Target Organ
↓
Hormone
↓
Physiologic Response

b. **Describe hormone receptors as recognizing and signaling mechanisms for hormonal action.**
   Refer to Figures 17-4 through 17-7 and Table 17-3.

MEMORY CHECK!

- Hormone receptors are located on the plasma membrane or in the intracellular compartment of a target cell. Water-soluble hormones, which include the protein hormones and epinephrine or norepinephrine, cannot cross the cell membrane and interact or bind with receptors located in or on the cell membrane. Fat-soluble hormones, steroids, vitamin D, and thyroid hormones diffuse freely across the plasma and nuclear membranes to bind primarily with nuclear receptors.

- In the plasma membrane model, the hormones are called "first messengers." The receptors for the water-soluble hormones first recognize the hormone on the plasma membrane and then bind with the hormone. Once recognition and binding have occurred, the hormone-receptor complex initiates the transmission of an intracellular signal by a "second messenger"; the second messenger relays the message inside the cell where a response can occur. The best-known second messenger is cyclic AMP (cAMP), although other substances are known as second messengers.

- For cells having cAMP as a second messenger, the purpose of these interactions is to activate the intracellular cyclic nucleotides such as adenylate cyclase. This enzyme converts adenosine triphosphate (ATP) to cAMP. Elevated levels of cAMP alter cell function in specific ways. An example of the function of cAMP as a second messenger can be seen in the action of epinephrine. The epinephrine-receptor complex interaction increases the synthesis of cAMP. Cyclic AMP, in turn, activates an elaborate enzyme cascade in which inactive enzymes are converted in sequence to active enzymes that lead to glycogen breakdown into glucose.

- In the lipid-soluble hormonal model, relatively small hydrophobic molecules cross the plasma membrane by simple diffusion. Once inside the cytosol, some hormones bind to receptor molecules in the cytoplasm and then diffuse into the nucleus. Hormones without cytoplasmic receptors diffuse directly into the nucleus and bind with an acceptor molecule. Once activated by hormones, the first messengers, the receptor likely binds to specific sites on the chromatin of the target cell. This causes RNA transcription and increased synthesis of specific proteins.

c. **Identify the origins and functions of hormones.**

Review the structure and function of endocrine glands in the summary of Chapter 17 on pages 469-471; refer to Tables 17-4 through 17-6.

MEMORY CHECK!

SITE OF ORIGIN AND EFFECTS OF HORMONES

Site	Hormone	Effect
Hypothalamus	Releasing hormones	Act on anterior pituitary to release specific hormones
Posterior pituitary	Antidiuretic hormone (ADH)	Causes conservation of body water by promoting water resorption by renal tubules
	Oxytocin	Stimulates uterine contraction and lactation
Anterior pituitary	Adrenocorticotropic hormone (ACTH)	Stimulates production of glucocorticoids by adrenal cortex
	Melanocyte-stimulating hormone (MSH)	Stimulates pigment production in skin
	Growth hormone (GH)	Promotes growth of body tissues
	Thyroid-stimulating hormone (TSH)	Stimulates production and release of thyroid hormones
	Follicle-stimulating hormone (FSH)	Initiates maturation of ovarian follicles; stimulates spermatogenesis
	Prolactin	Stimulates secretion of breast milk
	Luteinizing hormone (LH)	Causes ovulation and stimulates ovary to produce estrogen and progesterone; stimulates androgen production by interstitial cells of testes
Thyroid	Thyroxine (T_3, T_4)	Increases rate of cellular metabolism
	Calcitonin	Osteoblastic—lowers serum calcium
Parathyroid	Parathyroid hormone (PTH)	Osteoclastic—raises serum calcium
Pancreatic islets of Langerhans	Insulin	Promotes utilization of glucose; lowers serum glucose
	Amylin	Delays nutrient uptake and suppresses glucagon after meals
	Glucagon	Promotes utilization of glycogen; raises serum glucose
Adrenal cortex	Glucocorticoids, mostly cortisol	Antagonizes effects of insulin; inhibits inflammatory response and fibroblastic activity
	Mineralocorticoid, mostly aldosterone	Promotes retention of sodium by renal tubules
	Androgens and estrogens	Promotes secondary sex characteristics
Adrenal medulla	Catecholamines (epinephrine and norepinephrine)	Regulates blood pressure by effects on vascular smooth muscle and heart

Objectives

After studying this chapter, the learner will be able to do the following:

1. **Identify the mechanisms causing hormonal alterations.**
   Study pages 474-475; refer to Figure 18-1.

Any significantly elevated or depressed hormone levels have a variety of causes. Feedback systems may fail to function properly or may respond to inappropriate signals. Inadequate amounts of biologically free or active hormone occur when the secretory cells are unable to produce. A gland also may synthesize or release excessive amounts of hormone. Once in the circulation, hormones may be degraded too fast or too slow, or they may be inactivated by antibodies before reaching their target cell. Hormones produced by nonendocrine tissues also may result in abnormally elevated hormone levels.

The target cell may fail to respond to its hormone. The general types of abnormal target cell responses are receptor-associated disorders and intracellular disorders. **Receptor-associated disorders** may exhibit any of the following: decreased numbers of receptors, defective hormone-receptor binding, impaired receptor function with insensitivity to the hormone, presence of antibodies against specific receptors that either reduce available binding sites or mimic hormone action, or unusual expression by some tumor cells having abnormal receptor activity.

Intracellular disorders may involve inadequate synthesis of the second messenger, such as cAMP, needed to signal intracellular events. The target cell for water-soluble hormones such as insulin may not respond to hormone-receptor binding and thus fail to generate the required second messenger. The cell also may fail to respond to the second messenger if levels of intracellular enzymes or proteins are altered.

The target cell response for lipid-soluble hormones such as thyroid hormone are thought to occur less frequently than those affecting the water-soluble hormones. For lipid-soluble hormones, the number of intracellular receptors may be decreased or their receptors may have an altered affinity for hormones. Alterations of new messenger RNA or absence of substrates for new protein synthesis also may alter target cell response.

2. **Distinguish between SIADH and diabetes insipidus.**
   Study pages 475-477.

Diseases of the posterior pituitary are rare, but when they occur, they are usually related to abnormal antidiuretic hormone (ADH/vasopressin) secretion. **Syndrome of inappropriate ADH secretion (SIADH)** is characterized by high levels of ADH without normal physiologic stimuli for its release.

SIADH is associated with several forms of cancer because of the ectopic secretion of ADH by tumor cells. Tumors associated with SIADH include oat cell adenocarcinoma of the lung, carcinoma of the duodenum and pancreas, leukemia, lymphoma, and Hodgkin lymphoma. Transient SIADH may follow pituitary surgery as stored ADH is released in an unregulated fashion. SIADH may be seen in infectious pulmonary diseases because of the ectopic production of ADH by infected lung tissue or by increased posterior pituitary secretion of ADH in response to hypoxia. SIADH also may be associated with psychiatric disease and may occur after treatment with a variety of drugs that stimulate ADH release.

The main features of SIADH are water retention and solute loss, particularly sodium. This leads to hyponatremia and hypoosmolality. As ADH is released continually, water retention results from the normal action of ADH on the renal tubules and collecting ducts. This action increases their permeability to water, thus increasing water reabsorption. Hyponatremia suppresses renin and aldosterone secretion, thus decreasing proximal tubule reabsorption of sodium.

Thirst, impaired taste, anorexia, dyspnea on exertion, fatigue, and dulled consciousness occur when the serum sodium falls from 140 to 130 mEq/L. Vomiting and abdominal cramps occur with a drop in sodium levels from 130 to 120 mEq/L. With a serum sodium level below 113 mEq/L, confusion, lethargy, muscle twitching, and convulsions may occur. Symptoms usually resolve with correction of hyponatremia. The treatment of SIADH involves the correction of any underlying casual problems, correction of severe hyponatremia by administration of hypertonic saline, and careful fluid restriction. Resistant or chronic SIADH may be treated with demeclocycline, which causes development of tubular resistance to ADH.

Diabetes insipidus is related to an insufficiency of ADH leading to polyuria and polydipsia. There are three forms of diabetes insipidus: a neurogenic or central form, a nephrogenic form, and a psychogenic form. The **neurogenic form of diabetes insipidus** occurs when any organic lesion of the hypothalamus, infundibular stem, or posterior pituitary interferes with ADH synthesis, transport, or release. This results in too little ADH. **Nephrogenic diabetes insipidus** is an insensitivity of the renal tubule to ADH, particularly the collecting tubules. This diabetes is generally related to disorders and drugs that damage the renal tubules or inhibit the generation of cAMP in the tubules. The **psychogenic form** is caused by extremely large volume fluid intake.

The clinical manifestations of diabetes insipidus are due to the absence of ADH. These signs and symptoms include polyuria, nocturia, continuous thirst, polydipsia, low urine osmolality, and high-normal plasma osmolality. Individuals with longstanding diabetes insipidus develop a large bladder capacity and hydronephrosis.

Individuals who have excessive urine output and a low urine osmolality after a dehydration or water restriction test may require ADH replacement with a synthetic vasopressin analogue. Drugs that potentiate the action of otherwise insufficient amounts of endogenous ADH may be used to stimulate ADH release from the hypothalamus in less severely affected individuals.

3. **Describe the disorders of the anterior pituitary as either hypofunctions or hyperfunctions of the gland.**
   Study pages 477-480; refer to Figures 18-3 through 18-5.

Anterior pituitary hypofunction may develop from infarction of the gland, removal or destruction of the gland, or vasospasm of the artery supplying the gland. **Hyperfunction of the anterior pituitary** generally involves an adenoma composed of secretory pituitary cells. An adenoma may lead to hypersecretion of the hormone produced by the adenoma and hyposecretion of another hormone due to the compressive effects of the tumor.

The pituitary gland is extremely vascular and is therefore extremely vulnerable to infarction and subsequent hypopituitarism. The pituitary gland may be susceptible to necrosis because its blood supply through the portal system is already partially deoxygenated. The likelihood of infarction is increased during pregnancy. The primary pathologic mechanism in postpartum pituitary infarction, or **Sheehan syndrome,** is vasospasm of the artery supplying the anterior pituitary. Following tissue necrosis, edema occurs, which expands the pituitary within the fixed confines of the sella turcica. This further impedes blood supply to the pituitary and promotes hypofunction.

The signs and symptoms of hypofunction of the anterior pituitary are highly variable and depend on which hormones are affected. If all hormones are absent, a condition termed **panhypopituitarism** develops. The individual suffers from cortisol deficiency because of lack of ACTH, thyroid deficiency from lack of TSH, diabetes insipidus from lack of ADH, and gonadal failure and loss of secondary sex characteristics from absence of FSH and LH. Growth hormone and somatomedin levels are low and may affect children. These deficiencies do not generally develop in adults.

In cases of **hypopituitarism,** the underlying disorder should be corrected as quickly as possible. Thyroid and cortisol replacement therapy may need to be initiated and maintained. Sex steroid replacement may be required depending on the needs and desires of the individual.

Pituitary adenomas that cause **hyperpituitarism** are usually benign, slow-growing tumors. Effects from an increase in tumor size include nonspecific complaints of headache, fatigue, neck pain or stiffness, and seizures. Visual changes produced by pressure on the optic chiasma include visual field impairments. If the tumor infiltrates other cranial nerves, various neuromuscular functions are affected. Hypersecretion of hormones secreted by the adenoma leads to symptoms associated with the particular hormone that is affected.

Acromegaly occurs in adults who are exposed to continuously excessive levels of growth hormone (GH). Acromegaly is uncommon. The most common cause of acromegaly is a primary autonomous GH-secreting pituitary adenoma. Acromegaly occurs in adults and is a slowly progressive disease. If untreated, it is associated with a decreased life expectancy due to an increased occurrence of hypertension, congestive heart failure, and diabetes mellitus.

In the adult, after epiphyseal closure has occurred, increased amounts of GH and somatomedins cause connective tissue and cytoplasm increases. In children and adolescents whose epiphyseal plates have not yet closed, increased GH levels may cause **giantism.**

In the individual with acromegaly, bony proliferation involves periosteal vertebral growth and enlargement of the facial bones and the bones of the hands and feet. The associated growth results in protrusion of the lower jaw and forehead. Because somatomedins stimulate cartilaginous growth, there is elongation of ribs at the bone-cartilage junction, causing a barrel-chested appearance and increased proliferation of cartilage in joints. Because of bony and soft tissue overgrowth, nerves may be entrapped and damaged. This may be manifested by weakness, muscular atrophy, foot drop, and sensory changes in the hands. Because of a space-occupying lesion, central nervous system symptoms of headache, seizure activity, and visual disturbances may develop. The metabolic effects of GH hypersecretion include impaired carbohydrate tolerance and increased metabolic rate. Diabetes mellitus occurs when the pancreas is unable to secrete enough insulin to offset the effects of GH.

The goal of treatment is to protect the individual from the effects of tumor growth and to control hormone hypersecretion while minimizing damage to appropriately secreting portions of the pituitary. Surgery and radiation therapy are used, depending on the extent of tumor growth.

Prolactinomas are the most common hormonally active pituitary tumors. Pathologic elevated prolactin in

MANIFESTATIONS OF HYPOTHYROID AND HYPERTHYROID STATES

Characteristic	Hypothyroidism	Hyperthyroidism
Basal metabolic rate	Decreased	Increased
Sympathetic response	Decreased	Increased
Weight	Gain	Loss
Temperature tolerance	Cold intolerance	Heat intolerance
	Decreased sweating	Increased sweating
Gastrointestinal function	Constipation	Diarrhea
	Decreased appetite	Increased appetite
Cardiovascular function	Decreased cardiac output	Increased cardiac output
	Bradycardia	Tachycardia and palpitations
Respiratory function	Hypoventilation	Dyspnea
Muscle tone and reflexes	Decreased	Increased
General appearance	Myxedematous	Exophthalmos
	Deep voice	Lid lag
	Impaired growth (child)	Decreased blinking
		Enlarged thyroid gland
General behavior	Mental retardation (infant)	Restlessness, irritability, anxiety
	Mental and physical sluggishness	Hyperkinesis
	Somnolence	Wakefulness

NOTE: Hypothyroidism is more common than hyperthyroidism.

women results in amenorrhea, galactorrhea, hirsutism, and osteopenia due to estrogen deficiency. In men, hyperprolactinemia causes hypogonadism and erectile dysfunction.

4. **Characterize the manifestations of hypothyroidism and hyperthyroidism.**
   Refer to Tables 18-1 and 18-2.

5. **Describe the disorders of hyperthyroidism; note the progressive states of severity.**
   Study pages 480-482; refer to Figure 18-6.

Whenever thyroid hormones (TH) from any source exert greater-than-normal responses, **thyrotoxicosis** exists. **Hyperthyroidism** is a form of thyrotoxicosis in which excess thyroid hormones are secreted by the thyroid gland. Specific diseases of hyperthyroidism include Graves disease and toxic multinodular goiter. Thyrotoxicosis not associated with hyperthyroidism is seen in subacute thyroiditis, increased TSH secretion, ectopic thyroid tissue, and ingestion of excessive TH. All forms of thyrotoxicosis share some common characteristics because of increased circulating levels of thyroid hormones. The major types of therapy used to control the elevated levels of TH include drug therapy, radioactive iodine therapy, and surgery.

Graves disease is the most common form of hyperthyroidism and is likely associated with autoimmune abnormalities. Thyroid receptor antibody of the IgG class binds to the plasma membrane and initiates thyroid growth, vascularity, and hypersecretion of hormone. Ophthalmopathy is characterized by edema of the orbital contents, exophthalmos, and extraocular muscle weakness that sometimes leads to diplopia and pain, lacrimation, photophobia, and blurred vision.

Toxic multinodular goiter occurs when the thyroid gland enlarges in response to increased demand for TH. If hyperthyroidism develops, the manifestations are similar to those of Graves disease. Exophthalmos and myxedema usually do not occur.

Thyrotoxic crisis is rare but a dangerous worsening of the thyrotoxic state; death can occur within 48 hours without appropriate treatment. This condition occurs most often in individuals who have undiagnosed or partially treated severe hyperthyroidism and who are subjected to excessive stress from other causes. The systemic symptoms of thyrotoxic crisis include hyperthermia, tachycardia, high-output heart failure, agitation or delirium, and nausea, vomiting, or diarrhea contributing to fluid depletion. The symptoms may be attributed to increased beta-adrenergic receptors and catecholamines. The treatment is to reduce circulating TH levels by blocking thyroid hormone synthesis.

6. Describe the disorders of hypothyroidism.
Study pages 482 and 484-485; refer to Figures 18-7 and 18-8.

Deficient production of TH by the thyroid gland results in **hypothyroidism,** which may be either primary or secondary. Primary causes include congenital defects or loss of thyroid tissue following treatment for hyperthyroidism and defective hormone synthesis resulting from antithyroid antibodies or endemic iodine deficiency. Causes of the less common secondary hypothyroidism are insufficient pituitary stimulation of the normal gland and peripheral resistance to TH.

Hypothyroidism can result from several distinct rare disorders. **Acute thyroiditis** is caused by bacterial infection of the thyroid gland. **Subacute thyroiditis** is a nonbacterial inflammation of the thyroid often preceded by a viral infection. Both conditions are accompanied by fever, tenderness, and enlargement of the thyroid. **Autoimmune thyroiditis,** or **Hashimoto disease,** results in destruction of thyroid tissue by circulating thyroid antibodies and infiltration of lymphocytes. Autoimmune thyroiditis also may be caused by an inherited immune defect.

Myxedema coma is a medical emergency associated with severe hypothyroidism. Symptoms include hypothermia without shivering, hypoventilation, hypotension, hypoglycemia, and lactic acidosis. Older patients with severe vascular disease and with moderate or untreated hypothyroidism are particularly at risk for developing myxedema coma. It also may occur after overuse of narcotics or sedatives or after an acute illness in hypothyroid individuals.

Hypothyroidism in infants occurs because of absent thyroid tissue and hereditary defects in thyroid hormone synthesis. Signs may not be evident for at least 4 months after birth but include abdominal protrusion, umbilical hernia, subnormal temperature, lethargy, excessive sleeping, and slow pulse. Skeletal growth is stunted and the child will be dwarfed with short limbs if not treated. These signs constitute **cretinism.** Mental retardation in cretins is a function of the severity of hypothyroidism and the delay before initiation of thyroxine treatment.

Hypothyroidism is difficult to identify at birth, but high birth weight, hypothermia, delay in passing meconium, and neonatal jaundice are suggestive signs. There is a high probability of normal growth and intellectual function if treatment is started immediately after birth.

Thyroid carcinoma is the most common endocrine malignancy but is still relatively rare. The most consistent causal risk factor for the development of thyroid cancer is exposure to ionizing radiation. Changes in voice and swallowing and difficulty in breathing are related to tumor growth impinging on the esophagus or trachea. Treatment

for this rare entity may include partial or total thyroidectomy, TSH suppressive therapy, radioactive iodine therapy, postoperative radiation therapy, and chemotherapy.

7. Distinguish between primary and secondary hyperparathyroidism, and hypoparathyroidism.
Study pages 485-486.

Approximately 80% of **primary hyperparathyroidism** disorders result from a chief cell adenoma with an increased secretion of parathyroid hormone (PTH). This causes hypercalcemia and decreased serum phosphate levels.

Secondary hyperparathyroidism may be a compensatory response of the parathyroid glands to chronic hypocalcemia. Loss of calcium by failing kidneys leads to increased secretion of PTH.

Hypersecretion of PTH causes excessive osteoclastic and osteolytic activity resulting in bone resorption. Pathologic fractures, kyphosis of the dorsal spine, and compression fractures of the vertebral bodies may occur. Chronic hypercalcemia may be associated with kidney stones, gastrointestinal disturbances, and muscle weakness and lethargy.

Long-term management of hypercalcemia uses drugs that decrease resorption of calcium from bone. Definitive treatment requires the surgical removal of the hyperplastic parathyroid glands.

Hypoparathyroidism is most commonly caused by damage to the parathyroid glands during thyroid surgery. In the absence of PTH, the ability to resorb calcium from bone and to regulate calcium reabsorption from the renal tubules is impaired. Hypocalcemia lowers the threshold for nerve and muscle excitation. Muscle spasms, hyperreflexia, clonic-tonic convulsions, laryngeal spasms, and, in severe cases, death from asphyxiation are seen with hypocalcemia.

The treatment of hypoparathyroidism involves administration of calcium and vitamin D. Hypoplastic dentition, cataracts, bone deformities, and basal ganglia calcifications do not respond to the correction of hypocalcemia, but the other symptoms of hypocalcemia are reversible.

8. Describe the similarities and differences between insulin-dependent (type 1) and non-insulin-dependent (type 2) diabetes mellitus; note other types of diabetes mellitus.
Study pages 487-492; refer to Tables 18-3 through 18-6.

Diabetes mellitus encompasses many etiologically unrelated diseases and includes many different causes of disturbed glucose tolerance. Diabetes mellitus is a syndrome characterized by chronic hyperglycemia and other disturbances of carbohydrate, fat, and protein metabolism. The four major categories of diabetes mellitus are absolute insulin deficiency (type 1 diabetes mellitus), insulin resistance with an insulin secretory deficit (type 2 diabetes mellitus), other types of diabetes mellitus, and gestational diabetes mellitus (GDM). Types 1 and 2 are the most common.

The diagnosis of diabetes is based on several observations: (1) more than one fasting plasma glucose level greater than 110 and less than 126 mg/dl; (2) elevated plasma glucose levels (between 140 and 200 mg/dl) in response to an oral glucose tolerance test; and (3) the classic symptoms of polydipsia, polyphagia, and polyuria. In individuals with poorly controlled diabetes, increases in the quantities of glycosylated hemoglobins are seen. Once a hemoglobin molecule is glycosylated, it remains that way.

Type 1 diabetes mellitus is characterized by a lack of insulin and a relative excess of glucagon and is most commonly diagnosed in individuals < 18 years of age (peaks during puberty and is rare after age 30). In type 1 diabetes mellitus, beta cells are destroyed and islet cell antibodies appear. These antibodies tend to disappear with time. This disease seems to be caused by the gradual process of autoimmune destruction in genetically susceptible individuals. Because of decreased use of glucose, glucose accumulates in the blood and is subsequently released in the urine. This in turn causes polyuria and polydipsia resulting from osmotic diuresis. Manifestations of type 1 diabetes mellitus include ketoacidosis, caused by increased levels of circulating ketones without the inhibiting effects of insulin; increased levels of circulating fatty acids; and weight loss.

Type 2 diabetes mellitus, which is more common than type 1, is probably caused by genetic susceptibility triggered by environmental factors. It primarily affects individuals after the age of 40. The greatest risk factor for this type of diabetes is obesity. In the obese, insulin has a diminished ability to influence glucose uptake and metabolism. In type 2 diabetes, amyloid deposits in the islets, fatty atrophy of the pancreas and liver, and vascular sclerosis are generally present. Some insulin production continues in type 2 diabetes mellitus, but the mass and number of beta cells is decreased.

CLASSIFICATIONS OF DIABETES AND GLUCOSE INTOLERANCE STATES

Classification	Former Terminology	Characteristics
Diabetes mellitus (DM)		
Type 1 Absolute insulin deficiency	Insulin-dependent diabetes mellitus (IDDM) Juvenile-onset diabetes	Few islet cells, acute onset at puberty, long preclinical record, insulin-dependent, ketosis-prone, autoimmune and genetic-environment etiology
Type 2 Insulin resistance with an insulin secretory deficiency	Non-insulin-dependent diabetes mellitus (NIDDM) Adult-onset, maturity-onset diabetes (over age 40)	Usually not insulin-dependent, not ketosis-prone, often obese, strong familial pattern
Other types	Secondary diabetes	Presence of diabetes and associated conditions such as pancreatic disease, hormonal disease, use of drugs, and/or chemicals
Gestational diabetes mellitus (GDM)	Asymptomatic, chemical, subclinical, borderline, latent diabetes	Glucose intolerance develops during pregnancy (third trimester); increased risk of perinatal complications; increased risk of developing diabetes within 15 years after parturition

The treatment of individuals with either type 1 or type 2 diabetes requires appropriate meal planning to restrict total caloric intake, cholesterol, and saturated fats. Oral medication may be needed for optimal management of hyperglycemia. Insulin is required in type 1 and also may be required in the treatment of some individuals with type 2 diabetes. Exercise is an important aspect of treatment for the individual with type 2 diabetes. Exercise reduces after-meal blood glucose levels and diminishes insulin requirement. Also, exercise facilitates weight loss in the overweight individual.

9. **Identify the acute complications of diabetes mellitus; describe the features of each.**
   Study page 492; refer to Figure 18-9 and Table 18-7.

Acute complications of diabetes mellitus include hypoglycemia or insulin shock, diabetic ketoacidosis (DKA), and hyperosmolar hyperglycemic nonketotic syndrome (HHNS).

ACUTE COMPLICATIONS OF DIABETES MELLITUS

Variable	Hypoglycemia Insulin Shock	DKA	HHNS
Onset	Rapid	Slow	Slowest
Symptoms	Weak, anxious, confused	Nausea, vomiting, polyuria, polyphagia, polydipsia, headache, irritable, comatose	Similar to DKA; stuporous, focal motor seizures
Skin	Cold, moist, pale	Hot, flushed, dry	Very dry
Mucous membranes	Normal	Dry	Extremely dry
Respiration	Normal	Hyperventilation, "fruity" or acetone odor to breath	Normal
Those at risk	Type 1 and 2 DM, fluctuating blood glucose levels, insufficient food intake, excessive exercise, oral medication, excessive insulin	Type 1 DM, stressful situations, omission of insulin	Type 2 DM, high carbohydrate diets, diuresis, hyperosmolar dialysis
Blood sugar/dl	30 mg or less in newborns, 60 mg or less in adults	300-750 mg	500-2000 mg
Treatment	Fast-acting carbohydrate, intravenous glucose, subcutaneous glucagon	Low-dose insulin, electrolyte and fluid replacement	Fluid and electrolyte replacement

NOTE: The Somogyi effect occurs if an overdose of insulin induces hypoglycemia followed by rebound hyperglycemia because of release of hormones that stimulate lipolysis gluconeogenesis, and glycogenolysis leading to elevated serum glucose. The Dawn phenomenon is an early-morning hyperglycemia caused by nocturnal elevation of growth hormone.

10. **Describe the chronic complication of diabetes mellitus.**
    Study pages 492-497; refer to Figure 18-10.

CHRONIC COMPLICATIONS OF DIABETES MELLITUS

Chronic Hyperglycemia
involves

*Nonenzymatic glycosylation

*Shunting of glucose to polyol pathway

*Activation of protein kinase C

leading to:

Diabetic Neuropathies	Microvascular Disease	Macrovascular Disease	Infection
Axonal and Schwann cell degenerations, altered motor nerve conduction, sensory alterations	Retinopathy* Nephropathy* Capillary basement membrane thickening, decreased tissue perfusion or ischemia, hypertension	Coronary heart disease* CVA* Peripheral vascular disease* Proliferation of fibrous plaques, atherosclerosis because of high serum lipids, ischemia	Sensory impairment, atherosclerosis, ischemia, hypoxia, leukocytic impairment

*Major consequences.

11. **Describe the etiology, pathogenesis, and manifestations of hyperfunction and hypofunction of the adrenal cortex.**
    Study pages 497-501; refer to Figures 18-11 through 18-13 and Tables 18-8 and 18-9.

Cushing syndrome (chronic hypercortisolism) refers to excessive levels of circulating cortisol caused by hyperfunction of the adrenal cortex with or without pituitary involvement. **Cushing disease** refers specifically to pituitary-dependent hypercortisolism. Cushing-like syndrome also may develop as a result of the exogenous administration of cortisone. Elevated levels of pituitary ACTH and adrenal neoplasms account for many cases of hypercorticoadrenalism.

Two observations consistently apply to individuals with Cushing syndrome: (1) they lack diurnal or circadian secretion patterns of ACTH and cortisol and (2) they do not increase ACTH and cortisol secretion in response to a stressor.

Most of the clinical signs and symptoms of Cushing syndrome are caused by hypercortisolism. The most common feature is the accumulation of adipose tissue in the trunk, facial, and cervical areas. These have been de-

scribed as "truncal obesity," "moon face," and "buffalo hump." Protein wasting is commonly observed in hypercortisolism and is caused by the catabolic effects of cortisol on peripheral tissues. Muscle wasting is especially obvious in the muscles of the extremities. Loss of the protein matrix in bone leads to osteoporosis and accompanying pathologic fractures, vertebral compression fractures, bone and back pain, kyphosis, and reduced height. Loss of collagen also leads to thin, weakened integumentary tissues through which capillaries are more visible. This accounts for the characteristic purple striae observed in the trunk area. Loss of collagenous support around small vessels makes them susceptible to rupture and easy bruising.

With elevated cortisol levels, vascular sensitivity to catecholamines is significantly increased, which leads to vasoconstriction and hypertension. Chronically elevated cortisol levels also cause suppression of the immune system and increased susceptibility to infections.

Approximately 50% of individuals with Cushing syndrome experience irritability and depression. Without treatment, approximately 50% of individuals with Cushing syndrome die within 5 years of onset because of infection, suicide, complications from generalized arteriosclerosis, and hypertensive disease. Treatment is specific for the cause of hypercorticoadrenalism and includes medication, radiation, and surgery.

Hyperaldosteronism is characterized by excessive aldosterone secretion by the adrenal glands. An aldosterone-secreting adenoma or excessive stimulation of the normal adrenal cortex by substances such as angiotensin, ACTH, or elevated potassium may cause hypersecretion.

Conn disease, or **primary aldosteronism,** presents a clinical picture of hypertension, hypokalemia, renal potassium wasting, and neuromuscular manifestations. The most common cause of primary aldosteronism is the benign, single adrenal adenoma followed by multiple tumors or idiopathic hyperplasia of the adrenals.

Because aldosterone secretion is normally stimulated by the renin-angiotensin system, **secondary hyperaldosteronism** can result from sustained elevated renin release and activation of angiotensin. Increased renin-angiotensin secretion occurs with decreased circulating blood volume and decreased delivery of blood to the kidneys.

Hypertension and hypokalemia are the essential manifestations of hyperaldosteronism. Hypertension usually results from increased intravascular volume and from altered serum sodium concentrations. If hypertension is sustained, left ventricular hypertrophy and progressive arteriosclerosis develop. Aldosterone-stimulated potassium loss can result in the typical manifestations of hypokalemia.

Treatment manages hypertension and hypokalemia with correction of any underlying causal abnormalities. If an aldosterone-secreting adenoma is present, it must be surgically removed.

Hypersecretion of adrenal androgens and estrogens may be caused by benign or malignant adrenal tumors, Cushing syndrome, or defects in steroid synthesis. The clinical manifestations depend on the hormone secreted, the sex of the individual, and the age at which the hypersecretion occurs. Hypersecretion of estrogens causes **feminization,** or the development of female sex characteristics. Hypersecretion of androgens causes **virilization,** or the development of male sex characteristics.

The effects of an estrogen-secreting tumor are most evident in males and cause gynecomastia, testicular atrophy, and decreased libido. In female children, such tumors may lead to early development of secondary sex characteristics. Androgen-secreting tumor changes are more easily observed in females and include excessive face and body hair growth or hirsutism, clitoral enlargement,

deepening of the voice, amenorrhea, acne, and breast atrophy. In children, virilizing tumors promote precocious sexual development and bone aging. Treatment of androgen-secreting tumors usually involves surgical excision.

Hypocortisolism develops either because of inadequate stimulation of the adrenal glands by ACTH or because of an inability of the adrenals to produce and secrete the adrenal cortical hormones. Hypofunction of the adrenal cortex may affect glucocorticoid or mineralocorticoid secretion or a combination of both. Primary adrenal insufficiency is termed **Addison disease,** a relatively rare adult disease.

Addison disease is characterized by elevated serum ACTH levels with inadequate corticosteroid synthesis and output. The most common cause is idiopathic organ-specific autoimmune disease. The symptoms of Addison disease are primarily a result of hypocortisolism and hypoaldosteronism. These manifestations include weakness, gastrointestinal disturbances, hypoglycemia, hyperpigmentation from increased ACTH secretion, and hypotension.

The treatment of Addison disease involves glucocorticoid and possibly mineralocorticoid replacement therapy and dietary modifications to include adequate sodium. Hypocortisolism requires daily chronic glucocorticoid replacement therapy, and additional cortisol must be administered during acute stress.

12. **Characterize adrenal medulla hyperfunction.**
    Study pages 501-502.

The most prominent cause of adrenal medulla hypersecretion is a **pheochromocytoma.** Fewer than 10% of these rare tumors metastasize; if they do, they are usually found in the lungs, liver, bones, or paraaortic lymph glands. Pheochromocytomas cause excessive production of epinephrine and norepinephrine due to autonomous functioning of the tumor. The clinical manifestations of a pheochromocytoma include persistent hypertension associated with flushing, diaphoresis, tachycardia, palpitations, and constipation. Hypermetabolism may develop because of stimulation of the thyroid gland by the catecholamines. Glucose intolerance may occur because of catecholamine-induced inhibition of insulin release by the pancreas.

The usual treatment of pheochromocytoma is surgical excision of the tumor. Medical therapy with adrenergic blocking agents is used to stabilize blood pressure prior to surgery.

Practice Examination

1. Which laboratory values would be expected in an individual with SIADH?
   a. serum sodium = 150 mEq/L and urine hypoosmolality
   b. serum potassium = 5 mEq/L and serum hypoosmolality
   c. serum sodium = 120 mEq/L and urine hypoosmolality
   d. serum potassium = 3 mEq/L and serum hyperosmolality

2. Hypopituitarism in an adult male likely includes all of the following *except:*
   a. dwarfism.
   b. impotence.
   c. muscular mass decrease.
   d. skin pallor.

3. Excessive secretion of GH in an adult may cause:
   a. acromegaly.
   b. giantism.
   c. hypoglycemia.
   d. decreased metabolic rate.

4. A manifestation shared by both diabetes mellitus and diabetes insipidus is:
   a. elevated blood and urine glucose levels.
   b. inability to produce ADH.
   c. inability to produce insulin.
   d. polyuria.
   e. elevated blood urine and ketone body levels.

5. The manifestations of hyperthyroidism include all of the following *except:*
   a. diarrhea.
   b. constipation.
   c. heat intolerance.
   d. weight loss.
   e. wakefulness.

6. Hypothyroidism crisis is:
   a. myxedema coma.
   b. Addison disease.
   c. Cushing disease.
   d. Graves disease.
   e. cretinism.

7. Graves disease is:
   a. hyperthyroidism.
   b. associated with autoimmunity.
   c. manifested by ophthalmopathy.
   d. All of the above are correct.

8. Inadequate levels of thyroid hormones at birth may cause:
   a. mental retardation.
   b. immediate death.
   c. thyroid crisis.
   d. myxedema.
   e. dwarfism.

9. Hyperparathyroidism causes:
   a. increased osteoclastic activity.
   b. decreased plasma calcium.
   c. increased phosphorus absorption from GI tract.
   d. hypocalcemia.

10. A manifestation of hypocalcemia is:
    a. myopathy.
    b. lethargy.
    c. hypertension.
    d. tetany.
    e. bone cysts.

11. What is the most common cause of acromegaly?
    a. anterior pituitary adenoma
    b. overproduction of ACTH
    c. overproduction of TSH
    d. pituitary atrophy

12. If a 19-year-old woman were suffering from shortness of breath, weight loss, excessive sweating, exophthalmos, and irritability, which hormone would you expect to find elevated in her serum?
    a. cortisol
    b. thyroxine
    c. ACTH
    d. 17-ketosteroid

13. A 24-year-old female with a history of "juvenile-onset" diabetes is found in a stuporous state. She is hypotensive and has cold, clammy skin. What is the likely etiology of her condition?
    a. hyperglycemia
    b. insulin reaction
    c. renal failure
    d. peripheral neuropathy

14. A 10-year-old male was brought into the emergency room comatose, suffering from metabolic acidosis with a blood glucose of 800 mg/dl. The most probable disease causing his condition is:
    a. cretinism.
    b. type 1 diabetes mellitus.
    c. type 2 diabetes mellitus.
    d. IGT.
    e. GDM.

15. Your neighbor has not previously been diabetic but has gained 80 pounds in the past year and is able to produce some insulin. Her fasting blood sugar is always elevated. She is being treated with oral insulin-stimulating drugs. Your neighbor is most likely suffering from:
    a. diabetes insipidus.
    b. Type 1 diabetes mellitus.
    c. Type 2 diabetes mellitus.
    d. IGT.
    e. GDM.

16. Common symptoms and signs of diabetes mellitus include all of the following *except*:
    a. hyperglycemia.
    b. blurred vision.
    c. increased muscle anabolism.
    d. persistent infection.
    e. polyuria.

17. Which laboratory finding is *inconsistent* with a diagnosis of absolute insulin deficiency?
    a. FBS (fasting blood sugar) of 90 mg/dl
    b. ketonuria
    c. blood glucose of 210 mg/dl after 1 hour following ingestion of 100 g glucose
    d. decreased serum insulin level
    e. All of the above are consistent with type 1 diabetes mellitus.

18. Common complications to diabetes mellitus include all of the following *except*:
    a. retinopathy.
    b. peripheral neuropathy.
    c. nephropathy (kidney disease).
    d. None of the above is common.
    e. All of the above are common.

19. An individual with type 1 diabetes mellitus experiences hunger, lightheadedness, headache, confusion, and tachycardia while cross-country running. The likely cause of these manifestations is:
    a. hyperglycemia.
    b. eating a snack before running.
    c. hypoglycemia because of running.
    d. Both a and b are correct.
    e. None of the above is correct.

20. Which is/are expected during hyperinsulinism?
    a. excess insulin
    b. high serum glucose
    c. epinephrine release
    d. All of the above are correct.
    e. Both a and c are correct.

21. Long-term corticosteroid therapy may cause (more than one answer may be correct):
    a. delayed wound healing.
    b. osteoporosis.
    c. peptic ulcers.
    d. hyperkalemia.

22. Which electrolyte alteration occurs in Addison disease?
    a. hypokalemia
    b. hypernatremia
    c. hyponatremia
    d. hypocalcemia

23. A benign tumor of adrenal glands that causes hypersecretion of aldosterone is:
    a. Addison disease.
    b. a pheochromocytoma.
    c. Cushing disease.
    d. Cushing syndrome.
    e. Conn disease.

Match the hypersecretion with the consequence.

_____24. hypersecretion of aldosterone

_____25. hypersecretion of glucocorticoids

a. decreased cardiac output

b. hyperglycemia and/or osteoporosis

c. BMR (basal metabolic rate) increases

d. hypernatremia

e. hyponatremia

Case Study

Scott, a 17-year-old high school football player, was brought to the hospital emergency room in a coma. According to his mother, he had lost weight during the last month in spite of eating large amounts of food. Besides losing weight, he was excessively thirsty and had frequently awakened his younger brother as he noisily voided several times during the night. Physical examination was not significant except for tachycardia and hyperpnea.

Laboratory serum studies revealed the following:

Glucose on admission = 1000 mg/dl
pH = 7.25 (low)
pCO_2 = 30 mm Hg (low)
HCO_3^- = 12 mEq/L (low)
Glycosylated hemoglobin = 9% (high)

What do you think Scott's symptoms, signs, and diagnostic studies suggest?

19

Structure and Function of the Hematologic System

Objectives

After reviewing this chapter, the learner will be able to do the following:

1. **Identify the constituents of blood plasma.**
   Review pages 508-510; refer to Figure 19-1 and Table 19-1.

2. **Identify the structural characteristics, normal values, and functions of the cellular elements of blood.**
   Review pages 510-513; refer to Figures 19-2 through 19-5 and Table 19-2.

3. **Describe lymphoid organs and the mononuclear phagocyte system; note the effects of colony-stimulating factors (CSFs).**
   Review pages 513-515; refer to Figures 19-6 and 19-7 and Tables 19-3 and 19-4.

4. **Describe hematopoiesis and erythropoiesis and identify the CSFs and the nutritional requirements necessary for these processes.**
   Review pages 515-519 and 521-522; refer to Figures 19-8 through 19-15 and Table 19-6.

5. **Describe the mechanisms and the sequence of events in hemostasis.**
   Review pages 523 and 525-527; refer to Figures 19-16 though 19-19 and Table 19-7.

6. **Diagram the fibrinolytic system.**
   Review page 527; refer to Figure 19-20.

7. **Identify various hematologic values at different ages.**
   Refer to Table 19-8.

Practice Examination

1. Which does *not* constitute a plasma component?
   a. colloids
   b. electrolytes
   c. gases
   d. glucose
   e. platelets

2. Which is the most abundant protein in blood plasma?
   a. fibrinogen
   b. albumins
   c. globulins
   d. immunoglobulins
   e. hormones

3. Mast cell mediators are available to:
   a. vascular endothelial cells.
   b. nerves.
   c. immune system cells.
   d. only a and c are correct.
   e. a, b, and c are correct.

4. The progenitor of granulocytes is a:
   a. pronormoblast.
   b. promegakaryocyte.
   c. prolymphoblast.
   d. myeloblast.

5. Identify the correct sequence in the development of erythrocytes.
   a. polychromatophilic erythroblast, normoblast, reticulocyte
   b. normoblast, reticulocyte, basophilic erythroblast
   c. normoblast, committed proerythroblast, reticulocyte
   d. normoblast, basophilic erythroblast, reticulocyte

6. A differential count of WBCs includes all of the following *except:*
   a. granulocytes.
   b. agranulocytes.
   c. reticulocytes.
   d. monocytes.
   e. lymphocytes.

7. The purpose of erythropoietin is to:
   a. decrease maturation of erythroblasts.
   b. detect hypoxia.
   c. control erythrocyte production.
   d. control the size of platelets.

8. The main regulator of platelet circulating mass is:
   a. GP11b/111a complex.
   b. ADP.
   c. thrombopoietin.
   d. thromboxane.

9. About how many times more RBCs than WBCs are there in a mm³ of blood?
   a. 15
   b. 90
   c. 100
   d. 1000
   e. None of the above is correct.

10. If the total leukocytic count of an individual was 7000/mm³, about how many neutrophils would normally be present in a mm³ of blood?
    a. 400
    b. 700
    c. 2100
    d. 3000
    e. 4200

11. Which granulocyte functions in antibody-mediated defense against parasites?
    a. lymphocytes
    b. monocytes
    c. neutrophils
    d. eosinophils
    e. basophils

12. Erythropoietin:
    a. is secreted by the kidney.
    b. is a glycoprotein.
    c. causes recycling of iron for production of RBCs.
    d. is released by the kidney to stimulate erythrocyte and platelet formation.
    e. Both a and b are correct.

13. Which is *not* an agranulocyte?
    a. mast cell
    b. lymphocyte
    c. monocyte
    d. reticulocyte
    e. Both a and d are correct.

14. Which are the most effective phagocytes?
    a. neutrophils and basophils
    b. lymphocytes and eosinophils
    c. basophils and monocytes
    d. neutrophils and monocytes
    e. None of the above is correct.

15. Which vitamins are needed for erythropoiesis?
    a. C and E
    b. B_2 and B_{12}
    c. A and D
    d. Both a and b are correct.
    e. a, b, and c are correct.

Match the colony-stimulating factor with the cells that are stimulated.

_____16. IL-3

_____17. G-CSF

a. erythrocytes

b. macrophage, neutrophil

c. neutrophil, eosinophil, and basophil

d. normoblast

e. erythroblast

---

18. Which is *not* used to measure RBC indices?
    a. differential count
    b. reticulocyte count
    c. erythrocyte count
    d. hemoglobin determination

19. Which test reflects bone marrow activity?
    a. reticulocyte count
    b. hemoglobin mean
    c. hematocrit mean
    d. g/dl

20. As an individual ages:
    a. the erythrocyte life span is shortened.
    b. lymphocytic function decreases.
    c. platelet numbers decrease.
    d. All of the above are correct.

21. Hemostasis involves all of the following *except:*
    a. vasoconstriction.
    b. platelet plug formation.
    c. intrinsic pathway activities.
    d. clot formation.
    e. erythropoiesis.

22. When a blood vessel is damaged:
    a. subendothelial collagen is exposed.
    b. platelets are attracted to collagen.
    c. platelets degranulate.
    d. Both a and b are correct.
    e. a, b, and c are correct.

23. The biochemical mediators released by adhering platelets cause:
    a. vasodilation of the injured vessel.
    b. vasoconstriction of the injured vessel.
    c. the inflammatory process to proceed.
    d. All of the above are correct.

24. Which is the correct sequence in coagulation?
    a. X, tissue thromboplastin, XA
    b. prothrombin activator complex, X, XA
    c. fibrinogen, thrombin, stabilizer fibrin
    d. damaged tissue, VII, prothrombin

25. Which is the correct sequence in fibrinolysis?
    a. fibrin, plasminogen
    b. FDP, fibrinogen
    c. plasminogen, XIIa
    d. plasmin, fibrin

Alterations of Hematologic Function

a. **Identify the differentiation sequence, function, and normal values for erythrocytes.**
   Review pages 518-522; refer to Figure 19-10 and Table 19-2.

MEMORY CHECK!

DIFFERENTIATION OF ERYTHROCYTES

Uncommitted Pluripotential Stem Cell

⟵ Erythropoietin

Committed Proerythroblast (very large nucleus)

Several cell types (Hemoglobin synthesis begins)

Normoblast
(The nucleus shrinks and undergoes autolysis and resorption;
additional hemoglobin is synthesized)

Reticulocyte
(Larger than mature RBC; no nucleus; enters vascular circulation from
the bone marrow by diapedesis)

Erythrocyte
(Loses capacity for hemoglobin synthesis, disk shape achieved)

MEMORY CHECK!—cont'd

- The function of erythrocytes is to transport gas to and from the tissue cells and lungs. The normal adult range of values for circulating erythrocytes* in the blood is as follows:
  Number = 4.2–6.2 million/mm³
  Hematocrit = 42%–48%
  Hemoglobin = 12–16.5 g/dl

- The rate of erythropoiesis or formation of RBCs is measured by the reticulocyte count. A low count may indicate the inability of bone marrow to respond. A high count may indicate a good marrow response to low numbers of RBCs. Erythropoietin is secreted by the kidney in response to tissue hypoxia from anemia, high altitude, or pulmonary disease. Erythropoietin stimulates proliferation of stem cells in the marrow and accelerates maturation of erythroblasts.

*NOTE: Reticulocytes normally comprise less than 1% of the RBCs found in blood and 1 mm³ equals 1 μL, or one-millionth of a liter.

b. **Identify the differentiation sequence for granulocytes, agranulocytes, and platelets.**
   Refer to Figure 19-9.

MEMORY CHECK!

DIFFERENTIATION OF WBCs AND PLATELETS

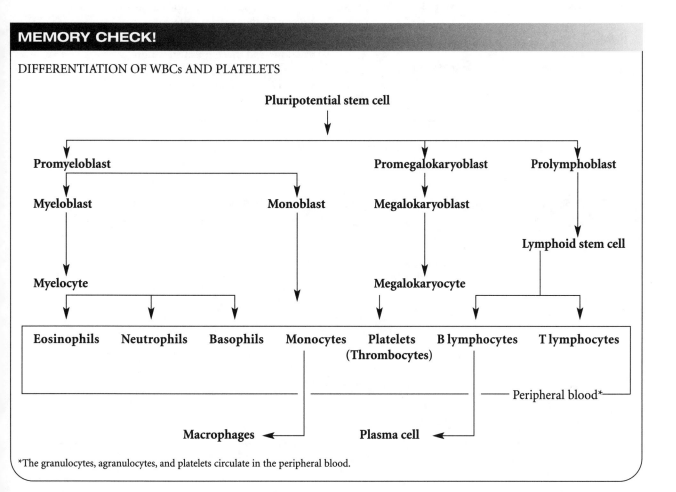

*The granulocytes, agranulocytes, and platelets circulate in the peripheral blood.

c. Identify the normal numbers in circulating blood, the function, and the life span of leukocytes and platelets.
    Refer to Table 19-2.

MEMORY CHECK!

CELLULAR COMPONENTS OF THE BLOOD

Cell	Normal Amounts	Function	Life Span
Leukocyte	5000-10,000/mm³	Bodily defense mechanisms	
Lymphocyte	25%-36% of leukocytes	Immunity	Days or years
Natural killer cell (Large granular lymphocyte)	5%-10% of circulating pool	Kill tumor cells and virus infected cells	Unknown
Monocyte and macrophage	3%-8% of leukocytes	Phagocytosis, mononuclear phagocyte system	Months or years
Eosinophil	1%-4% of leukocytes	Phagocytosis, antibody-mediated defense against parasites, allergic reactions, recovery phase of infection	Unknown
Neutrophil	57%-67% of leukocytes	Phagocytosis, particularly during early phase of inflammation/infection	4 days
Basophil	0%-0.75% of leukocytes	Unknown, but associated with allergic reactions and mechanical irritation	Unknown
Platelet	140,000-340,000/mm³	Hemostasis following vascular injury, normal coagulation and clot formation/reactions	8-11 days

---

d. Briefly diagram the coagulation cascade and the fibrinolytic system.
    Refer to Figures 19-16 through 19-20.

MEMORY CHECK!

COAGULATION CASCADE

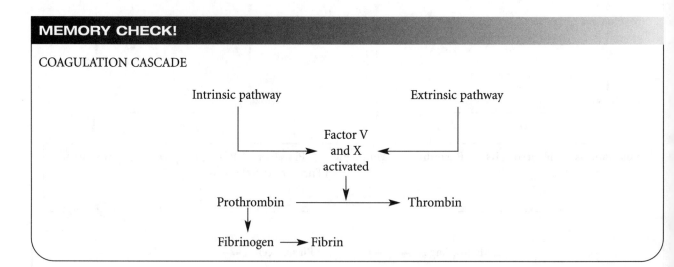

FIBRINOLYTIC SYSTEM

Plasminogen + activator

↓

Plasmin

Fibrinogen   Fibrin
(plasma)   (clot)

Fibrin degradation products

Objectives

After studying this chapter, the learner will be able to do the following:

1. **Define and classify anemia.**
   Study page 538; refer to Figures 20-2 through 20-5 and Tables 20-1 and 20-2.

Anemia is a reduction in the total number of circulating erythrocytes or a decrease in the quality or quantity of hemoglobin. Anemic conditions are usually a result of impaired erythrocyte production, blood loss, increased erythrocyte destruction, or a combination of the three.

Whether there is decreased/defective production or destruction of erythrocytes, anemias are classified according to either their **etiologic basis** or the **morphologic appearance** of the erythrocytes. Descriptions of anemias based on erythrocyte cellular structure refer to the cell's size and hemoglobin content. The morphologic classification is widely used. Terms that refer to cellular size end with –*cytic.* Terms that describe hemoglobin content end with –*chromic.* An erythrocyte can be **macrocytic,** meaning abnormally large, or **microcytic,** meaning abnormally small, and **hyperchromic,** containing an unusually high concentration of hemoglobin within its cytoplasm, or **hypochromic,** containing an abnormally low concentration of hemoglobin. For comparison, cells of normal size are termed **normocytic** and cells with normal amounts of hemoglobin are termed **normochromic.** In some anemias, the erythrocytes take on various sizes or they have various shapes; this is **anisocytosis** and **poikilocytosis,** respectively.

2. **Describe the pathophysiology of the clinical manifestations of anemias.**
   Study pages 538-539 and 541; refer to Figure 20-1.

Compensation for reduced oxygen-carrying capacity of the blood requires the cardiovascular, respiratory, and hematologic systems to respond. A reduction in the number of circulating erythrocytes after hemorrhage affects the consistency and volume of the blood. To compensate for reduced blood volume, fluids from the interstitium move into the blood vessels and plasma volume expands. The thinner, less viscous blood flows faster and more turbulently than normal blood. Increased blood flow within the heart can cause ventricular dysfunction, cardiac dilation, and heart valve insufficiency.

Hypoxemia of anemia causes arterioles, capillaries, and venules to dilate, which speeds blood flow even more. As venous return to the heart increases, the heart must pump harder and faster to meet normal oxygen demand and to prevent cardiopulmonary congestion. Congestive heart failure can develop.

Tissue hypoxia also causes the rate and depth of breathing to increase in an attempt to make more oxygen available to the remaining erythrocytes. When anemia is severe or sudden in onset, peripheral blood vessels constrict to direct available blood flow to the vital organs. A number of systemic symptoms occur subsequent to this shunting of blood.

Decreased blood flow is sensed by the kidneys, and in an effort to improve kidney perfusion, the renal renin-angiotensin response is activated. This results in salt and water retention, causing increased workload for the heart. The individual will experience shortness of breath or dyspnea, a rapid pounding heartbeat, dizziness, and fatigue even when at rest.

The skin, mucous membranes, lips, nail beds, and conjunctivae become pale because of reduced hemoglobin concentration or yellowish as a result of an accumulation in the skin of products of red blood cell breakdown or hemolysis. Decreased oxygen delivery to the skin results in impaired healing and loss of elasticity. Thinning and early graying of the hair can occur.

If the anemia is due to vitamin B_{12} deficiency, the nervous system is affected. Myelin degeneration may occur with loss of nerve fibers in the spinal cord. Paresthesias, gait disturbances, extreme weakness, spasticity, and reflex abnormalities may then result.

Decreased oxygen supply to the gastrointestinal tract often produces abdominal pain, nausea, vomiting, and anorexia. Low-grade fever, less than 101° F, occurs in some anemic individuals and may be the result of leukocytic pyrogens being released from ischemic tissues. Therapeutic intervention for any anemic condition requires treatment of the underlying disorder and palliation of symptoms. Therapies for anemia include transfusions, dietary corrections, and administration of supplemental vitamins or iron.

3. **Develop a comparative chart of the macrocytic-normochromic, microcytic-hypochromic, and normocytic-normochromic anemias.**
   Study pages 541 and 543-536; refer to Figures 20-2 through 20-6 and Tables 20-1, 20-3, and 20-4.

ANEMIAS

Anemia	Etiology	High-Risk Groups	Symptoms
Macrocytic-normochromic			
Pernicious	Insufficient influence of vitamin B_{12} on developing cells because of deficient IF; antibodies develop against parietal cells; gastrectomy or ileectomy therapies; chronic gastritis	Anglo-Saxon and Scandinavian populations	Typical;* digestive symptoms from lack of HCl and enzymes; glossitis; peripheral neuropathy: tingling numbness, loss of vibratory sense
Folate (folic acid)	Dietary deficiency inhibits DNA synthesis	Alcoholics; chronically malnourished persons	Typical,* similar to pernicious except no neurologic disorders
Microcytic-hypochromic			
Iron deficiency (IDA)	Excessive bleeding, which depletes iron; poor diet; no meat; possible *H. pylori* infection	Pregnant women; adolescents, children; elderly; those with chronic blood loss	Typical*
Sideroblastic (SA)	Dysfunctional iron uptake by erythroblasts; decreased heme synthesis, enzymes, etc.; genetic factors	Acquired from drugs: ethanol, lead, chloramphenicol; hereditary via recessive X-linked	Typical,* mild hepatomegaly and splenomegaly; erythropoietic hemochromatosis
Normocytic-normochromic			
Aplastic (AA)	Radiation; drugs; lesions within red bone marrow; immune response that halts erythropoiesis (Fanconi anemia)	Anyone	Typical;* petechiae; ecchymosis; bleeding; infection; pancytopenia
Posthemorrhagic	Sudden and acute blood loss	Surgery; trauma	Shock; acidosis
Hemolytic	Premature dysfunction or destruction of mature erythrocytes in circulation; genetics resulting in fragile cells; acquired from infections, drugs, autoimmunity, warm IgG, or cold IgM, antibodies	Anyone	Splenomegaly; jaundice

ANEMIAS—cont'd

Anemia	Etiology	High-Risk Groups	Symptoms
Normocytic-normochromic—cont'd			
Anemia of chronic disease (ACD)	Bacterial toxins; cytokines from activated macrophages and lymphocytes; suppressed progenitor cells; reduced iron in blood	AIDS; autoimmunity; neoplasms	Mild because of disability caused by chronic condition

*Typical signs and symptoms: fatigue, weakness, dyspnea, and pallor.
Treatment: Removing cause, if possible, and replacing the deficient element; marrow transplants; or immunosuppression.

4. **Describe the types, causes, manifestations, and treatment of polycythemia.**
   Study pages 547-548; refer to Table 20-5.

   Polycythemia is an unusual disease—considered a myeloproliferative, nonmalignant disease—that causes excessively large numbers of erythrocytes in the blood. It is typically accompanied by increased circulating platelets and granulocytes. There are essentially two types of polycythemia: (1) primary and secondary absolute or (2) relative. Relative polycythemia results from hemoconcentration of blood associated with dehydration. The primary form of absolute polycythemia is relatively rare and tends to occur in men between the ages of 40 and 60 of Jewish or European ancestry. Rarely is polycythemia found in children or multiple members of a single family. Secondary polycythemia, the more common form, is essentially a physiologic response to hypoxia. It is not uncommon to find an increased red cell count in individuals living at high altitudes, in smokers, and in individuals with congestive heart failure or chronic obstructive pulmonary disease.

   The clinical signs of polycythemia include ruddy, red color of the face, hands, feet, ears, and mucous membranes; engorgement of retinal and sublingual veins; elevated blood pressure; splenomegaly; and hepatomegaly. Symptoms include headache, a feeling of fullness in the head, dizziness, weakness, itching, sweating, epigastric distress, fatigue on exertion, backache, and visual disturbances. The clinical manifestations of vascular disease likely predominate. Angina pectoris, calf pain associated with vasospasms during walking, thrombosis, and cerebral insufficiency can occur.

   Treatment for polycythemia consists of reducing erythrocytosis and blood volume, controlling symptoms, and preventing thrombosis. Erythrocytosis and blood volume are reduced by phlebotomy, wherein a vein is opened and blood is removed according to need. Radioactive phosphorus is also used to suppress erythro-poiesis. Smokers should be urged to quit, and patients with congestive heart failure and chronic obstructive pulmonary disease require appropriate pharmaceutical intervention.

5. **Describe terms associated with high or low leukocyte counts and the causes of the alterations.**
   Study pages 548-549 and 551; refer to Tables 20-6 and 20-7.

   Leukocytosis exists when the leukocyte count is higher than normal; leukopenia is a condition in which the leukocyte count is lower than normal. Leukocytosis is a normal, protective response to invading microorganisms, strenuous exercise, emotional changes, temperature changes, anesthesia, surgery, pregnancy, some drugs, hormones, and toxins. Malignancies and hematologic disorders also cause leukocytosis. Increased levels of circulating neutrophils, eosinophils, basophils, and monocytes are chiefly a physiologic response to infection. Elevations also can occur as a result of polycythemia and chronic myelocytic leukemia that increase stem cell proliferation in the bone marrow.

   Leukopenia is never beneficial. As the leukocyte count falls below 1000 per cubic millimeter, the individual is at risk for infection. The risk for very serious life-threatening infections develops with counts below 500/mm^3. Leukopenia can be caused by radiation, anaphylactic shock, systemic lupus erythematosus, and certain chemotherapeutic agents. Decreased leukocytic counts occur when infectious processes delete the circulating granulocytes and monocytes. Infectious agents draw them out of the circulation and into infected tissues faster than they can be replaced. Decreases also can be caused by disorders that suppress marrow function.

   Granulocytosis or **neutrophilia** is prevalent in the early stages of infection or inflammation when stored neutrophils from the venous sinuses are released into the circulating blood. Emptying of the venous sinuses stimulates formation of granulocytes in the marrow. When the demand for neutrophils exceeds the circulatory supply, the marrow releases immature neutrophils and other leukocytes into the blood; this is called a **shift to the left.** The shift to the left is sometimes called a *leukemoid reaction* because the morphologic findings in blood smears are similar to those of individuals with leukemia. As infection or inflammation diminishes and granulopoiesis replenishes the circulating granulocytes, a **shift to the right** or back to normal occurs. **Neutropenia,** or low neutrophilic count, may be caused by decreased or ineffective neutrophil production because the marrow is producing other formed elements. Also, autoimmunity, reduced neutrophil survival, and abnormal neutrophil distribution and sequestration in tissues lead to neutropenia. Neutropenia exists when the neutrophil count is less than 2000/mm³. If neutrophils are reduced to below 500/mm³ and the entire granulocyte count is extremely low, a very serious condition called **agranulocytosis** results. The usual cause of agranulocytosis is interference with hematopoiesis in the bone marrow or increased cell destruction in the circulation. Chemotherapeutic agents used in the treatment of hematologic disorders and other malignancies and some drugs cause bone marrow suppression. Clinical manifestations of agranulocytosis include respiratory infection, general malaise, septicemia, fever, tachycardia, and ulcers in the mouth and colon. If untreated, sepsis caused by agranulocytosis can result in death within 3 to 6 days.

Eosinophilia is an absolute increase in the total numbers of circulating eosinophils. Allergic disorders associated with asthma, hay fever, parasitic invasion, and drug reactions are often the cause of eosinophilia. Chemotactic factor of anaphylaxis (CTF-A) and histamine released from mast cells attract eosinophils to the area. **Eosinopenia** is a decrease in circulating eosinophils generally due to migration of eosinophils into inflammatory sites. It also may be seen in Cushing syndrome as a result of stress due to surgery, shock, trauma, burns, or mental distress.

Basophilia is quite rare and is generally seen as a response to inflammation and hypersensitivity reactions of the immediate type. An increase in basophils also is seen in chronic myeloid leukemia and myeloid metaplasia. **Basopenia** is seen in hyperthyroidism, acute infection, and long-term therapy with steroids, as well as during ovulation and pregnancy.

Monocytosis, an increase in monocytes, is often transient and correlates poorly with disease states. When present, it is most commonly associated with bacterial infections during the late stages of recovery when needed to phagocytize any surviving microorganisms and debris. Monocytosis is seen in chronic infections such as tuberculosis and subacute bacterial endocarditis. **Monocyto-**

penia, a decrease in monocytes, is rare but has been identified with hairy cell leukemia and prednisone therapy.

A **lymphocytosis** is rare in acute bacterial infections and occurs most often in acute viral infections, especially those caused by the Epstein-Barr virus (EBV). **Lymphocytopenia** may be associated with neoplasias, immune deficiencies, and destruction by drugs. It may be that the lymphocytopenia associated with heart failure and other acute illnesses is caused by elevated levels of cortisol. Lymphocytopenia is a major problem in AIDS. The lymphocytopenia seen with this condition is caused by the HIV virus, which is cytopathic for T helper lymphocytes.

6. **Describe the pathogenesis of infectious mononucleosis.**
   Study pages 551-552.

Infectious mononucleosis is an acute infection of B lymphocytes. The most common etiologic virus is the Epstein-Barr virus (EBV); however, cytomegalovirus (CMV) and other viruses, as well as *Toxoplasma gondii*, have been identified as causative agents for this disease.

Infectious mononucleosis usually affects young adults between the ages of 15 and 30 years. The proliferation of clones of B and T cells and removal of dead and damaged leukocytes are largely responsible for the swelling of cervical lymphoid tissues. The incubation period for infectious mononucleosis is approximately 30 to 50 days. The accompanying sore throat is caused by inflammation at the site of viral entry. Splenomegaly occurs in affected individuals.

Serologic tests to determine a heterophile antibody response are necessary for diagnosis. These heterophilic antibodies are IgM agglutinins against nonhuman red blood cells (sheep or horse).

Infectious mononucleosis is usually self-limiting with recovery occurring in a few weeks. Treatment consists of rest and alleviation of symptoms with analgesics. Streptococcal pharyngitis is treated with penicillin or erythromycin. Steroids are used when airway obstruction or other organ involvement is evident.

7. **Classify, contrast, and describe the manifestations of leukemia.**
   Study pages 552-554 and 556; refer to Figures 20-6, 20-7, and 20-10, and Tables 20-8 and 20-9.

Leukemia is a malignant disorder of the blood and blood-forming organs, exhibiting an uncontrolled proliferation of dysfunctional leukocytes. The excessive proliferation of leukemic cells crowds the bone marrow and causes decreased production and function of normal hematopoietic cells.

The two major forms of leukemia are acute and chronic. They are classified by predominant cell type; the type is named according to the point of arrested cell maturation. Acute leukemia is characterized by undifferentiated and immature or blastic cells. The onset of disease is abrupt and rapid, and the affected individual usually has a short survival time. In chronic leukemia, the predominant cell appears mature but does not function normally. The onset of disease is gradual and the prolonged clinical course results in a relatively longer survival time. Leukemia occurs with varying frequencies at different ages and is about ten times more frequent in adults than in children in the United States.

Causal risk factors acting together with a genetic predisposition can alter the nuclear DNA of a single cell, and then the resulting leukemic cell proliferates. The leukemic cell is unable to mature and respond to normal regulatory mechanisms. Abnormal chromosomes are reported in 40% to 50% of patients with acute leukemia. Studies indicate a significant tendency for leukemia to recur in families. Hereditary abnormalities are also associated with an increased incidence of leukemia.

Acquired disorders that progress to acute leukemia include chronic myelocytic leukemia (CML), polycythemia, Hodgkin lymphoma, multiple myeloma, ovarian cancer, chronic lymphocytic leukemia (CLL), and sideroblastic anemia. Large doses of ionizing radiation also are associated with an increased incidence in myelogenous leukemia. Drugs such as chloramphenicol and certain alkylating agents cause bone marrow depression and also can predispose an individual to leukemia. Acute myelogenous leukemia (AML) is the most frequently reported secondary cancer following high doses of chemotherapy used for some other cancers.

LEUKEMIAS

	Myelocytic		Lymphocytic	
	AML	**CML or CGL**	**ALL**	**CLL**
Origin	Unknown	Myeloid stem cell	80% B cells; 20% T cells	B cells
Onset	Acute	Gradual	Acute	Gradual
Signs/symptoms	Pallor, petechial hemorrhage, lymphadenopathy	Splenomegaly, hepatomegaly, Philadelphia syndrome	Splenomegaly, hepatomegaly, lymphadenopathy, bleeding	Splenomegaly, fatigue, weight loss, night sweats
Presence of blasts	High	Low	High	Rare
Treatment	Chemotherapy, marrow transplants	No cure: chemotherapy, marrow transplants	Chemotherapy, marrow transplants	No cure: chemotherapy, marrow transplants
Survival	20% to 50% long-term survival	Months to years	5-year survival rate about 70%; long term is 40%	Years

NOTE: Death is usually caused by hemorrhage and infections.

8. Differentiate multiple myeloma from the leukemias.
   Study pages 557-559; refer to Figures 20-8 and 20-9.

Multiple myeloma is a B cell cancer arising from a hematopoietic stem cell associated with mature plasma cell structure and function. Multiple myelomas involve chromosomal translocations, which occur in many individuals. One chromosome partner is chromosome 14, the site of immunoglobulin genes, which recombines with other chromosomal sites. This disorder likely originates in the bone marrow and moves through the circulation to lymph nodes; then the myeloma cells return to the bone marrow or soft tissue sites. Development of myeloma is governed by cytokines; IL-6 is likely the major myeloma growth factor.

Chemotherapy, radiation therapy, plasmapheresis, blood stem cell transplantation, and marrow transplant have been used for treatment. With chemotherapy and aggressive management of complications, a median survival of 24 to 30 months and a 10-year survival rate of 3% can be achieved. After conventional chemotherapy relapse, thalidomide can be used because it suppresses tumor necrosis factor and has antiangiogenesis ability.

MULTIPLE MYELOMA/COMMON LEUKEMIAS

Characteristic	Multiple Myeloma	Common Leukemias
Malignant proliferation of WBC in the bone marrow	Yes	Yes
Anemia	Yes	Yes
Bleeding	Yes	Yes
Recurrent infections	Yes	Yes
Plasma cells	Yes	No
Ineffective immunoglobulins/M-protein	Yes	No
Bence-Jones protein in urine	Yes	No
Pathologic bone fractures	Yes	No
WBC blood elevation	No	Yes
Osteocytic lesions	Yes	Possible
Elevated calcium serum	Yes	Possible
Bone pain	Yes	Possible
Renal disease	Yes	Possible

9. **Compare Hodgkin and non-Hodgkin lymphomas.**
Study pages 559-564; refer to Figures 20-11 through 20-14 and Tables 20-10 through 20-12.

Lymphomas are tumors of (1) primary lymphoid tissue or the thymus and bone marrow and (2) secondary lymphoid tissue or lymph nodes, spleen, tonsils, and intestinal lymphoid tissue. Most lymphomas are neoplasms of secondary lymphoid tissue involving lymph nodes and/or spleen. The major types of malignant lymphomas are **Hodgkin** and **non-Hodgkin lymphomas.** Bone marrow involvement occurs more often in non-Hodgkin lymphoma than in Hodgkin lymphoma. Hodgkin lymphoma uses one of four histologic subtypes for classification. The subtypes are based on the appearance of the nonmalignant cells and the specific type of cytokine involved. Non-Hodgkin lymphoma has a lack of Reed-Sternberg cells seen in Hodgkin lymphoma and other cellular changes not characteristic of Hodgkin lymphomas. In both lymphomas, the genetic alterations involve mutation of proto-oncogenes and inactivation or disruption of tumor suppressor genes.

MALIGNANT LYMPHOMAS

	Hodgkin	Non-Hodgkin
Cause	Proto-oncogenes	Mutations on oncogenes and immunoglobulin genes
Cellular deviation	B cells, monocytes, Reed-Sternberg cells*	Other than Hodgkin
Age of onset	2 peaks: 20s and 30s 60s and 70s	After 50 years
Nodes involved	Single node or chain: cervical, inguinal, axillary, retroperitoneal	Multiple nodes: cervical, axillary, inguinal, femoral
Extranodal involvement	Uncommon	More common
Symptoms	Painless mass, fever, night sweats, weakness, weight loss (likely localized)	Similar to Hodgkin plus pleural effusion, abdominal pain, splenomegaly (generalized)
Treatment	Radiotherapy or surgery for localized, chemotherapy for generalized	Chemotherapy and radiotherapy; possible autologous marrow transplantation
Curability	More than 75%; cure is possible, but relapse after chemotherapy within 2 years has poor prognosis	Long-term, nodular lymphoma has better prognosis than diffuse disease

*Reed-Sternberg cells are malignant tissue macrophages that are scattered among normal cells.

10. Describe thrombocytopenia and thrombocythemia.

Study pages 565-567.

Thrombocytopenia exists when the platelet count is below 100,000 platelets per cubic millimeter of blood. Hemorrhage from minor trauma can occur with counts of 50,000 or less. Spontaneous bleeding can occur with counts between 15,000 and 10,000. Severe bleeding results if the count is below 10,000. Such bleeding can be fatal if it occurs in the gastrointestinal tract, respiratory system, or central nervous system.

Immune thrombocytopenic purpura (ITP) is usually a chronic condition more prevalent in females. It is thought to be an autoimmune disorder in which an IgG autoantibody is formed that binds to and destroys the platelets. The individual most commonly presents with mucosal or skin bleeding, which often is manifested as menorrhagia, hematuria, purpura, and petechiae.

In **thrombotic thrombocytopenia purpura (TTP)**, platelets aggregate and occlude the microcirculation. Platelet aggregation occurs without activation of the coagulation cascade and is related to other thrombotic microangiopathic conditions, including hemolytic syndromes and low platelet syndromes.

Thrombocythemia has a platelet count greater than 400,000 per cubic millimeter of blood. It is usually asymptomatic until the count exceeds 1 million/mm^3. Then, intravascular clot formation or thrombosis, hemorrhage, or other abnormalities can occur.

Primary or **essential thrombocythemia** is a myeloproliferative disorder in which megakaryocytes in the marrow are produced in excess of 600,000/mm^3 of blood. Clinical manifestations of primary thrombocytosis include thrombosis of peripheral blood vessels or, in severe cases, thrombosis of hepatic, mesenteric, or pulmonary vessels. Splenomegaly and easy bruising also occur. In individuals with thrombotic and hemorrhagic complications, the platelet count is lowered by use of chemotherapy agents.

Secondary thrombocythemia occurs following splenectomy because platelets that normally would be stored in the spleen remain in circulating blood. Secondary thrombocytosis may be seen in conjunction with treatment of rheumatoid arthritis and cancers.

11. Identify the causes of coagulation disorders; characterize disseminated intravascular coagulation.

Study pages 567-573; refer to Figure 20-15.

Disorders of coagulation are usually caused by defects or deficiencies of one or more of the clotting factors. Two common inherited disorders are the **hemophilias** and **von Willebrand disease.** These are caused by deficiencies of clotting factor, hemophilia by a single clotting factor and von Willebrand disease by multiple clotting factor deficiencies.

Other coagulation defects are acquired and usually result from deficient synthesis of clotting factors by an impaired liver. A deficiency of vitamin K, which is necessary for normal synthesis of the clotting factors by the liver, is an acquired coagulation defect.

Disseminated intravascular coagulation (DIC) is an acquired coagulation disorder having a variety of predisposing conditions. DIC is a paradoxical condition in which clotting and hemorrhage occur within the vascular system simultaneously. The development of DIC is generally associated with endothelial damage, exposure to tissue factor (TF), which complexes with factor VII, and direct activation of factor X. Gram-negative sepsis, septic shock, hypoxia, and low flow states associated with cardiopulmonary arrest can damage the endothelium and precipitate DIC by activating the intrinsic clotting pathway. Endotoxins of gram-negatives activate both intrinsic and extrinsic clotting pathways.

Release of tissue factor is associated with normal tissue breakdown. Excessive amounts of tissue factor in the circulation activate both clotting pathways. When either system is activated, widespread, unrestricted coagulation occurs throughout the body, leading to thrombic events within the vasculature.

The amount of thrombin that enters the systemic circulation during DIC greatly exceeds the ability of the body's naturally occurring antithrombins. The obstruction that results from circulatory deposition of thrombin interferes with blood flow and causes widespread organ hypoperfusion that can lead to ischemia, infarction, and necrosis with manifestations of multisystem organ dysfunction. The clotting factors are consumed as widespread clotting develops. Thrombosis in the presence of hemorrhage comprises this paradoxical alteration.

Plasmin, which is present because of overstimulation of the clotting cascade, begins to degrade fibrin before a stable clot can develop. As fibrin is broken down by plasmin, fibrin degradation products (FDPs) are released into the circulation; these are potent anticoagulants. The macrophage system likely is unable to clear the blood of FDPs because of lack of fibronectin. The clearance of particulate matter or fibrin clumps is mediated by the adhesive properties of fibronectin.

Treatment of DIC attempts to remove the underlying pathology, restore hemostasis, and maintain organ viability. Organ viability is treated primarily by adequate fluid replacement to ensure adequate circulating blood volume so that optimal tissue perfusion can be maintained.

Practice Examination

1. Anemia refers to a deficiency of:
   a. blood plasma.
   b. erythrocytes.
   c. platelets.
   d. hemoglobin.
   e. Both b and d are correct.

2. Morphologic classification of anemia is based on all
   of the following *except:*
   a. size.
   b. color.
   c. shape.
   d. cause.

3. Hypoxemia causes:
   a. arterioles, capillaries, and venules to dilate.
   b. the heart to contract more forcefully.
   c. the rate and depth of breathing to increase.
   d. Both a and b are correct.
   e. a, b, and c are correct.

Match the etiology of the anemia with RBC morphologic appearance.

_____ 4. vitamin B_{12} deficiency   a. macrocytic-normochromic

_____ 5. iron deficiency   b. microcytic-hypochromic

_____ 6. folic acid deficiency   c. normocytic-normochromic

_____ 7. excessive bleeding

8. Which symptoms are consistent with aplastic anemia but *not* with pernicious anemia?
   a. hemorrhage into the tissues
   b. pallor
   c. fatigue
   d. hypoxia
   e. neuropathy

9. A cause of macrocytic-normochromic anemia is:
   a. iron deficiency.
   b. antibodies against parietal cells.
   c. an enzyme deficiency.
   d. inheritance of abnormal hemoglobin structure.
   e. None of the above is correct.

10. An individual having chronic gastritis and tingling
    in the fingers requires which of the following for
    treatment?
    a. oral B_{12}
    b. B_{12} by intramuscular injection
    c. ferrous fumarate by intramuscular injection
    d. oral folate
    e. transfusions

11. Secondary polycythemia may be caused by:
    a. dehydration.
    b. chronic obstructive pulmonary disease.
    c. living at high altitudes.
    d. Both b and c are correct.
    e. a, b, and c are correct.

12. The symptoms of polycythemia are essentially
    caused by:
    a. fewer erythrocytes than normal.
    b. decreased blood volume.
    c. increased blood viscosity.
    d. increased rate of blood flow.

Match the leukocytic alteration with its cause.

_____13. eosinophilia   a. pregnancy

_____14. leukopenia   b. allergic disorders

                                c. radiation

                                d. early stage of infection

                                e. surgical stress

15. Leukocytosis is found in all of the following *except:*
    a. inflammatory responses.
    b. allergic responses.
    c. bacterial infections.
    d. bone marrow depression.

16. What is the most notable characteristic of infectious
    mononucleosis?
    a. It has a short incubation period of less than 1
       week.
    b. It usually affects preteens.
    c. The presence of heterophil antibody is diagnosti-
       cally helpful.
    d. Lymphocytosis persists for less than 1 week.

17. Which likely does *not* play a role in leukemia?
    a. radiation
    b. Down syndrome
    c. polycythemia
    d. chloramphenicol
    e. diet

18. CML is characterized by its:
    a. acute onset.
    b. high incidence in children.
    c. presence of the Philadelphia chromosome.
    d. survival time of days to months.

19. Clinical manifestations of multiple myeloma in-
    clude all of the following *except:*
    a. bone pain.
    b. decreased serum calcium.
    c. m-protein.
    d. renal damage.
    e. pathologic fractures.

Match the characteristic with the malignant lymphoma.

_____20. Epstein-Barr virus   a. Hodgkin lymphoma

_____21. Reed-Sternberg cell   b. non-Hodgkin lymphoma

_____22. more frequent extranodal involvement

23. A thrombocytopenia with a platelet count below 50,000/mm³ likely will cause:
    a. hemorrhage from minor trauma.
    b. spontaneous bleeding.
    c. death.
    d. polycythemia.

24. Thromboembolic disease can be caused by all of the following *except:*
    a. injured vessel walls.
    b. tissue damage that releases excessive tissue factor.
    c. obstructed blood flow.
    d. deficient dietary intake of vitamin K.
    e. polycythemia.

25. DIC is associated with:
    a. endothelial damage.
    b. activation of factor X.
    c. release of tissue factor.
    d. Both a and c are correct.
    e. a, b, and c are correct.

Case Study 1

Ann is a healthy 26-year-old white female. Since the beginning of this current golf season, she has noted increased shortness of breath and low levels of energy and enthusiasm. These seem worse during her menses. Today, while playing poorly in a golf tournament at a high, mountainous course, she became lightheaded and was taken by her golfing partner to the emergency clinic of a multispecialty medical group.

The attending physician's notes indicated a temperature of 98° F, an elevated heart rate and respiratory rate, and low blood pressure. Ann states that heavy menstrual flow has been a problem for 10 to 12 years and she takes 1000 mg of aspirin every 3 to 4 hours for 6 days during menstruation. During the summer months while playing golf, she also takes aspirin to avoid "stiffness in my joints."

Laboratory values are as follows:
 Hemoglobin = 8 g/dl
 Hematocrit = 32%
 Erythrocyte count = 3.1×10^6/mm³
 RBC smear showed microcytic and hypochromic cells.
 Reticulocyte count = 1.5%
 Other laboratory values were within normal limits.

Considering the circumstances and the preliminary work-up, what type of anemia is most likely for Ann? Which clinical sign shows her body is attempting to compensate for anemia?

Case Study 2

L.L., a 9-year-old male, was brought to his dentist for a regular preschool check-up. The dentist and mother were having a chatty conversation when L.L.'s mother stated that her son recently had stopped showing interest in sports and complained of fatigue. During the dental examination, the dentist noted gingival bleeding whenever the tissue was lightly probed. Three nontender lymph nodes were palpable in the submandibular nodes. No other abnormalities were noted. The dentist advised the mother to take L.L. to the medical clinic next door.

The physical examination showed L.L.'s skin to be pale with ecchymoses and petechiae of the trunk. The spleen and liver were not palpable, and the remaining examination was unremarkable. A sample of blood was withdrawn.

The CBC revealed the following:

Hemoglobin = 9.2 g/dl	Eosinophils = 445/mm^3
Hematocrit = 30%	Monocytes = 1900/mm^3
RBCs = 3 × 10^6/mm^3	Lymphocytes = 4500/mm^3
WBCs = 16 × 10^3/mm^3	Blasts = much higher than normal
Neutrophils = 8 × 10^3/mm^3	Platelets = 30 × 10^3/mm^3
Basophils = 250/mm^3	

Considering the examinations and CBC, what would the physician likely conclude and do?

Alterations of Hematologic Function in Children

Foundational Objective

a. **Identify the postnatal changes occurring in the blood throughout childhood.**
   Refer to Table 19-8.

MEMORY CHECK!

- Blood cell counts tend to rise above adult levels at birth and then decline gradually throughout childhood. The immediate rise in values is the result of accelerated hematopoiesis during fetal life, the trauma of birth, and cutting of the umbilical cord. The presence of large numbers of immature erythrocytes and leukocytes in peripheral blood is found in the neonate. Within the first 2 weeks to 3 months of life, up to 1 year, normal values for adults are approached. Platelet counts in full-term neonates are comparable to those of adults and remain so throughout infancy and childhood. Average blood volume in the full-term neonate is slightly above that of older children and adults, 85 ml/kg of body weight compared with 75 ml/kg, respectively.

Objectives

After studying this chapter, the learner will be able to do the following:

1. **Describe the etiology of childhood iron deficiency anemia and identify appropriate diagnostic and treatment measures.**
   Study pages 580-581; refer to Table 21-1.

   Iron deficiency anemia is the most common childhood anemia and is caused by poor dietary iron intake, gastrointestinal blood loss, or both. Early exposure to cow's milk protein often causes hemorrhagic bowel inflammation and occult blood loss in the infant. The onset of menstruation in females also is a contributor. Poor socioeconomic status can be a significant casual factor. The highest incidence of iron deficiency anemia occurs at 6 months to 2 years of age and peaks again in adolescence during rapid growth periods.

   There are few symptoms in infants and young children until moderate anemia develops. General irritability, activity intolerance, and weakness are indicators of anemia. When hemoglobin falls below 5 g/dl, systolic murmurs may occur. Iron stores are best measured by serum ferritin and total iron-binding capacity. Treatment for iron deficiency anemia is iron supplements; oral supplements are preferred.

2. Compare and contrast the two major causes of hemolytic disease of the newborn.
Study pages 581-583; refer to Figure 21-1.

The two major causes of **hemolytic disease of the newborn (HDN)** are **blood type incompatibility** and **Rh factor incompatibility.** Blood type incompatibility is a mild form of hemolytic disease. Rh incompatibility is potentially much more severe. Blood type incompatibility in the mother occurs when maternal antibodies to fetal erythrocytes are formed because of a prior incompatible pregnancy or exposure of the mother to fetal erythrocytes during pregnancy. Incompatibility in the infant occurs when sufficient antibody, usually IgG, crosses the placenta from the mother to the infant or when maternal antibodies attach to and damage fetal erythrocytes. ABO incompatibility occurs in 20% to 25% of pregnancies, with only one in ten cases producing HDN. Usual causes are a type O mother with a type A or B fetus, a type A mother with a type B fetus, or a type B mother with a type A fetus. Hemolysis in the newborn is usually limited, resolves after birth, and requires limited treatment; however, mild hemolysis may contribute to hyperbilirubinemia.

Rh incompatibility occurs in less than 10% of pregnancies and rarely is a problem during the first pregnancy; the first pregnancy initiates sensitization. Rh incompatibility becomes a greater problem with subsequent pregnancies. It should be noted that HDN caused by Rh incompatibility occurs in only 5% of pregnancies after five or more pregnancies. In the most severe form, Rh incompatibility can lead to severe anemia, edema, central nervous system damage, and fetal death. It may also contribute to severe hyperbilirubinemia.

Blood typing in mothers and infants reveals those at risk. Indirect Coombs' test reveals antibodies in mothers, and direct Coombs' test reveals antibodies bound to fetal erythrocytes. In patients with a prior history of HDN, diagnostic tests to determine risk include maternal antibody titers, fetal blood sampling, amniotic fluid spectrophotometry, and fetal ultrasound. Immunoprophylaxis with Rh immunoglobulin (RhoGAM) for at-risk mothers has been very successful.

3. Describe childhood sickle cell disease and identify its most common forms of presentation.
Study pages 583-585 and 587; refer to Figures 21-2 through 21-4 and Table 21-2.

Sickle cell disease is an inherited, autosomal recessive disorder most common in the United States among blacks. The disease is characterized by the presence of **hemoglobin S (HbS)** within the erythrocytes. This hemoglobin becomes elongated and sickle-shaped whenever it is deoxygenated or dehydrated.

The parent's medical history and clinical findings may generate an index of suspicion about the child's condition. The sickle solubility test and hemoglobin electrophoresis are used to assist in diagnosis. Prenatal chorionic villus sampling is now available.

Acute complications or crises occur in sickle cell disease and may be provoked by infection, exposure to cold, low PO_2, acidosis, or localized hypoxemia. Infections are frequent in childhood and may generate various degrees of other triggers.

Vasoocclusive crises result from a "log-jam" effect produced by stiff, sickled erythrocytes in the microcirculation. Symptoms include symmetric swelling of the hands and feet, which may be the first clinical manifestation in infancy. In older children, swollen painful joints, priapism, severe abdominal pain from infarctions of abdominal organs, and strokes may occur. Other complications include sickle cell retinopathy, renal necrosis, and necrosis of the femoral head.

Sequestration crises occur only in the young child. Large amounts of blood may pool in the liver and spleen, which can contain as much as one-fifth of the blood volume and, thus, precipitate shock. Up to a 50% mortality rate has been reported with these crises. **Hyperhemolytic crises,** although unusual, may occur with some drug use or with infections.

Aplastic crises may occur because of the decreased survival of sickled erythrocytes; fewer erythrocytes peak at 10 to 20 days after initiation of the crisis. This development may lead to aplastic anemia if compensatory mechanisms are not intact. Most sickle cell deaths are due to overwhelming infection and sepsis.

4. Describe the thalassemias.
Study pages 587-588; refer to Figures 21-5 and 21-6.

The alpha- and beta-thalassemias are inherited autosomal recessive disorders that cause an impaired rate of synthesis of one of the two chains—alpha or beta—of adult hemoglobin. Beta-thalassemia is more common that alpha-thalassemia.

Beta-thalassemia involves slowed or defective synthesis of the beta globin chain and is prevalent among Greeks, Italians, some Arabs, and Sephardic Jews. Alpha-thalassemia, wherein the alpha chain is affected, is most common among Chinese, Vietnamese, Cambodians, and Laotians. Both thalassemias are common among blacks. The effects range from mild microcytosis to death in utero, and the pathophysiology depends on the number of defective genes and mode of inheritance.

The fundamental defect in beta-thalassemia is the uncoupling of alpha and beta chain synthesis. The free alpha chains are unstable and easily precipitated in the cell. Most erythroblasts that contain precipitates are destroyed by mononuclear phagocytes in the marrow, resulting in ineffective erythropoiesis and anemia. Individuals with beta-thalassemia minor, the mild form, are usually asymptomatic. Persons with beta-thalassemia major, the severe form, may become quite ill. Anemia is severe and results in significant cardiovascular overload with high output congestive heart failure. Today, blood transfusion can increase life span by a decade or two. Death is usually caused by hemochromatosis.

There are four forms of **alpha-thalassemia,** with each dependent on the number of defective genes. The severity is variable. Individuals who inherit the mildest form of alpha-thalassemia, the alpha trait, usually are symptom-free or have mild microcytosis. Alpha-thalassemia major causes hydrops fetalis and fulminant intrauterine congestive heart failure. The fetus has a grossly enlarged heart and liver. Diagnosis usually is made postmortem. In children with thalassemia major, cardiovascular compromise causes death by 5 to 6 years of age if untreated.

Individuals who are carriers or have thalassemia minor generally have few symptoms and require no specific treatment. For thalassemia major, therapies to support and prolong life are necessary. There is no cure for either condition.

5. **Describe childhood hemophilias and their complications.**
   Study pages 588-590; refer to Tables 21-3 and 21-4.

Hemophilia, or spontaneous bleeding, is rare in the first year of life, although significant bleeding may occur during circumcision. However, this is an unusual complication, because hemostasis in these infants is achieved through the extrinsic pathway that does not require factors VIII, IX, or XI, which are responsible for 90% to 95% of bleeding if they are absent. **Hematoma** formation is a more common problem during the first year of life and may be caused by injections, firm holding, or the many accidents that occur in the development of movement in children. These accidents also may precipitate bleeding in the joints. Spontaneous hematuria and epistaxis are bothersome but rarely serious. Life-threatening intracranial and cervical bleeding may result from normal childhood injury. The administration of blood products to replace deficient or absent factors has enhanced the physical capabilities of individuals suffering hemophilic defects.

6. **Describe the pathophysiology of idiopathic thrombocytopenic purpura and identify its most likely etiology.**
   Study pages 590-591.

Idiopathic thrombocytopenic purpura (ITP, autoimmune [primary] thrombocytopenia purpura) is the most common thrombocytopenic purpura of childhood. Antiplatelet antibodies attach to platelets that are then sequestered in the spleen, where they are destroyed by mononuclear phagocytes.

Classic symptoms of bruising and petechiae are usually preceded by viral illness occurring 1 to 4 weeks earlier that may cause sensitization of the platelets, which triggers an antibody response; high levels of IgG have been found on the platelets of affected children.

The prognosis is excellent. The acute phase lasts 1 to 2 weeks, although thrombocytopenia may persist longer. Complete recovery occurs in approximately 75% of individuals at 3 months after onset, with 90% of afflicted children recovering by 9 to 12 months. Although serious complications are few, severe intracranial bleeding does occur in about 1% of cases and can be serious.

7. **Describe proposed causative factors and common manifestations for childhood leukemias.**
   Study pages 591-593; refer to Figure 21-7 and Table 21-6.

Leukemia, in its various forms, is the most common childhood malignancy; it comprises 33% of the neoplasms of children. Acute lymphoblastic leukemia (ALL) represents 80% to 85% of all childhood leukemias. Peak incidence of ALL occurs at between 2 and 6 years of age and is twice as common in white children as in nonwhite children. The etiology of leukemia is probably multifactorial, with genetic predisposition, environment, and viruses playing a role. Exposure to high levels of ionizing radiation also has become an established etiologic factor.

The appearance of the **blast cell** in the bone marrow with a reduction of red blood cells and granulocytes is the hallmark of acute leukemia. Symptoms may be rapid or slow but generally reflect the effects of bone marrow failure. Findings include decreased red blood cells and platelets and changes in white blood cells. Pallor, fatigue, petechiae, purpura, and fever are generally present. Fever may be due to a hypermetabolic state brought on by the rapid production and destruction of leukemic cells or because of a secondary infection due to neutropenia. Renal failure may ensue because of high uric acid levels that produce precipitates of urates in the renal tubules. Other symptoms, such as bone and joint pain, may be due to infiltration of leukemic cells into other organs. The central nervous system is a common site of extramedullary infiltration, although few children have this problem at diagnosis; it occurs later in the course of the disease.

8. **Distinguish between non-Hodgkin lymphoma and Hodgkin lymphoma.**
   Study pages 593-594; refer to Figures 21-8 through 21-10.

Non-Hodgkin lymphoma (NHL) and **Hodgkin lymphoma** comprise approximately 11% of all childhood cancers; NHL is the most common. Either group of disease is rare before the age of 5 years, and the relative incidence increases throughout childhood. Males are affected more often than females. At particular risk are children with inherited or acquired immunodeficiency syndromes. A viral etiology is suggested; a strong correlation between the Epstein-Barr virus and lymphoma exists.

Childhood non-Hodgkin lymphoma is a diffuse rather than nodular disease. Disease sites commonly involve extranodal sites such as brain, lung, bone, and skin. Rapidly enlarging lymphoid tissue and painless lymphadenopathy are common with abdominal sites. Symptoms often include abdominal pain and vomiting, but a palpable mass is not always present. An anterior mediastinal mass, with or without pleural effusion, may be present. If the mass is large, respiratory compromise, tracheal compression, and superior vena cava syndrome may arise. CNS involvement is common.

Most children with NHL are cured. Optimal treatment is evolving, but combination chemotherapy with or without radiation therapy is successful.

Besides a viral etiology for **Hodgkin lymphoma** in children, genetic susceptibility has been suggested as a cause. Hodgkin lymphoma incidence gradually rises through the age of 11 years. There is a marked increase through adolescence that continues into the thirties. Histologically, the tumor consists of neoplastic Reed-Sternberg cells typically surrounded by small lymphocytes, macrophages, neutrophils, and plasma cells.

Painless lymphadenopathy in the lower cervical chain, with or without fever, is the most common symptom. Mediastinal involvement can lead to airway obstruction. Extranodal primary involvement is rare in Hodgkin lymphoma.

Treatment for Hodgkin lymphoma includes chemotherapy and radiation therapy. The survival rate for children with Hodgkin lymphoma is high; 70% to 90% is common.

Practice Examination

True/False

_____ 1. Early initiation of iron-rich cow's milk in an infant's diet is an excellent preventive measure against iron deficiency anemia.

_____ 2. Although a frequent problem, ABO incompatibility seldom results in significant disease.

_____ 3. Sequestration crisis is a serious complication of sickle cell disease unique to childhood.

_____ 4. Rh incompatibility is a problem only of an Rh-positive woman bearing an Rh-negative fetus during a second pregnancy.

_____ 5. Because hemostasis in the newborn is chiefly attained through the extrinsic pathway, serious bleeding in the newborn period usually is not a problem in hemophiliacs.

_____ 6. Idiopathic thrombocytopenic purpura is a genetically transmitted disease.

_____ 7. Leukemias are multifactorial diseases with genetic disposition, environment, and bacterial infections playing a role in their etiologies.

8. Which is the most common blood disorder of infancy and childhood?
   a. iron deficiency anemia
   b. pernicious anemia
   c. folate deficiency anemia
   d. sideroblastic anemia

9. Maternal-fetal blood incompatibility may exist in which condition?
   a. Rh-positive mother, Rh-negative fetus
   b. Rh-negative mother, Rh-positive fetus
   c. Rh-negative father, Rh-positive mother
   d. Rh-negative father, Rh-negative mother

10. Beta-thalassemia is:
    a. common among Italians.
    b. an X-linked recessive disorder.
    c. an autosomal recessive disorder.
    d. Both a and b are correct.
    e. Both a and c are correct.

11. Which statement is correct?
    a. Sickle cell disease is an autosomal dominant disorder.
    b. Sickle cell disease is an X-linked recessive disorder.
    c. Sickle cell disease is an X-linked dominant disorder.
    d. Sickle cell disease is an autosomal recessive disorder.

12. Idiopathic thrombocytopenic purpura involves antibodies against:
    a. neutrophils.
    b. eosinophils.
    c. platelets.
    d. basophils.

13. Which are factors associated with iron deficiency anemia?
    a. rapid growth
    b. low socioeconomic status
    c. cow's milk for infants
    d. Both a and c are correct.
    e. a, b, and c are correct.

14. What is the most likely cause of idiopathic thrombocytopenic purpura?
    a. stress and fatigue
    b. genetic predisposition
    c. prolonged occult bleeding
    d. viral sensitization
    e. Both b and c are correct.

15. Hodgkin lymphoma has:
    a. extensive extranodal involvement.
    b. rare extranodal involvement.
    c. painless cervical lymphadenopathy.
    d. Both a and c are correct.
    e. Both b and c are correct.

16. In sickle cell disease, vasoocclusive crisis is the result of:
    a. damage to platelets due to IgG.
    b. "plugging" of peripheral blood vessels by "stiff" sickled erythrocytes.
    c. ingestion of sulfa drugs.
    d. sequestration of large numbers of erythrocytes in the spleen.

17. Which factor may play a part in the development of childhood leukemia?
    a. genetic predisposition
    b. environmental factors
    c. viral infections
    d. radiation
    e. All of the above are correct.

18. Which statement is true about acute lymphocytic leukemia?
    a. It is the most common childhood leukemia.
    b. It usually occurs between 2 and 6 years of age.
    c. It is uniformly fatal.
    d. It is easily predicted through genetic testing.
    e. Both a and b are correct.

Match the circumstance with the alteration.

_____19. leukocyte counts approaching 100,000/mm³   a. leukemia

_____20. low platelet counts   b. ITP

_____21. lack of coagulation factors VIII, IX, and XI   c. sickle cell disease

_____22. may present early as symmetric, painful swelling of hands and feet   d. Rh incompatibility

_____23. may cause severe hemolysis in the newborn period   e. hemophilia

_____24. may result in aplastic crises

_____25. may result in fetal death

Case Study

Steven D. is a 10-year-old white male seeking medical attention because of possible physical abuse observed by his gym teacher. The teacher noticed severe bruising over much of his upper body when his shirt "rode up" during an exercise. Steven emphatically states that he has never been abused by anyone. He denies any accidents and didn't tell anyone about his bruises because he thought they might "get me into trouble." His mother cannot explain the bruises either and did not see them before today because her son does all of his own hygiene and is quite modest about revealing his body even to family members. Steven's physical examination is benign except for multiple, irregular dark purple bruises over most of his torso and lower extremities. His complete blood count is well within normal limits except for a low platelet count of 18,000/mm^3.

What is Steven's diagnosis?

22

Structure and Function of the Cardiovascular and Lymphatic Systems

Objectives

After reviewing this chapter, the learner will be able to do the following:

1. Describe the function of the circulatory system; distinguish between pulmonary and systemic circulation.
   Review page 598; refer to Figure 22-1.

2. Describe the heart wall and the chambers, fibrous skeleton, valves, and great vessels of the heart; trace the blood flow through the heart.
   Review pages 598 and 601-602; refer to Figures 22-2 through 22-8.

3. Describe the coronary arteries, veins, and lymphatic vessels.
   Review pages 602-603 and 605; refer to Figure 22-9.

4. Describe the initiation of and conduction sequence of electrical impulses through the heart; identify the autonomic innervation and its effects on the heart.
   Review pages 605-609; refer to Figures 22-10 through 22-12.

5. Identify the structure and characteristics of myocardial cells.
   Review pages 609-610 and 612-613; refer to Figures 22-13 through 22-16.

6. Use the Frank-Starling law and Laplace law to demonstrate interrelationships that affect cardiac function; indicate the influence of reflexes on heart rate.
   Review pages 613-616; refer to Figures 22-17 through 22-20.

7. Contrast the structure and function of arteries, capillaries, and veins.
   Review pages 617 and 621-622; refer to Figures 22-21 through 22-27 and Table 22-2.

8. Describe the determinants of blood flow.
   Review pages 622-625; refer to Figures 22-28 through 22-31.

9. Identify the factors that regulate arterial and venous blood pressure.
   Review pages 626-628 and 630; refer to Figures 22-32 through 22-35 and Table 22-3.

10. Describe the regulation of coronary circulation.
    Review pages 631-632.

11. Describe the normal structure and function of the lymphatic system.
    Review pages 632-633; refer to Figures 22-36 through 22-38.

12. Note the changes that aging causes in the cardiovascular system.
    Review page 617.

Practice Examination

1. Oxygenated blood flows through the:
   a. superior vena cava.
   b. pulmonary veins.
   c. pulmonary arteries.
   d. coronary veins.
   e. None of the above is correct.

2. The hepatic vein:
   a. carries blood from the vena cava to the liver.
   b. carries blood from the liver to the vena cava.
   c. carries blood from the aorta to the liver.
   d. carries blood from the liver to the aorta.

3. The position of the heart in the mediastinum is:
   a. inferior to the diaphragm and between the lungs.
   b. between the lungs, superior to the diaphragm.
   c. posterior to the trachea, anterior to the esophagus.
   d. posterior to the lungs and anterior to the diaphragm.

4. The pericardial space is found between the:
   a. myocardium and parietal pericardium.
   b. endocardium and visceral pericardium.
   c. visceral and parietal pericardium.
   d. visceral and epicardial pericardium.

5. In the normal cardiac cycle, which of the following occurs? (More than one answer may be correct.)
   a. The right atrium and right ventricles contract simultaneously.
   b. The two atria contract simultaneously, whereas the two ventricles relax.
   c. The two ventricles contract simultaneously, whereas the two atria relax.
   d. Both the ventricles and atria contract simultaneously to increase cardiac output.

6. The QRS complex of the EKG represents:
   a. atrial depolarization.
   b. ventricular depolarization.
   c. atrial contraction.
   d. ventricular repolarization.
   e. atrial repolarization.

7. A person having a heart rate of 100, a systolic blood pressure of 200, and a stroke volume of 40 ml would have an average cardiac output of:
   a. 0.5 ml/min.
   b. 5 l/min.
   c. 4 ml/min.
   d. 8000 ml/min.
   e. None of the above is correct.

8. During atrial systole, the:
   a. AV valves are open.
   b. atria are filling.
   c. ventricles are emptying.
   d. semilunar valves are open.

9. Which does *not* significantly affect heart rate?
   a. sympathetic nerves
   b. parasympathetic nerves
   c. atrioventricular valves
   d. acetylcholine

10. One cardiac cycle:
    a. has a duration that changes if the heart rate changes.
    b. usually requires less than 1 second to complete.
    c. is equal to stroke volume times heart rate.
    d. pumps approximately 5 liters of blood.
    e. Both a and b are correct.

11. Compared with arteries, veins:
    a. have a larger diameter.
    b. are thick-coated.
    c. recoil quickly after distension.
    d. Both a and b are correct.

12. Normal systolic pressure within the left ventricle is in the range of:
    a. 100–140 mm Hg.
    b. 15–30 mm Hg.
    c. 0–10 mm Hg.
    d. None of the above is correct.

13. Backflow of blood from the arteries into the relaxing ventricles is prevented by the:
    a. venous valves.
    b. pericardial fluid.
    c. semilunar valves.
    d. atrioventricular valves.

14. Adrenomedullin (ADM):
    a. exhibits powerful vasoconstriction activity.
    b. is present only in cardiovascular tissue.
    c. mediates sodium reabsorption.
    d. exhibits powerful vasodilatory activity.

15. The Frank-Starling law of the heart concerns the relationship between:
    a. the length of the cardiac muscle fiber and the strength of contraction.
    b. stroke volume and arterial resistance.
    c. rapidity of nerve conduction and stroke volume.
    d. systolic rate and cardiac output.

16. How does cardiac muscle differ from skeletal muscle? (More than one answer may be correct.)
    a. It is arranged in parallel units.
    b. It is arranged in branching networks.
    c. It is multinucleated.
    d. It is single-nucleated.
    e. It is more accessible to sodium and potassium ions.

17. Blood pressure is measured by the:
    a. pressure exerted on the ventricular walls during systole.
    b. pressure exerted by the blood on the wall of any blood vessel.
    c. pressure exerted on arteries by the blood.
    d. product of the stroke volume times heart rate.

18. Identify the correct sequence of the portions of the pulmonary circulation.
    a. 1, 5, 3, 2, 4   1. pulmonary veins
    b. 4, 2, 3, 1, 5   2. pulmonary arteries
    c. 4, 1, 3, 2, 5   3. lungs
    d. 5, 2, 3, 1, 4   4. right ventricle
    e. 5, 1, 3, 2, 4   5. left atrium

19. The heartbeat is initiated by the:
    a. coronary sinus.
    b. atrioventricular bundle.
    c. right ventricle.
    d. SA node.
    e. AV node.

20. If the sympathetic nervous system stimulation of the heart predominates over parasympathetic nervous system stimulation, the heart will:
    a. increase its rate.
    b. contract with greater force and at a slower rate.
    c. decrease its rate and force of contraction.
    d. contract with less force and at a higher rate.

21. When fluids exhibit a turbulent flow:
    a. resistance increases.
    b. it is a sign of greater blood viscosity.
    c. the fluids have greater velocity than with laminar flow.
    d. there is greater hydrostatic pressure than if the fluids had laminar flow.

22. Identify the normal sequence of an electrical impulse through the heart's conduction system.
    a. 4, 1, 2, 5, 3   1. atrioventricular bundle
    b. 4, 2, 5, 1, 3   2. AV node
    c. 2, 4, 1, 5, 3   3. Purkinje fibers
    d. 4, 2, 1, 5, 3   4. SA node
                           5. right and left bundle branches

23. Which factor might increase resistance to the flow of blood through the blood vessels?
    a. an increased inner radius of diameter of blood vessels
    b. decreased numbers of capillaries
    c. decreased blood viscosity
    d. decreased numbers of red blood cells

24. Depolarization of cardiac muscle cells occurs because of:
    a. the cell's interior becoming more negatively charged.
    b. the cell's interior becoming less negatively charged.
    c. impermeability of the cell membrane to sodium.
    d. impermeability of the cell membrane to potassium.

25. Which statement is true?
    a. Lymphatic walls consist of multiple layers of flattened endothelial cells.
    b. Lymph from the entire body, except for the upper right quadrant, eventually drains into the thoracic duct.
    c. The thoracic duct has approximately the same diameter as the great veins.
    d. Lymph contains more proteins than does blood plasma.
    e. The lymphatic system, like the circulatory system, is a closed circuit.

23

Alterations of Cardiovascular Function

a. Describe the flow of blood through the heart and identify the coronary vessels.
Refer to Figures 22-5 and 22-9.

MEMORY CHECK!

- The pumping action of the heart consists of contraction and relaxation of the myocardial layer of the heart wall. During relaxation, termed *diastole,* blood fills the chambers. The contraction that follows, termed *systole,* forces the blood from the chamber into the pulmonary, or systemic, circulation. During diastole, blood from the veins of the systemic circulation enters the thin-walled right atrium from the superior vena cava and the inferior vena cava. Venous blood from the coronary circulation enters the right atrium through the coronary sinus. The right atrium fills, and its fluid pressure pushes open the right atrioventricular or tricuspid valve. Blood fills the right ventricle. The same sequence of events occurs a fraction of a second earlier in the left heart. The four pulmonary veins, two from the right lung and two from the left lung, carry oxygenated blood from the pulmonary circulation to the left atrium. As the left atrium fills, its fluid pressure pushes the cusps of the mitral valve open and blood flows into the left ventricle. Blood circulates from the left ventricle and returns to the right atrium because of a progressive fall in pressure from the left ventricle to the right atrium of approximately 120 mm Hg. Blood always flows from a higher pressure area toward a lower pressure area.

- The blood within the heart chambers does not supply oxygen and other nutrients to the cells of the heart. Like all other organs, heart structures are nourished by vessels of the systemic circulation. The coronary circulation consists of coronary arteries and cardiac veins. The right and left coronary arteries traverse the epicardium and branch several times. The left coronary artery arises from a single opening behind the left cusp of the aortic semilunar valve. It divides into two branches, the left anterior descending artery and the circumflex artery. The left anterior descending artery delivers blood to portions of the left and right ventricles and much of the interventricular septum. The circumflex artery supplies blood to the left atrium and the lateral wall of the left ventricle, and often branches to the posterior surfaces of the left atrium and left ventricle. The right coronary artery originates from an opening behind the right aortic cusp. Three major branches of the right coronary artery supply blood to the right atrium, upper right ventricle, and both ventricles.

Continued

MEMORY CHECK!—cont'd

- Collateral arteries are connections, or anastomoses, between two branches of the same coronary artery or connections of branches of the right coronary artery with branches of the left. They are particularly common within the interventricular and interatrial septa, at the apex of the heart, over the anterior surface of the right ventricle, and around the sinus node. The heart has an extensive capillary network with about one capillary per muscle cell. Blood travels from the arteries to the arterioles, then into the capillaries, where exchange of oxygen and other nutrients takes place.

- Blood from the coronary arteries drains into the cardiac veins, which travel alongside the arteries. The cardiac veins feed into the great cardiac vein and then into the coronary sinus located between the atria and ventricles. The coronary sinus empties into the right atrium.

b. **Describe the conduction system of the heart.**
   Review pages 605-609; refer to Figures 22-10 through 22-12.

MEMORY CHECK!

- Continuous, rhythmic repetition of the cardiac cycle or systole and diastole depends on the continuous, rhythmic transmission of electrical impulses. As an electrical impulse passes from cell to cell in the myocardium, muscular contraction or systole occurs. After the action potential passes, the fibers relax and return to their resting length; this relaxation is diastole.

- The myocardium differs from other muscle tissues; it contains its own intrinsic conduction system. It can generate and transmit action potentials without stimulation from the nervous system. These cells are concentrated at certain sites in the myocardium called *nodes*. Although the heart is innervated by both sympathetic and parasympathetic fibers, neural impulses are not needed to maintain the cardiac cycle.

- Normally, electrical impulses arise in the sinoatrial node or SA node, often called the *pacemaker* of the heart. There are numerous autonomic nerve endings within the node that enable the node to respond to the nervous system. In the resting adult, the SA node generates about 75 action potentials per minute. Each action potential travels rapidly from cell to cell and through special pathways in the atrial myocardium, which causes both atria to contract. Atrial contraction initiates systole. Transmission of the action potential from the atrial to the ventricular myocardium occurs through muscle fibers of the conduction system. The action potential travels first to the atrioventricular node or AV node, then to the atrioventricular bundle, then to the common bundle, and finally through the bundle branches of the interventricular septum to Purkinje fibers in the heart wall.

- The extensive network of Purkinje fibers enables the rapid spread of the impulse to the ventricular apices.

- Electrical activation of the muscle cells, or depolarization, is caused by the movement of electrically charged solutes, primarily sodium and potassium, across cardiac cell membranes. Deactivation, or repolarization, occurs by ion movement in the opposite direction. Movement of ions into and out of the cell creates an electrical or voltage difference across the cell membrane. This difference or potential of charged ions causes the impulse to flow within cells and from cell to cell.

- Sympathetic neural stimulation of the myocardium and coronary vessels depends on the presence of adrenergic receptors that are able to bind specifically with neurotransmitters of the sympathetic nervous system. Norepinephrine binding to receptors increases the rate of impulse generation and conduction and also the strength of myocardial contraction during systole. Also, coronary arterioles dilate to supply the heart with more oxygen and nutrients. These effects enable the heart to pump more blood. Parasympathetic or vagus nerve activity decreases the heart rate. The vagus nerve releases acetylcholine.

c. **Describe the interrelationships between myocardial stretch and chamber wall dimensions and the contractible force of the heart.**
   Review pages 613-616; refer to Figures 22-17 through 22-20.

MEMORY CHECK!

- Cardiac muscle, like other muscle, increases its strength of contraction within certain limits when it is stretched. The Frank-Starling law of the heart states that there is a direct relationship between the volume of blood in the heart and stretch or length of cardiac fibers at the end of diastole and the force of contraction during the next systole. The greater the stretch from preload blood volume, the stronger the contraction.

- Laplace law states the relationships between wall thickness, pressure, and wall tension. Wall tension is related directly to the product of intraventricular pressure and internal radius and inversely to the wall thickness. Stated another way, the pressure or contractible force is directly related to wall thickness and wall tension and indirectly related to the radius. The thicker the wall and greater the wall tension and smaller the radius, the greater the force of contraction.

d. **Establish the determinants of blood flow.**
   Review pages 622-625; refer to Figures 22-28 and 22-31.

MEMORY CHECK!

- Blood flow is determined primarily by two factors: pressure and resistance. Pressure in a liquid system is the force exerted on the liquid per unit area. Fluid moves from the arterial "side" of the capillaries, which is a region of greater pressure, to the venous side, which is a region of lesser pressure. Resistance opposes force. In the cardiovascular system, most opposition to blood flow is because of the diameter and length of the blood vessels themselves.

- The relationship between blood flow, pressure, and resistance can be stated as Q equals P divided by R, where Q is blood flow, P is the pressure difference, and R is resistance.

- Resistance to fluid flow considers the length of the tube or vessel, the viscosity of the fluid, and the radius of the lumen. According to the Poiseuille formula, the resistance equals viscosity of blood times length of vessel divided by the fourth power of the lumen's radius.

- Because this equation was derived using straight, rigid tubes with steady, streamlined flow, it cannot be applied exactly to the vascular system. Nevertheless, it is a useful model for vascular resistance assessment. Small changes in the lumen's radius lead to large changes in vascular resistance. Because vessel length is relatively constant, length is not as important as lumen size in determining flow through a single vessel. However, blood flowing through the distributing arteries encounters more resistance than blood flowing through the capillary bed. In the capillary bed, flow is distributed among many short, tiny branches.

- If "R equals viscosity times length divided by the fourth power of radius" is substituted into the formula "Q equals P divided by R," a helpful summary of likely factors affecting blood flow rate can be expressed. Now, blood flow equals pressure times radius to the fourth power divided by the viscosity times the length. The higher the pressure and greater the vessel radius and the less the viscosity of blood and length of vessel, the greater the flow of blood.

e. **Establish the determinants of blood pressure.**
Review pages 622-628 and 630; refer to Figures 22-32 through 22-35 and Table 22-3.

MEMORY CHECK!

- The mean arterial pressure, which is the average pressure in the arteries throughout the cardiac cycle, depends on the elastic properties of the arterial walls and the mean volume of blood in the arterial system. The main determinants of venous blood pressure are the volume of fluid within the veins and the compliance or distensibility of their vessel walls. The venous system accommodates approximately 60% of the total blood volume at any given moment with a venous pressure averaging less than 10 mm Hg. Conversely, the arteries accommodate about 15% of the total blood volume with a pressure of about 100 mm Hg. Some important relationships are as follows:

- Mean blood pressure equals cardiac output times peripheral resistance.

- Cardiac output equals heart rate times stroke volume.

- Peripheral resistance equals blood viscosity times vessel length divided by vessel radius raised to the fourth power.

- Blood pressure equals heart rate times stroke volume times viscosity times length divided by the radius to the fourth power. The higher the heart rate, stroke volume, blood viscosity, and vessel length and the less the vessel radius to the fourth power, the greater the blood pressure.

Objectives

After studying this chapter, the learner will be able to do the following:

1. **Distinguish between arteriosclerosis and atherosclerosis; describe the development of atheromatous plaque and its manifestations.**
Study pages 640-642 and 644; refer to Figures 23-1 through 23-5.

Arteriosclerosis is a chronic disease of the arterial system characterized by abnormal thickening and hardening of the vessel walls. Smooth muscle cells and collagen fibers migrate into the tunica intima, causing it to stiffen and thicken; this decreases the artery's ability to change lumen size.

Atherosclerosis is a form of arteriosclerosis in which the thickening of vessel walls is caused by hardening of soft deposits of intraarterial fat and fibrin that reduce lumen size. Atherosclerosis can take several forms depending on the anatomic vessel location, the individual's age and genetic and physiologic status, and the risk factors to which each individual may have been exposed. It is the leading contributor to coronary artery and cerebrovascular disease.

Atherogenesis begins with injury to the endothelial cells of arteries. Injured endothelial cells are unable to produce normal amounts of antithrombic and vasodilating cytokines. Macrophages adhere to injured endothelial cells and release oxygen radicals that result in oxidation of low-density lipoprotein (LDL). The oxidized LDL is engulfed by macrophages; lipid-laden macrophages are called **foam cells,** which accumulate to form the fatty streak. The lesions of atherosclerosis occur primarily within the tunica intima, or the innermost layer. These lesions include the fatty streak, fibrous plaque, and the complicated lesion. The early **fatty streak** is a flat, yellow, lipid-filled smooth muscle cell that causes no obstruction of the affected vessel.

Fibrous plaque is the characteristic lesion of advancing atherosclerosis and consists of lipid-laden smooth muscle cells surrounded by collagen, elastic fibers, and a mucoprotein matrix. The lesion is elevated and protrudes into the lumen of the artery. The growing mass fixes to the inner wall of the tunica intima and may invade the muscular tunica media. Fibrous plaques likely develop from fatty streaks. The core of the fibrous plaque consists of lipids and debris from cellular necrosis caused by insufficient blood supply. If the lesion progresses sufficiently, it occludes the arterial lumen at arterial bifurcations, curves, or regions where the arteries taper.

Complicated lesions occur as the fibrous plaques are altered by hemorrhage, calcification, cellular necrosis, and blood clots throughout the intimal layer. As the altered complex structure becomes rigid, it causes extensive vascular occlusion.

The signs and symptoms of atherosclerosis result from inadequate tissue perfusion because of obstruction of vessels that supply the tissues. Atherosclerosis may have many different manifestations. High blood pressure develops if atherosclerosis elevates systemic vascular resistance. Cerebral or myocardial ischemia is a life-threatening manifestation of atherosclerosis that occurs in the vessels of the brain or heart respectively.

Management focuses on removing the initial causes of vessel injury and preventing further lesion progression. This includes exercise, smoking cessation, and control of hypertension and diabetes.

Fat intake should be reduced to less than 30% of daily caloric intake with no more than 10% saturated fats. Daily cholesterol intake must be reduced to 250 to 300 mg. See flow chart on page 158.

2. **Distinguish between primary, secondary, complicated, and malignant hypertension.**
    Study pages 644-650; refer to Figures 23-6 through 23-8 and Tables 23-1 and 23-2.

Adult hypertension begins when the systolic pressure exceeds 140 mm Hg and the diastolic pressure exceeds 90 mm Hg. Increasing pressures in both systolic and diastolic pressure categorize hypertension from stage 1 (mild) to stage 3 (severe). Stage 1 (mild) exists when systolic is 140-159 mm Hg and diastolic is 90-99 mm Hg, stage 2 (moderate) is when systolic is 160-179 mm Hg and diastolic is 100-109 mm Hg, and stage 3 (severe) is when systolic is more than or equal to 180 mm Hg and diastolic is more than or equal to 110 mm Hg. **Isolated systolic hypertension** is elevated systolic blood pressure accompanied by normal diastolic pressure (below 90 mm Hg).

Hypertension is caused by increases in cardiac output, total peripheral resistance, or both. Cardiac output is increased by any condition that increases heart rate or stroke volume, whereas peripheral resistance is increased by any factor that increases blood viscosity or reduces vessel diameter.

Primary hypertension, which is also called *essential* or *idiopathic hypertension,* has a combination of genetic and environmental factors likely responsible for its development. Primary hypertension affects 92% to 95% of hypertensive individuals.

The exact cause of primary hypertension is unknown, although several hypotheses are proposed, including (a) overactivity of the sympathetic nervous system, (b) overactivity of the rennin-angiotensin-aldosterone system, (c) sodium and water retention by the kidneys, (d) hormonal inhibition of sodium-potassium transport across cell walls, and (e) complex interactions involving insulin resistance and endothelial function.

Secondary hypertension is caused by any systemic disease process that raises peripheral vascular resistance or cardiac output. Causes include renal disease, adrenal disorders, vascular disease, and drugs (corticosteroids, oral contraceptives, and antihistamines). Fortunately, if the cause is identified and removed before permanent structural changes occur, blood pressure can return to normal. Rigidity of the aorta is the chief vascular cause of isolated systolic hypertension.

Complicated hypertension is sustained primary hypertension that causes pathologic effects in addition to hemodynamic alterations and fluid and electrolyte imbalances. Complicated hypertension compromises the structure and function of vessels, the heart, kidneys, eyes, and the brain.

Cardiovascular complications include left ventricular hypertrophy, angina pectoris, congestive heart failure or left heart failure, coronary artery disease, myocardial infarction, and sudden death.

Malignant hypertension is a rapidly progressive hypertension in which diastolic pressure is usually above 140 mm Hg. It can cause profound cerebral edema that disrupts cerebral function and causes loss of consciousness. High hydrostatic pressures in the capillaries cause vascular fluid to move into the interstitial space. If blood pressure is not reduced, cerebral edema and dysfunction increase until death occurs.

The early stages of hypertension have no clinical manifestations; thus, hypertension is called a "silent disease." Some hypertensive individuals never have signs, symptoms, or complications; others become very ill and their hypertension can cause death. Others have anatomic and physiologic damage caused by past hypertensive disease even if current blood pressure is within normal ranges. Most of the clinical manifestations of hypertensive disease are caused by complications that damage organs and tissues other than the vascular system. Besides elevated blood pressure, the signs and symptoms are specific for the organs or tissues affected. Heart disease, renal insufficiency, central nervous system dysfunction, impaired vision, impaired mobility, vascular occlusion, or edema can be caused by sustained hypertension.

Atherosclerosis

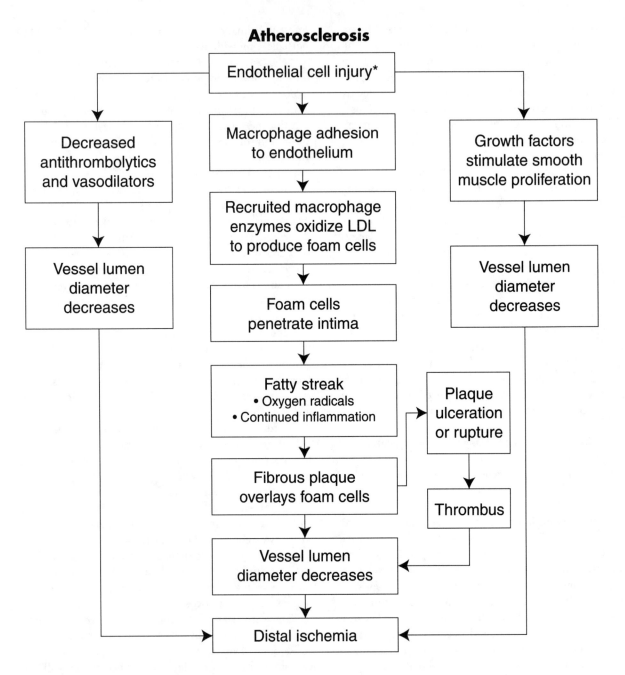

*There is increasing evidence that inflammation and infection may be causes of endothelial injury.

Hypertension is usually managed with both pharmacologic and nonpharmacologic methods. Treatment begins with reducing or eliminating risk factors. The usual recommendations are to restrict sodium intake, increase physical training, and discontinue cigarette smoking.

Four groups of drugs are used to manage hypertension: diuretics, angiotensin inhibitors, vascular smooth muscle relaxants, and adrenergic blockers. Diuretics and B-blockers are initially used because they reduce morbidity and mortality. If the response is inadequate, others are added.

3. **Define and identify the causes of orthostatic or postural hypotension.**
   Study pages 650-651.

Orthostatic or **postural hypotension** is a drop in both systolic and diastolic arterial blood pressure on standing from a reclining position. The normal or compensatory vasoconstrictor response to standing is replaced by a marked vasodilation and blood pooling in the muscle vasculature and in the splanchnic and renal beds. Acute orthostatic hypotension may be the result of (1) anatomic variation, (2) altered body chemistry, (3) antihypertensive and antidepressant therapy, (4) prolonged immobility caused by illness, (5) starvation, (6) physical exhaustion, (7) fluid volume depletion (dehydration), and (8) venous pooling.

Chronic orthostatic hypotension may be secondary to a specific disease. The diseases that may cause secondary orthostatic hypotension are adrenal insufficiency, diabetes mellitus, intracranial tumors, cerebral infarcts, and peripheral neuropathies.

4. Define aneurysm and list the types.
Study pages 651-652; refer to Figures 23-9 through 23-11.

An **aneurysm** is a localized dilation or outpouching of a vessel wall or cardiac chamber. The tension on the wall increases as the vessel becomes thinner, so the possibility of rupture increases. This is an example of the law of Laplace. The stretching produces infarct expansion, a weak and thin layer of necrotic muscle, and fibrous tissue that bulges with each systole. With time, the aneurysm can leak, cause pressure on surrounding organs, impair blood flow, or rupture.

The aorta is particularly susceptible to aneurysm formation because of the constant stress on its vessel wall and the absence of penetrating vasa vasorum in its adventitial layer. Three-fourths of all aneurysms occur in the abdominal aorta.

True aneurysms are fusiform and circumferential in nature and involve all three layers of the arterial wall; there is weakening of the vessel wall. **False aneurysms** or **saccular aneurysms** are usually the result of trauma. These aneurysms are caused by a break in the wall or a dissection of the layers of the arterial wall; blood is contained at the point of aneurysm by the adventitial layer.

Treatment of aneurysms is nearly always surgical. Leaking cerebral aneurysms are treated with clot-stabilizing drugs and a number of clinical measures designed to reduce intracranial pressure and promote hemodynamic stability before surgical intervention.

5. Distinguish between a thrombus and an embolus.
Study pages 652-653; refer to Table 23-3.

A **thrombus** is a blood clot that remains attached to a vessel wall. Thrombi tend to develop wherever intravascular conditions promote activation of the coagulation cascade.

In the arteries, activation of the coagulation cascade is usually caused by roughening of the tunica intima by atherosclerosis. Infectious agents also roughen the normally smooth lining of the artery, which causes platelets to adhere readily. Pooling of arterial blood within an aneurysm can stimulate thrombus formation. In the veins, thrombus formation is more often associated with inflammation. Thrombi also form on heart valves if there is inflammation of the endocardium or rheumatic heart disease.

A thrombus poses two threats to the circulation. First, the thrombus may be large enough to occlude the artery and cause ischemia in the tissue supplied by the artery. Alternatively, the thrombus may dislodge and travel through the vascular system until it occludes flow into a distal systemic or pulmonic vascular bed.

Pharmacologic treatment includes the administration of heparin, warfarin, and streptokinase. A balloon-tipped catheter can be used to remove or compress a thrombus.

Embolism is the obstruction of a vessel by an **embolus**, or a bolus of matter that circulates in the bloodstream. The embolus may be a dislodged thrombus, an air bubble, or an aggregate of fat, bacteria, or cancer cells. An embolus travels in the bloodstream until it reaches a vessel through which it cannot pass; an embolus will eventually lodge in a systemic or pulmonary vessel. Pulmonary emboli originate mostly from the deep veins of the legs or in the heart. Systemic emboli most commonly originate in the left heart and are associated with thrombi after myocardial infarction, valvular disease, left heart failure, endocarditis, and dysrhythmias.

Embolism of a coronary or cerebral artery is an immediate threat to life if the embolus severely obstructs these important vessels. Occlusion of a coronary artery will cause a myocardial infarction, whereas occlusion of a cerebral artery will cause a stroke or CVA.

6. Distinguish between arterial and venous occlusive disease.
Study pages 653-655; refer to Figures 23-12 and 23-13.

Thromboangiitis obliterans, or Buerger disease, tends to occur in young men who are heavy cigarette smokers. It is an inflammatory disease of the peripheral arteries. Inflammation, thrombus formation, and vasospasm can eventually occlude and obliterate portions of small and medium-sized arteries in the feet and sometimes in the hands. The pathogenesis of thromboangiitis obliterans is unknown.

The chief symptom of thromboangiitis obliterans is pain and tenderness of the affected part. Clinical manifestations are caused by sluggish blood flow and include rubor caused by dilated capillaries under the skin and cyanosis caused by blood that remains in the capillaries after its oxygen has diffused into the interstitium.

The most important part of treatment is cessation of cigarette smoking. Vasodilators may alleviate vasospasm. If vasospasm persists, sympathectomy may be performed and gangrene necessitates amputation.

Raynaud phenomenon and **Raynaud disease** are characterized by attacks of vasospasm in the small arteries and arterioles of the fingers and, less commonly, the toes. Raynaud phenomenon is secondary to systemic diseases such as collagen vascular disease, pulmonary hypertension, thoracic outlet syndrome, myxedema trauma, serum sickness, or long-term exposure to environmental conditions such as cold or vibrating machinery in the workplace. Raynaud disease is a primary vasospastic disorder of unknown origin tending to affect young women. It consists of vasospastic attacks triggered by brief exposure to cold or by emotional stress. Genetic predisposition may play a role in its development.

The vasospastic attacks of either disorder cause changes in skin color and sensation because of ischemia. Vasospasm occurs with varying frequency and severity and causes pallor, numbness, and the sensation of cold in the digits. Also, sluggish blood flow resulting from ischemia may cause the skin to appear cyanotic. Rubor follows as vasospasm ends and the capillaries become engorged with oxygenated blood.

Treatment for Raynaud phenomenon consists of removing the stimulus or treating the primary disease process. Treatment of Raynaud disease is limited to prevention or alleviation of vasospasm itself. Exposure to cold temperatures, emotional stress, and cigarette smoking are avoided. Exercises that build centrifugal force in the extremities are also helpful in the early stages of vasospasm for either entity.

A **varicose vein** is a vein in which blood has pooled. Varicose veins are distended, tortuous, and palpable. Varicose veins in the legs are caused by trauma to the saphenous veins that damages one or more valves or by venous distention from a combination of standing for long periods and the action of gravity on blood within the legs. If a valve is damaged and permits backflow, a section of the vein is subjected to the pressure exerted by a larger volume of blood under the influence of gravity. The vein swells as it becomes engorged, and surrounding tissue becomes edematous because increased hydrostatic pressure pushes plasma through the stretched vessel wall.

Varicose veins and valvular incompetence can progress to **chronic venous insufficiency (CVI)**. This condition is characterized by chronic pooling of blood in the veins of the lower extremities and leads to hyperpigmentation of the skin over the feet and ankles. Edema of the feet and ankles may progress proximally to the knees.

Any trauma or pressure lowers the oxygen supply by further reducing blood flow into the area. Cell death occurs and necrotic tissue develops into **venous stasis ulcers.** Persistent ulceration develops because the high metabolic demands of healing tissue cannot be met by the existing compromised circulation.

Venous thrombi are more common than arterial thrombi because flow and pressure are lower in the veins than in the arteries. With aging, the deep veins in the lower extremities become especially susceptible to thrombus formation. This is notable in individuals with long-term bed rest or those wearing constrictive clothing. Genetic abnormalities increase the risk for venous thrombosis and occur in persons having conditions predisposing them to blood flow stasis, endothelial injury, or hypercoagulability.

The inflammatory response triggered by the clotting cascade causes extreme tenderness, swelling, and redness in the area of thrombus formation. With venous occlusion, the skin is discolored rather than pale, edema is prominent, and pain is most marked at the site of occlusion. Treatment of varicose veins and chronic venous insufficiency begins conservatively. If conservative treatment is ineffective, saphenous vein stripping may be performed.

Superior vena cava syndrome (SVCS) is a progressive occlusion of the superior vena cava (SVC) that leads to venous distention in the upper extremities and head. The leading cause of SVCS is bronchogenic cancer, followed by lymphomas and metastasis of other cancers. The SVC is a relatively low-pressure vessel that lies in the closed thoracic compartment; therefore, tissue expansion within the thoracic compartment can easily compress the SVC.

Clinical manifestations of SVCS include edema and venous distension in the upper extremities and face including the ocular beds. Cerebral and central nervous system edema may cause headache, visual disturbance, or impaired consciousness. Respiratory distress may be present because of edema of the bronchial structures or compression of the bronchus by a carcinoma.

SVCS is generally not a vascular emergency but rather an oncologic problem. Treatment consists of radiotherapy for the neoplasm and the administration of diuretics, steroids, and anticoagulants.

7. **Characterize coronary artery disease; distinguish between myocardial ischemia and myocardial infarction and list complications of each.**
Study pages 655-666; refer to Figures 23-14 through 23-24 and Tables 23-4 and 23-5.

Coronary artery disease, myocardial ischemia, and **myocardial infarction** all impair the pumping ability of the heart by depriving the heart muscle of oxygen and nutrients. **Coronary artery disease (CAD)** diminishes the myocardial blood supply until deprivation impairs myocardial metabolism. The myocardial cells remain alive but are unable to function normally. Persistent ischemia or the complete occlusion of a coronary artery causes acute coronary syndromes including infarction or death.

In the United States, coronary artery disease is responsible for one-third of deaths in persons. The risk factors for CAD are classified as either modifiable or nonmodifiable. The **nonmodifiable risk factors** are variables that cannot be altered by persons wishing to decrease their risk of cardiovascular disease. These include genetic predispositions and diabetes mellitus. The **modifiable risk factors** include hyperlipidemia, hypertension, cigarette smoking, obesity, sedentary lifestyle, postmenopausal hormone therapy (presently controversial), and heavy alcohol consumption. Other risk factors include serum fibrinogen and C-reactive protein and possible infections.

The most common cause of **myocardial ischemia** is atherosclerosis. The growing mass of plaque, platelets, fibrin, and cellular debris can eventually narrow the coronary artery lumen enough to impede blood flow. Platelet aggregations are known to release a prostaglandin that is a potent vasoconstrictor capable of causing spasm of the coronary arteries. This prostaglandin, thromboxane A_2, also promotes platelet aggregation, so a vicious positive feedback cycle of vasoconstriction and platelet buildup occurs in the vessel walls.

Imbalances between blood supply and myocardial demand cause myocardial ischemia. Supply is reduced by increased resistance in coronary vessels, hypotension, decreased blood volume, valvular incompetence, or anemia. Demand is increased by high systolic blood pressure, increased ventricular volume, left ventricular hypertrophy, increased heart rate, and hyperviscosity of the blood. Ischemia occurs whenever demand exceeds supply.

Ischemia can be asymptomatic; if so, it is referred to as **silent ischemia.** The absence of angina may be caused by an abnormality in left ventricular symptomatic afferent innervation. Silent ischemia may result in less local inflammation which suggests that a high level of inflammatory cytokines may be essential to induce anginal pain. Myocardial ischemia induced by mental stress can exist without angina.

Myocardial cells become ischemic within 10 seconds of coronary occlusion. After several minutes, the heart cells lose their ability to contract. Anaerobic processes take over and lactic acid accumulates. Cardiac cells remain viable for approximately 20 minutes under ischemic conditions. If blood flow is restored, aerobic metabolism resumes, and contractility is restored. If the coronary arteries cannot compensate for lack of oxygen, **myocardial infarction** occurs.

The number and severity of postinfarction complications depend on the location and extent of necrosis, the individual's physiologic condition before the infarction, and the therapeutic intervention. Dysrhythmias or arrhythmias, which are disturbances of cardiac rhythm, are the most common complication of acute myocardial infarction and affect more than 90% of individuals. Sudden death resulting from cardiac arrest is often caused by dysrhythmias, particularly ventricular fibrillation. Acute myocardial infarction is usually accompanied by left ventricular failure characterized by pulmonary congestion, reduced myocardial contractility, and abnormal heart wall motion. Inflammation of the pericardium, or pericarditis, is a common complication of acute myocardial infarction. Dressler postinfarction pericarditis syndrome is thought to be an antigen-antibody response to the necrotic myocardium. Pain, fever, friction rub, pleural effusion, and arthralgias may accompany this syndrome. Transient ischemic attacks or an outright cerebrovascular accident may result from thromboemboli that have broken loose from coronary arteries or cardiac valves to occlude cerebral vessels. Pulmonary emboli are especially common. Rupture of the wall of the infarcted ventricle may be a consequence of aneurysm formation because of decreased muscle mass at the infarcted site.

Myocardial Ischemia/Infarction

| | | Acute Coronary Syndromes (Thrombus Formation) | |
Stable Angina	Prinzmetal Angina	Unstable Angina	Infarction
Cause			
Temporary ischemia, exertion, vessels cannot dilate in response to increased demand	Vasospasm, with or without atherosclerosis; occurs at night and at rest	Advanced reversible ischemia; occurs at rest	Irreversible ischemia, cellular necrosis with repair or scarring
Electrocardiography			
Normal, transient ST depression and T wave inversion	Transient ST elevation	Normal, transient ST depression and T wave inversion	Irreversible abnormal, pronounced Q waves
Plasma Enzyme Levels			
Negative	Negative	Negative	CPK-MB fraction, LDH, and SGOT or AST elevation; monoclonal antibodies against troponin I
Pain Relief and Treatment*			
Rest and nitroglycerin, beta blockers, calcium antagonists	Nitroglycerin, beta blockers, calcium antagonists	Rest and nitroglycerin ineffective, beta blockers, calcium antagonists, anticoagulant therapy	Narcotics, anticoagulant therapy (aspirin), thrombolytic agents, ACE inhibitors, beta blockers, statins, surgery

*When medical therapy fails to relieve angina, percutaneous transluminal intervention (PTCI) or coronary artery bypass grafting (CABG) may be required.

NOTE: The first symptom of myocardial ischemia or infarction is usually sudden, severe chest pain. The pain of infarction is more severe and persistent than the pain of ischemia; it may be heavy and crushing and radiating to neck, jaw, back, shoulder, or left arm. Exercise stress testing is useful in differentiating angina from other types of chest pain. Radioisotope imaging with thallium-201 is another diagnostic test to detect CAD. Single photon emission computerized tomography (SPECT) is able to identify ischemia and coronary risk.

8. **Characterize the terms associated with pericardial disease.**
   Study pages 667-669; refer to Figures 23-25 through 23-27.

Pericardial disease is often a localized manifestation of another disorder. Infection, trauma or surgery, neoplasms, or metabolic, immunologic, or vascular disorders can elicit a pericardial response. Pericarditis, pericardial effusion, or constrictive pericarditis are the consequences of the elicited response.

Acute pericarditis, although idiopathic, is commonly caused by infection, connective tissue disease, or radiation therapy. The pericardial membranes become inflamed and roughened, and an exudate may develop.

Symptoms include sudden onset of severe chest pain that worsens with respiratory movements. Individuals with acute pericarditis also may report dysphagia, restlessness, irritability, anxiety, weakness, and malaise. Friction rub or a short, scratchy, grating sensation similar to the sound of sandpaper may be heard at the cardiac apex and left sternal border and is pathognomonic for pericarditis. Treatment for uncomplicated acute pericarditis consists of relieving symptoms.

Pericardial effusion is the accumulation of fluid in the pericardial cavity and is possible with all forms of pericarditis. The fluid may be a transudate or an exudate. Pericardial effusion indicates an underlying disorder. If the fluid creates sufficient pressure to cause cardiac compression, it becomes a serious condition known as **tam-**

ponade. The danger of tamponade is that pressure exerted by the pericardial fluid will eventually equal diastolic pressure within the heart chambers. The first structures to be affected by tamponade are the right atrium and ventricle because diastolic pressures are normally lowest therein. Subsequent decreased atrial filling leads to decreased ventricular filling, decreased stroke volume, and reduced cardiac output. Life-threatening circulatory collapse may develop.

The most significant clinical finding in tamponade is **pulsus paradoxus.** In this circumstance, arterial blood pressure during expiration exceeds arterial pressure during inspiration by more than 10 mm Hg. There is impairment of diastolic filling of the left ventricle plus reduction of blood volume within all cardiac chambers.

Treatment of pericardial effusion or tamponade generally consists of aspiration of the excessive pericardial fluid. Persistent pain is treated with analgesics, antiinflammatory agents, or steroids. Surgery may be required if the tamponade cause is trauma or aneurysm.

Constrictive pericarditis is either idiopathic or associated with radiation exposure, rheumatoid arthritis, uremia, or coronary artery bypass graft. In constrictive pericarditis, fibrous scarring with occasional calcification of the pericardium causes the visceral and parietal pericardial layers to adhere; thus, there is obliteration of the pericardial cavity. Like tamponade, constrictive pericarditis compresses the heart and eventually reduces cardiac output. Unlike tamponade, however, constrictive pericarditis always develops gradually.

Symptoms are exercise intolerance, dyspnea on exertion, fatigue, anorexia, weight loss, edema, distention of the jugular vein, and hepatic congestion. Chest x-ray films often show prominent pulmonary vessels and calcification of the pericardium.

Initial treatment for constrictive pericarditis involves digitalis glycosides, diuretics, and sodium restriction. Surgical removal of the pericardium may be indicated because its removal does not compromise cardiac function.

9. **Compare the cardiomyopathies.**
   Study page 669; refer to Figure 23-28 and Tables 23-6 and 23-7.

The **cardiomyopathies** are a diverse group of diseases that primarily affect the myocardium itself and are not secondary to the usual cardiovascular disorders such as coronary artery disease, hypertension, or valvular dysfunction. They may be secondary to infectious disease, exposure to toxins, systemic connective tissue disease, infiltrative and proliferative disorders, or nutritional deficiencies; most cases of cardiomyopathy are idiopathic.

Characteristics of Cardiomyopathies

	Dilated	Hypertrophic	Restrictive
Hemodynamic changes			
Cardiac output	Decreased	Normal	Normal or decreased
Stroke volume	Decreased	Normal or increased	Normal or decreased
Ventricular filling pressure	Increased	Normal or increased	Increased
Ejection fraction	Decreased	Increased	Normal or decreased
Structural changes			
	Chamber size increased, decreased mitral valve competence	Hypertrophy of left ventricle and interventricular septum, chamber size normal or decreased, decreased mitral valve competence	Reduced ventricular compliance, infiltration of myocardium with amyloid or hemosiderin or glycogen deposits, chamber size decreased, decreased mitral valve competence
Manifestations			
	Dyspnea, fatigue, pulmonary congestion, palpitations	Angina, syncope, palpitations, left heart failure	Cardiomegaly, dysrhythmias, right heart failure

Valvular Stenosis and Regurgitation

Valvular Disorders	Causes	Manifestations
Aortic stenosis	Rheumatic heart disease, congenital malformation, calcification degeneration	Decreased stroke volume, left ventricular failure, dyspnea, angina, systolic murmur
Mitral stenosis	Acute rheumatic heart fever, bacterial endocarditis	Decreased stroke volume, right ventricular failure, chest pain, orthopnea, pulmonary hypertension, dysrhythmia, palpitations, induced thrombi, ascites, diastolic murmurs
Aortic regurgitation	Bacterial endocarditis, hypertension, connective disease disorders	Congestive left heart failure, dyspnea, throbbing peripheral pulse, palpitations, chest pain, diastolic and systolic murmurs
Mitral regurgitation	Rheumatic heart disease, mitral valve prolapse, CAD, infective endocarditis, connective tissue disorders	Left heart failure, pulmonary hypertension, dyspnea, hemoptysis, palpitations, murmur throughout systole
Tricuspid regurgitation	Congenital, high blood pressure in pulmonary circulation or right ventricle	Right heart failure, peripheral edema, ascites, hepatomegaly, murmur throughout systole
Mitral valve prolapse	Autosomal dominant pattern, hyperthyroidism-related	Regurgitant murmur, fatigue and lethargy, greater risk for infective endocarditis

10. **Identify the causes and manifestations of valvular dysfunction.**
    Study pages 670-671 and 673-674; refer to Figures 23-29 through 23-31 and Table 23-8.

In **valvular stenosis,** the valve orifice is constricted or narrowed. This impedes the forward flow of blood and increases the workload of the cardiac chamber "in front" of or before the diseased valve. Increased volume and pressure cause the myocardium to work harder and myocardial hypertrophy develops.

In **valvular regurgitation,** known also as insufficiency or incompetence, the valve leaflets or cusps fail to close completely. This permits blood flow to continue even when the valve should be closed. During systole, some blood leaks back into the atrial "upstream" chamber. This increases the workload of both atrium and ventricle. Increased volume leads to chamber dilation; increased workload leads to hypertrophy. Although all four heart valves may be affected, those of the left heart are more commonly affected than those of the right heart.

11. **Distinguish between rheumatic heart disease and infective endocarditis.**
    Study pages 674-679; refer to Figures 23-32 through 23-35 and Table 23-9. (See table on page 165.)

12. **Characterize dysrhythmias of the heart.**
    Study page 679; refer to Tables 23-10 and 23-11.

Dysrhythmias or arrhythmias can be caused by either an abnormal rate of impulse generation or an abnormal conduction of impulses. Dysrhythmias can impair the pumping of the heart and cause heart failure. One kind of dysrhythmia is a **heart block.** In AV node block, impulses are prevented from reaching the ventricular myocardium; the ventricles contract at a slower rate than normal.

Bradycardia is a slow heart rhythm below 60 beats per minute. Bradycardia can result from vagal hyperactivity. Pacemakers can assist in blocks and bradycardia.

Tachycardia is a very rapid heart rhythm over 100 beats per minute. Tachycardia results with improper autonomic control mechanisms of the heart, lung disease, shock, and fever.

Sinus dysrhythmia is a variation in heart rate during breathing. The causes of sinus dysrhythmia are unknown. This phenomenon is common in young people and infrequently requires treatment.

Premature contractions or extrasystoles are contractions that occur before the next expected contraction. Premature contractions may occur with hyperkalemia or hypercalcemia. Frequent premature contractions can lead to fibrillation during which cardiac muscle fibers contract

Rheumatic Heart Disease and Infective Endocarditis

Cause	Pathophysiology	Manifestations	Treatment
RHD			
Sequel to pharyngeal infection with group A beta-hemolytic streptococci, immune response to streptococcal cell membrane antigens	Carditis of all three layers of heart wall, endocardial inflammation and vegetative growth on valves, valvular stenosis, Aschoff bodies	Fever, lymphadenopathy, acute migratory polyarthritis, chorea, erythema marginatum or truncal rash, history of streptococcal pharyngeal infection, high antistreptolysin O titer, ECG abnormalities	Oral penicillin or erythromycin, salicylates, surgical repair of damaged valves; to prevent recurrence—continuous prophylactic antibiotic therapy for as long as 5 years
Infective Endocarditis			
Staphylococcus aureus followed by viridans streptococci, viruses, fungi, rickettsiae	Prior endothelial damage to valves, mitral valve prolapse, prosthetic valves, septal defects, bloodborne microbial colonization to damaged valve; adhered microbes multiply and form endocardial vegetations	Fever, cardiac murmur, petechial lesions of skin and mucosa, positive blood cultures, ECG abnormalities	Long-term antimicrobial therapy—penicillin and streptomycin, prophylactic antibiotics for procedures increasing risk of transient bacteremia

out of sequence with each other. In fibrillation, the affected heart chambers do not effectively pump blood, so tissue and organ perfusion is impaired. **Ventricular fibrillation** is a life-threatening condition because the ventricle cannot fill or eject blood to vital tissues because contractions are so rapid. If fibrillation is not corrected immediately by defibrillation or some other method, death may occur within minutes.

13. **Discuss contractility, preload, and afterload as mechanisms for heart failure.**
    Study pages 684 and 687-688; refer to Figures 23-36 through 23-40.

According to the Frank-Starling law of the heart, contractility is optimal within a certain range of myocardial cell lengths; the more the myocardium is stretched, the harder it contracts. Normally, an increase of diastolic stretch results in a larger systolic ejection force and a larger stroke volume. Increases of preload or left ventricular end-diastolic volume (LVEDV) increase myocardial oxygen consumption by requiring a greater force of contraction to accomplish systole. The increased force of cardiac contraction is accompanied by increased metabolic demand in the myocardium, and more oxygen is required to support myocardial metabolism. Unfortunately, increased myocardial stretch decreases myocardial capillary perfusion by mechanically narrowing coronary capillary lumina. Also, if preload increases beyond the ventricle's ability to empty, the coronary artery blood supply will drop as the ejection fraction decreases. These two factors will cause the overworked and overstretched myocardium to become hypoxic. Myocardial ischemia results in **ventricular remodeling,** which causes progression of myocyte contractile dysfunction.

Afterload is the force or pressure against which a cardiac chamber must eject blood during systole. Increased afterload is associated with increased systemic vascular resistance or pulmonary vascular resistance such as occurs in systemic or pulmonary hypertension. The ventricle responds to the resistance by developing hypertrophy. The hypertrophied ventricular myocardium must use greater force during ejection and consume more oxygen with each contraction. Thickened myocardium changes the myocytes; ventricular remodeling and the hypertrophy deposits collagen between the myocytes. This decreases contractility, leading to dilation and heart failure.

Left Side Failure (Congestive Heart Failure)

Pathology sequence

Systolic or diastolic ventricular dysfunction

↓

Decreased left ventricular emptying
(end-diastolic volume and preload increases)

↓

Increased volume and pressure in left ventricle

↓

Increased volume and pressure in left atrium
(increased preload)

↓

Increased volume in pulmonary veins

↓

Increased volume in pulmonary capillary bed

↓

Fluid transudation from capillaries to alveoli

↓

Aleveolar space fluid

↓

Pulmonary edema

↓

Increased pulmonary vascular resistance

↓

Right ventricular failure

Manifestations of the left side heart failure

- Exertional and nocturnal dyspnea
- Blood-tinged sputum
- Orthopnea
- Cough
- Cyanosis
- Decreased urinary output
- Rales
- Fatigue
- S_3 gallop

NOTE: Treatment for left heart failure is to correct the underlying cause. Valvular dysfunction may require surgery. Vasodilators can improve coronary artery perfusion. The hypotension associated with left ventricular failure is usually treated with a cardiotonic antihypotensive. Oxygen is administered continuously to increase the supply of oxygen to the myocardium. Diuretics are given to decrease pulmonary edema and blood volume, and sodium and fluid intake are restricted. ACE inhibitors reduce preload and afterload by decreasing aldosterone levels and peripheral vascular resistance. Morphine sulfate dilates the pulmonary and systemic vessels, which decreases pulmonary and systemic capillary hydrostatic pressure. Also, morphine sulfate is an analgesic and an opiate, which improves the emotional state of the individual and may limit the cerebrally mediated release of epinephrine. Surgery or heart transplant may be necessary.

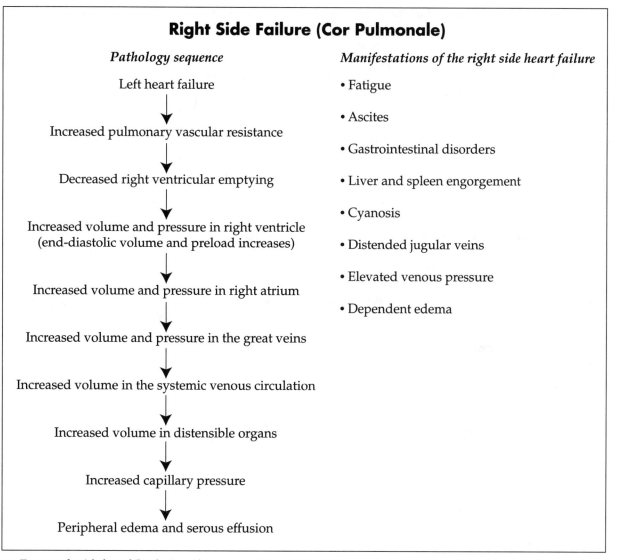

Right Side Failure (Cor Pulmonale)

Pathology sequence	*Manifestations of the right side heart failure*
Left heart failure	• Fatigue
↓	• Ascites
Increased pulmonary vascular resistance	• Gastrointestinal disorders
↓	• Liver and spleen engorgement
Decreased right ventricular emptying	• Cyanosis
↓	• Distended jugular veins
Increased volume and pressure in right ventricle (end-diastolic volume and preload increases)	• Elevated venous pressure
↓	• Dependent edema
Increased volume and pressure in right atrium	
↓	
Increased volume and pressure in the great veins	
↓	
Increased volume in the systemic venous circulation	
↓	
Increased volume in distensible organs	
↓	
Increased capillary pressure	
↓	
Peripheral edema and serous effusion	

NOTE: Treatment for right heart failure begins with treatment of the underlying left heart failure or pulmonary disease. Diuretics and restricted water and sodium intake are used to reduce venous blood volume or preload. Myocardial contractility is enhanced with digoxin or other cardiotonic medications.

14. Describe high-output heart failure.
Study page 688; refer to Figure 23-41.

High-output failure is the inability of the heart to adequately supply the body with bloodborne nutrients, despite adequate blood volume and normal or elevated myocardial contractility. In high-output failure, the heart increases its output but the body's metabolic needs are still not met. Common causes of high-output failure are anemia, septicemia, hyperthyroidism, and beriberi.

Anemia decreases the oxygen-carrying capacity of the blood. Metabolic acidosis occurs as the body's cells switch to anaerobic metabolism (see Chapter 4). In response to metabolic acidosis, heart rate and stroke volume increase in an attempt to circulate blood faster. If anemia is severe, however, even maximum cardiac output does not supply the cells with enough oxygen for metabolism.

In **septicemia**, disturbed metabolism, bacterial toxins, and the inflammatory process cause systemic vasodilation and fever. Faced with a lowered systemic vascular resistance (SVR) and an elevated metabolic rate, cardiac output increases to maintain blood pressure and prevent metabolic acidosis. In overwhelming septicemia, however, the heart may not be able to raise its output enough to compensate for vasodilation. Body tissues show signs of inadequate blood supply despite a very high cardiac output.

Hyperthyroidism accelerates cellular metabolism through the actions of elevated levels of thyroxine from the thyroid gland. This may occur chronically (thyrotoxicosis) or acutely (thyroid storm). Because the body's demand for oxygen threatens to cause metabolic acidosis, cardiac output increases. If blood levels of thyroxine are high and the metabolic response to thyroxine is quite vigorous, even an abnormally elevated cardiac output may be inadequate.

In the United States, **beriberi** (thiamine deficiency) usually is caused by malnutrition secondary to chronic alcoholism. Beriberi actually causes a mixed type of heart failure. Thiamine deficiency impairs cellular metabolism in all tissues, including the myocardium. In the heart, impaired cardiac metabolism leads to insufficient contractile strength. In blood vessels, thiamine deficiency leads mainly to peripheral vasodilation, which decreases SVR. Heart failure ensues as decreased SVR triggers increased cardiac output, which the impaired myocardium is unable to deliver. The strain of demands for increased output in the face of impaired metabolism may deplete cardiac reserves until low-output failure begins.

15. **Characterize impaired cellular metabolism because of shock.**
    Study pages 689 and 691; refer to Figure 23-42.

The final outcome of any type of shock is impaired cellular metabolism and cellular lysis. The following diagram is illustrative of these events:

16. **Classify the different types of shock by etiology.**
    Study pages 691-693, 695, and 697-698; refer to Figures 23-43 through 23-47 and Table 23-12.

Shock is a condition in which the cardiovascular system fails to perfuse the tissues adequately. This failure results in widespread impairment of cellular metabolism. Any factor that alters heart function, blood volume, or blood pressure can cause shock.

Ultimately, shock, irrespective of its cause, progresses to organ failure and death unless compensatory mechanisms or clinical intervention reverse the process. Shock causes many diverse signs and symptoms. The individual may feel sick, weak, cold, hot, nauseated, dizzy, confused, afraid, thirsty, and short of breath. Blood pressure, cardiac output, and urinary output are usually decreased. Respiratory rate is usually increased.

Shock's Impairment of Cellular Metabolism

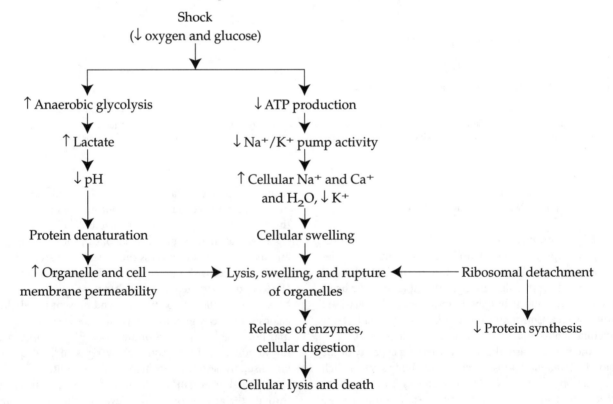

Types of Shock

Type	Etiology
Cardiogenic (heart failure)	Myocardial ischemia, myocardial infarction, congestive heart failure, myocardial or pericardial infections, dysrhythmias, excessive right ventricular afterload, drug toxicity
Hypovolemic (insufficient intravascular fluid volume)	Loss of whole blood plasma or interstitial fluid, fluid sequestration
Neurogenic (neural alterations of vascular smooth muscle tone)	Loss of sympathetic stimulation or parasympathetic overstimulation motor tone to vascular smooth muscle with ensuing vasodilation, decreased systemic vascular resistance
Anaphylactic (immunologic alterations)	Hypersensitivity leads to vasodilation and peripheral pooling
Septic (infectious processes)	Bacteremia and triggering substances released by the bacteria including endotoxins from gram-negatives, lipoteichoic acids and peptidoglycans from gram-positives, and superantigens cause the host to initiate a proinflammatory response; many **proinflammatory mediators*** promote vasodilation; then a compensatory host antiinflammatory response with its mediators follows; next, a mixed antagonistic response between inflammatory and antiinflammatory mediators leads the host into multiple organ dysfunction syndrome (MODS)

*Proinflammatory mediators include tumor necrosis factor, IL-1, IL-6 , and IL-8, platelet activating factor, arachidonic acid metabolites, leukemia inhibitory factor, nitric oxide, and many kinins. Antiinflammatory mediators include IL-4, IL-10, IL-11, IL-13, transforming growth factor B, colony-stimulating factors, soluble tumor necrosis factor receptor, IL-1 receptor antagonist, protein C, and endogenous glucocorticoids.

NOTE: The consequence of shock is reduced tissue perfusion and impaired cellular metabolism. Treatment of shock requires removing the underlying cause. After cause correction, supplemental oxygen is always given. Intravenous fluid is given to expand the intravascular volume except in cardiogenic shock, which requires preload reduction by diuresis.

17. **Briefly diagram the common events found in all types of shock and relate the events to the signs and symptoms of shock.**
    Refer to Figures 23-43 through 23-47.

Events, Signs, and Symptoms of Shock

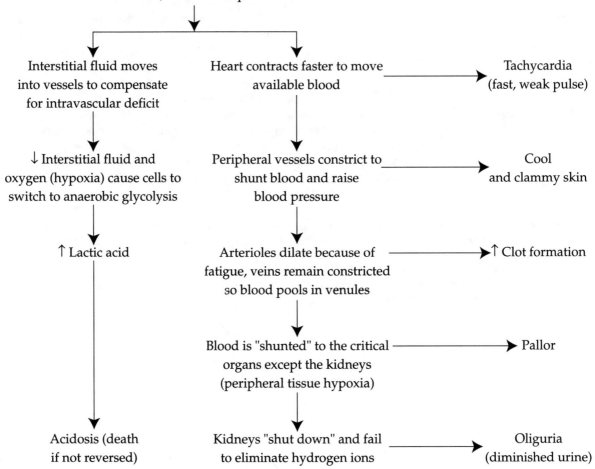

Low cardiac output, intravascular fluid deficit, vasodilation, and fluid sequestration

Interstitial fluid moves into vessels to compensate for intravascular deficit

Heart contracts faster to move available blood → Tachycardia (fast, weak pulse)

↓ Interstitial fluid and oxygen (hypoxia) cause cells to switch to anaerobic glycolysis

Peripheral vessels constrict to shunt blood and raise blood pressure → Cool and clammy skin

↑ Lactic acid

Arterioles dilate because of fatigue, veins remain constricted so blood pools in venules → ↑ Clot formation

Blood is "shunted" to the critical organs except the kidneys (peripheral tissue hypoxia) → Pallor

Acidosis (death if not reversed)

Kidneys "shut down" and fail to eliminate hydrogen ions → Oliguria (diminished urine)

18. Illustrate the pathogenic sequence of multiple organ dysfunction syndrome (MODS) because of shock.
Study pages 698-700; refer to Figure 23-48 and Table 23-13.

Sepsis and septic shock are the most common causes of MODS. Severe trauma, burns, and respiratory or renal failure also contribute to MODS. The following diagram is illustrative of the pathogenesis of MODS:

Pathogenesis of Multiple Organ Dysfunction Syndrome (MODS)

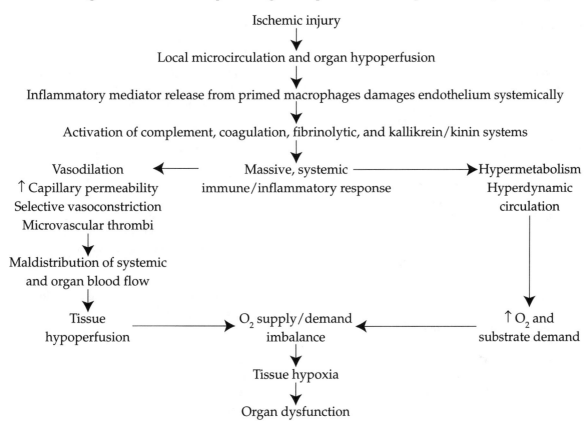

Practice Examination

1. Arteriosclerosis raises the systolic blood pressure by:
   a. increasing arterial distensibility and vessel lumen radius or diameter.
   b. increasing arterial distensibility and decreasing vessel lumen radius or diameter.
   c. decreasing arterial distensibility and increasing vessel lumen radius or diameter.
   d. decreasing arterial distensibility and lumen diameter.
   e. None of the above is correct.

2. Events in the development of atherosclerotic plaque include all of the following *except*:
   a. accumulation of LDL (low-density lipoprotein).
   b. smooth muscle proliferation.
   c. calcification.
   d. decreased elasticity.
   e. complement activation.

3. G.P. is a 50-year-old male who was referred for evaluation of blood pressure. If he has a high diastolic blood pressure, which reading belongs to G.P.?
   a. 140/82 mm Hg
   b. 160/72 mm Hg
   c. 130/95 mm Hg
   d. 95/68 mm Hg
   e. 140/72 mm Hg

4. The complications of uncontrolled hypertension include all of the following *except:*
   a. cerebrovascular accidents.
   b. anemia.
   c. renal injury.
   d. cardiac hypertrophy.
   e. All of the above are complications.

5. Primary hypertension:
   a. is essentially idiopathic.
   b. can be caused by renal disease.
   c. can be caused by hormone imbalance.
   d. results from arterial coarctation.
   e. b, c, and d are correct.

6. Orthostatic hypotension is caused by all of the following *except:*
   a. increased age.
   b. increased blood volume.
   c. autonomic nervous system dysfunction.
   d. bed rest.
   e. severe varicose veins.

7. Localized outpouching of a vessel wall or heart chamber is a/an:
   a. thrombus.
   b. embolus.
   c. thromboembolus.
   d. aneurysm.
   e. vegetation.

8. Which is a possible cause of varicose veins?
   a. gravitational forces on blood
   b. long periods of standing
   c. trauma to the saphenous veins
   d. Both b and c are correct.
   e. a, b, and c are correct.

9. A 76-year-old male came to the emergency room after experiencing chest pain while shoveling snow. Laboratory tests revealed essentially normal blood levels of SGOT or AST, CPK, and LDH enzymes. The chest pain was relieved following rest and nitroglycerin therapy. The most probable diagnosis is:
   a. myocardial infarct.
   b. emphysema.
   c. angina pectoris.
   d. hepatic cirrhosis.
   e. acute pancreatitis.

10. Complications of an infarcted myocardium likely could include which of the following? (More than one answer may be correct.)
    a. emphysema
    b. heart failure
    c. endocarditis
    d. death
    e. systemic thromboembolism

11. In pericardial effusion:
    a. fibrotic lesions obliterate the pericardial cavity.
    b. there is associated rheumatoid arthritis.
    c. tamponade compresses the right heart before affecting other structures.
    d. arterial blood pressure during expiration exceeds that during inspiration.
    e. Both c and d are correct.

12. Chamber volume increase is observed in _____ cardiomyopathy.
    a. dilated
    b. hypertrophic
    c. restrictive
    d. Both a and b are correct.
    e. a, b, and c are correct.

Match the valvular dysfunction with its characteristic.

_____13. aortic stenosis

_____14. tricuspid regurgitation

_____15. mitral stenosis

_____16. mitral regurgitation

a. right ventricular hypertrophy

b. left ventricular hypertrophy

c. right atrial hypertrophy

d. left atrial hypertrophy

e. left atrial/right ventricular hypertrophy

f. right and left ventricular/left atrial hypertrophy

g. hypertrophy of all chambers

---

17. Which statement is true regarding rheumatic heart disease? (More than one answer may be correct.)
  a. It is caused by staphylococcal infections.
  b. It is caused by hypersensitivity/immunity to streptococci.
  c. It damages the tricuspid valve most often.
  d. It usually damages a mitral valve.

18. Which is *not* an expected finding in acute rheumatic fever?
  a. elevated ESR (erythrocyte sedimentation rate)
  b. elevated ASO titer (antistreptolysin O)
  c. leukopenia
  d. fever

19. Bacterial (or infective) endocarditis differs from rheumatic heart disease because of which of the following? (More than one answer may be correct.)
  a. Bacterial endocarditis is an infection of the heart, endocardium, and valves.
  b. It always follows rheumatic fever.
  c. It may occur following dental or bladder catheterization procedures.
  d. It commonly involves the vena cava valve.
  e. It is caused by a type III hypersensitivity.

20. Individuals with only left heart failure would exhibit which of the following? (More than one answer may be correct.)
  a. hepatomegaly
  b. dyspnea
  c. ankle swelling
  d. pulmonary edema
  e. peripheral edema

21. In congestive heart failure, the pump or myocardium itself fails because of which of the following? (More than one answer may be correct.)
  a. loss of contractile force of the heart
  b. hypertension
  c. cardiac dysrhythmias
  d. intermittent claudication from occlusive vascular disease

22. Shock is a complex pathophysiologic process involving all of the following *except:*
  a. decreased blood perfusion to kidneys.
  b. acidosis.
  c. rapid heart rate.
  d. hypertension.
  e. anaerobic glycolysis.

23. Systemic inflammatory response syndrome (SIRS) begins with an infection that progresses to:
  a. bacteremia.
  b. sepsis.
  c. septic shock
  d. multiple organ dysfunction syndrome (MODS).
  e. All of the above are correct.

24. Which statement is *incorrect* concerning hypertension?
  a. Malignant hypertension is characterized by a diastolic pressure of over 140 mm Hg.
  b. More than 90% of cases are of the essential or primary type.
  c. Headache is the most reliable symptom.
  d. When left untreated, the major risks include CVAs and cardiac hypertrophy.

25. A 53-year-old male was admitted to the emergency room after experiencing shortness of breath, weakness, cardiac dysrhythmias, and chest pain that did not subside after nitroglycerin therapy. Laboratory tests revealed the patient had an elevated serum CPK and SGOT or AST level. EKG tracings revealed a prominent Q wave and an elevated ST segment. The most probable diagnosis is:
   a. a transient ischemic attack.
   b. an acute myocardial infarct.
   c. an attack of unstable angina pectoris.
   d. Prinzmetal angina.
   e. coronary artery vasospasm.

Case Study

W.S., a 51-year-old white male, was assisting in the launching of his best friend's water-ski boat from a faulty boat trailer when he began to experience chest discomfort. At first, he believed his discomfort was because of the extreme July heat. Gradually, the discomfort became a crushing pain in his sternal area that radiated into his left arm and lower jaw. His friend suspected an ensuing heart attack and convinced W.S. to check into an emergency room. During the drive down a canyon with steep, winding curves, W.S. collapsed.

On arrival at the emergency room, W.S. was unconscious. His skin was cool, clammy, and very pale. His blood pressure was very low and his pulse was weak and irregular. Established resuscitation procedures were followed. After W.S.'s return to consciousness, an electrocardiogram showed evidence of myocardial injury and blood was drawn to check enzyme and electrolyte levels. When history was obtained, W.S. stated he is a harassed advertising executive and denied significant illnesses. However, he is being treated for primary hypertension. He acknowledged smoking three packs of cigarettes a day for 30 years. His father died of a heart attack at the age of 47.

W.S.'s subsequent electrocardiograms and serum levels of CPK, LDH, and SGOT or AST verified anterior myocardial infarction.

Knowing the diagnosis, identify W.S.'s risk factors, the early causes and precipitating events of his infarction, and the justification for using anticoagulant therapy.

Alterations of Cardiovascular Function in Children

Foundational Objective

a. **Describe the chambers, valves, and great vessels of the heart.**
   Review pages 598 and 601-602; refer to Figures 22-2 through 22-8.

MEMORY CHECK!

- The heart has four chambers, the left and right atria and the right and left ventricles. The atria are smaller than the ventricles and have thinner walls. Their walls are thin because they are low-pressure chambers that serve as conduits for blood rather than as pumps that must forcefully eject blood. The ventricles propel blood all the way through the pulmonary or systemic circulation and so must pump against pressure throughout these systems. Pressure is greatest in the systemic circulation, which is driven by the left ventricle.

- The right ventricle ejects large volumes of blood through a very small valve into the low-pressure pulmonary system. The left ventricle is larger and ejects blood through a relatively large valve into the high-pressure systemic circulation.

- The atria are separated by the interatrial septum and the ventricles by the interventricular septum. Indentation of the endocardium for valves occurs to separate the atria from the ventricles and the ventricles from the aorta and pulmonary arteries. One-way blood flow through the heart is ensured by the four heart valves, the atrioventricular (mitral and tricuspid) and the semilunar (pulmonary and aortic). The valve openings are guarded by flaps of tissue called *leaflets* or *cusps,* which are attached to the papillary muscles by the chordae tendineae cordis. The papillary muscles are extensions of the myocardium that pull the cusps together and downward at the onset of ventricular contraction, thus preventing backward flow of blood.

- The right heart atrium receives venous blood from the systemic circulation through the superior and inferior venae cavae. The pulmonary artery leaves the right ventricle, and its branches enter the pulmonary circulation. Oxygen and carbon dioxide exchange occurs at the alveolocapillary membrane, and four pulmonary veins carry oxygenated blood from the lungs to the left side of the heart. The oxygenated blood moves through the left atrium and ventricle into the aorta, which delivers blood to systemic vessels to supply the body.

Objectives

After studying this chapter, the learner will be able to do the following:

1. **Identify the most common congenital defects that obstruct outflow and describe their pathophysiology.**
   Study pages 712-713; refer to Figures 24-3 through 24-5.

   Coarctation of the aorta is caused by a narrowing of the aorta anywhere between the origin of the aortic arch and the abdominal bifurcation. This defect may be considered in terms of its proximity to the ductus arteriosus. A narrowing near the ductus arteriosus results in increased blood flow to the head and upper extremities and decreased blood flow to the lower extremities. There are signs of left heart failure in some infants. Surgical correction includes resection of the affected site on the aorta with various grafts and closure of the ductus.

   Aortic stenosis is a narrowing or stricture of the aortic valve, causing resistance to blood flow in the left ventricle, decreased cardiac output, left ventricular hypertrophy, and pulmonary vascular congestion.

   Children with aortic stenosis show signs of exercise intolerance, chest pain, and dizziness when standing for long periods. There is a characteristic murmur. Individuals are at risk for bacterial endocarditis, coronary insufficiency, and ventricular dysfunction.

   Aortic valvotomy is a palliative procedure. A valve replacement may be required as a subsequent procedure.

   Pulmonic stenosis is caused by the restriction or thickening of the leaflets of the pulmonary valve. Outflow is restricted from the right ventricle, resulting in increased afterload, and, if severe, may cause right ventricular hypertrophy and dilation. If pressures are high enough, the foramen ovale may reopen, resulting in a right-to-left shunt and cyanosis. Mild cases result in little or no symptomatology, while severe cases may require surgical correction.

2. **Describe the congenital defects with increased pulmonary blood flow and their pathophysiology and treatment.**
   Study pages 713-716; refer to Figures 24-6 and 24-7.

   Patent ductus arteriosus (PDA) results from the failure of the ductus arteriosus to close within the first weeks of life. Continued patency permits blood to flow from the higher-pressure aorta to the lower-pressure pulmonary artery, causing a left-to-right shunt to develop. Clinical manifestations are usually without cyanosis and include a "machinery" murmur and pulmonary vascular obstructive disease in later life. Treatment is usually by surgical ligation.

   Atrial septal defects (ASDs) are abnormal communications across the interatrial septum. The size of the ASD determines the direction of flow. If small, the shunt is left-to-right; if large, the pressures in the atria are equal, and shunt direction is determined by resistance of the ventricles. At birth, atrial size and resistance are generally equal; as the infant grows, the left ventricle thickens, and systemic pressure rises and causes a left-to-right shunt. These defects may be so mild that they go undetected until preschool age. A soft murmur is often heard at the second intracostal space, and a fixed splitting of the second heart sound also may be heard; this finding is indicative of right ventricular overload. Treatment is generally surgical correction.

   Ventricular septal defect (VSD) is essentially a defect in the intraventricular septum that leads to blood flow between the ventricles of the heart. Small defects have very little associated pathology and often close on their own, with the shunt usually flowing left-to-right. Large defects are a different matter. In a large VSD, pressures may become equal in both chambers, with blood flow again being left-to-right due to higher systemic pressures. In this case, large amounts of blood flow into the lungs through the pulmonary artery and back to the left heart and cause a great deal of left ventricular stress; heart failure may eventually result. Treatment ranges from observation in mild cases to surgical correction in more serious cases.

   Atrioventricular canal (AVC) defect consists of a low atrial septal defect that is continuous with a high ventricular septal defect and clefts of the mitral and tricuspid valves. A large central atrioventricular defect allows blood to flow between all four chambers of the heart. The directions of flow are determined by pulmonary and systemic resistance, left and right ventricular pressures, and the compliance of each chamber. Flow is generally from left to right.

   There is usually moderate to severe left heart failure and a characteristic murmur. There may be little to mild cyanosis; the cyanosis increases with crying.

   Complete surgical repair can be performed in infants. If the mitral valve defect is severe, a valve replacement may be needed.

3. **Describe the congenital defects with decreased pulmonary blood flow and their pathophysiology and treatment.**
   Study pages 716-717; refer to Figures 24-8 and 24-9.

   Tetralogy of Fallot is a syndrome of four defects. The associated defects that comprise tetralogy are (1) a ventricular septal defect (VSD), (2) an overriding aorta that straddles the VSD, (3) pulmonic stenosis, and (4) right ventricular hypertrophy. The pathophysiology associated with tetralogy may be varied and is dependent on the degree of pulmonary stenosis as well as the size of the VSD and pulmonary and systemic pressures. The shunt may be either left-to-right or right-to-left. In any event, these defects result in hypoxia in the systemic circulation while the body attempts to compensate by increasing red blood cell production and increasing blood flow to the lungs through collateral bronchial vessels. Cyanotic episodes also may be accompanied by syncope or seizures due to hypoxia. Surgical treatment is usually accomplished by various surgical procedures.

Tricuspid atresia is the failure of the tricuspid valve to develop. Thus there is no communication from right atrium to right ventricle. Blood flows through an atrial septal defect or a patent foramen ovale to the left heart and through a ventricular septal defect to the right ventricle and then to the lungs. It is often associated with pulmonic stenosis and transposition of the great arteries. There is complete mixing of unoxygenated and oxygenated blood in the left heart.

Cyanosis is usually seen in the newborn period. There may be tachycardia and dyspnea. Older children exhibit chronic hypoxemia with clubbing. Individuals are at risk for bacterial endocarditis, brain abscess, and stroke.

Palliative treatment is the placement of a shunt to increase blood flow to the lungs. Corrective repair consists of a surgical connection between the right atrium and the pulmonary artery.

4. **Describe defects that permit mixing of pulmonary and systemic blood.**
   Study pages 717-720; refer to Figures 24-10 through 24-13.

Complete transposition of the great vessels results in the effective switching of the aorta and pulmonary arteries so the pulmonary artery leaves the left ventricle and the aorta leaves the right ventricle. This creates two separate circulatory systems with no communication between them. Children with minimum communication are severely cyanotic. If large septal defects exist, cyanosis may be less but symptoms of left heart failure occur. Cardiomegaly develops a few weeks after birth. Switching procedures to make the left ventricle the systemic pump may be the best alternative of the various surgical corrections.

Total anomalous pulmonary venous connection (TAPVC) is a disorder in which the pulmonary circulation enters the right atrium instead of the left. TAPVC has four different variations with the same resultant patho-

physiology, all of which are associated with atrial septal defects (ASD). The most common forms of this anomaly are (1) drainage of the pulmonary veins into the superior vena cava and right atrium, (2) drainage into the right atrium through the coronary sinus, and (3) drainage into the right atrium through the inferior vena cava. TAPVC in any form results in a mixture of oxygenated and unoxygenated blood being pumped to the systemic circulation. The shunt is usually right-to-left. The amount of cyanosis generated by this anomaly is dependent on the mixture of unoxygenated and oxygenated blood. Thus the greater the pulmonary blood flow, the less the cyanosis. Congestive heart failure is a common complication. Most infants die by 2 months of age without surgical correction.

Truncus arteriosus is failure of normal septation and division of the embryonic vessel trunk into the pulmonary artery and the aorta; the resulting single vessel overrides both ventricles. Blood from both ventricles mixes in the common great artery and causes desaturation and hypoxemia. Blood ejected from the heart flows to the lower-pressure pulmonary arteries and causes increased pulmonary blood flow and reduced systemic blood flow.

Most infants have moderate to severe left heart failure and variable cyanosis, poor growth, and activity intolerance. There is a characteristic murmur, and children are at risk for brain abscess and bacterial endocarditis.

Corrective surgery involves closing the defect so that the truncus arteriosus receives the outflow from the left ventricle, excising the pulmonary arteries from the aorta, and attaching them to the right ventricle by a homograft.

Hypoplastic left heart syndrome is underdevelopment of the left heart, which results in a hypoplastic left ventricle and aortic atresia. Most blood from the left atrium flows across the patent foramen ovale to the right atrium, to the right ventricle, and out the pulmonary artery.

There is mild cyanosis and signs of left heart failure until the patent ductus arteriosus closes. Then there is progressive deterioration with cyanosis and decreased cardiac output, which leads to cardiovascular collapse. Without intervention, it is usually fatal in the first months of life.

A several-stage surgical repair approach is used for correction of this condition. Some believe that heart transplantation in the newborn period is the best option for these infants.

5. **Relate congestive heart failure (CHF) to congenital heart disease in children; describe the manifestations of left heart failure.**
   Study page 720; refer to Table 24-3.

Congestive heart failure is a common complication of many congenital heart defects. The most common causes of CHF in infancy are pressure and volume overloads secondary to congenital disease.

Dyspnea on exertion is often manifested in infants, as is difficulty with feeding. When the infant tries to suck and swallow, breathing is interrupted and the child easily becomes exhausted. Poor feeding and failure to thrive are primary indicators of left CHF or heart failure in infants. The infant's respiratory rate may be greater than 40 breaths per minute. In severe left heart failure, tachypnea may be accompanied by retractions, grunting, nasal flaring, wheezing, coughing, and rales. Hepatomegaly is typically attributable to systemic venous congestion caused by right ventricular failure. In left heart failure in infants, the liver has a dull, rounded edge that is felt more than 3 cm below the costal margin and may be tender. Fluid retention in infants is usually manifested by weight gain without any increase in caloric intake.

6. Describe the pathophysiology related to Kawasaki disease.
Study pages 721-722.

Kawasaki disease is an acute, self-limiting vasculitis that may result in cardiac sequelae. Eighty percent of cases occur in children younger than 5 years of age; a peak incidence is in the toddler age group. Currently, it is the leading cause of pediatric acquired heart disorders in the United States. This disease tends to cluster in miniepidemics and may be related to an infectious process with an autoimmune component. The disease process progresses through four clinical states:

Stage 1   Onset to 12 days: Small venules, arterioles, and the heart become inflamed.
Stage 2   12 to 25 days: Inflammation of larger vessels occurs and coronary artery aneurysms appear.
Stage 3   26 to 40 days: Medium-sized arteries begin granulation, and inflammation subsides in the microcirculation.
Stage 4   Day 40 and beyond. The vessels develop scarring, thickening of the intima, calcification, and formation of thrombi; arteritis is most often in the coronaries but may occur in a variety of arteries; 10% to 20% of children develop aneurysms in this process.

Diagnosis is made by evaluating six major findings, five of which must be present for diagnosis. These findings include (1) fever greater than 104° F, (2) bilateral conjunctivitis, (3) erythema of the oral mucosa, (4) erythema with desquamation of the palms and soles, (5) polymorphous erythematous rash, and (6) cervical lymphadenopathy. These may be accompanied by arthritis and abdominal pain. Later complications include coronary thrombosis.

Echocardiography may monitor the disease in the coronary arteries. Treatment is nonspecific, supportive, and preventive of coronary artery thrombosis.

7. Describe susceptibility and manifestations of systemic hypertension in children.
Study pages 722 and 724; refer to Figure 24-14 and Tables 24-4 through 24-7.

In the past, most hypertension in children was considered to be secondary to other diseases. **Systemic hypertension** is now known to exist in children. Hypertension-causing arterial disease can begin very early in life. Autopsies on infants have shown fatty streaks, the earliest lesions of atherosclerosis, in the intimal lining of blood vessels.

Obesity and smoking are risk factors for hypertension in children. In all primary hypertensive children, genetic correlates are strong, accompanied by inability of the peripheral vascular bed to adjust its resistance to meet tissue perfusion demands. Secondary hypertension has an underlying disease as its contributing factor.

Diagnosis of systemic hypertension in children is difficult because early stages may be asymptomatic and blood pressures vary from child to child and change as the child grows. Ambulatory blood pressure monitoring is becoming an important tool in both evaluation and management of childhood hypertension. The preventive efficacy of antihypertensive therapy during childhood is debatable, and some clinicians prefer to control or eliminate risk factors.

Practice Examination

True/False

_____ 1. Shunts are usually independent of systemic or pulmonary pressures and are due solely to heart defects.

_____ 2. A patent ductus arteriosus or VSD is sometimes helpful when it is associated with other cardiac defects.

_____ 3. VSDs always require surgical closure.

_____ 4. In ASDs or VSDs, murmurs indicate defects.

_____ 5. Cyanosis is not a major finding in transportation of the great vessels, because the blood is free to travel normally to the lungs.

Fill In the Blanks

6. Abnormal blood flow within the heart is usually referred to as a _____.

7. In VSD, the shunt is generally _____-to-_____.

8. Cyanotic defects usually shunt _____-to-_____.

9. Cyanosis due to cardiac defects is usually caused by mixture of _____ and _____ blood.

10. Some cardiac defects are not obvious at birth because of the fact that systemic and pulmonary pressures are nearly _____ at that point.

11. The patent ductus arteriosus has a _____-to-_____ shunt.

12. The ductus arteriosus should be totally closed within the _____ of life.

13. Thickening or restriction of the valve from the right ventricle is known as _____.

14. Defects that obstruct outflow from the ventricles tend to cause increased _____, which may lead to _____.

15. Narrowing of the great vessel leading to the systemic circulation is known as _____.

Match the description with the alteration.

_____16. associated with dyspnea when feeding

_____17. likely associated with an infectious etiology and an autoimmune response

_____18. vasculitis associated with aneurysm

_____19. if mild, often self-correcting

_____20. "blue spells"

_____21. ASD, overriding aorta, pulmonic stenosis, right ventricular hypertrophy

_____22. common complication of congenital heart defects

_____23. immediate cyanosis and distress after birth

_____24. two separate circulatory systems

_____25. may be associated with coronary thrombosis

a. Kawasaki disease

b. VSD

c. tetralogy of Fallot

d. transposition of the great vessels

e. left heart failure

Case Study

David M. is a 7-year-old requiring a routine physical examination at the nurse practitioner's office. David's past medical and family history is not unusual. His activity level is normal, and his mother verbalizes that he is quite healthy.

David's physical examination is normal until the cardiovascular system is evaluated. He is noted to have a systolic murmur. There are also bounding pulses in the arms and severely decreased pulses in the legs. A pediatric cardiology consultation is requested.

Which cardiac defect causes such a striking discrepancy in blood flow to the upper and lower extremities?

25

Structure and Function of the Pulmonary System

Objectives

After reviewing this chapter, the learner will be able to do the following:

1. Identify the sequence of structures of the pulmonary system as air moves into and out of the lungs; list the defense mechanisms of the pulmonary system.
   Review pages 730-731 and 734-735; refer to Figures 25-1 through 25-7 and Table 25-1.

2. Describe lung volumes and capacities.
   Refer to Figures 25-9 and Table 25-2.

3. Describe the neurochemical control of ventilation.
   Review pages 736-738; refer to Figure 25-10.

4. Relate changes in the thoracic volume to muscular contractions, alveolar surface tension, elastic properties of the lungs and chest wall, and conducting airway resistance.
   Review pages 738-741; refer to Figures 25-11 and 25-12.

5. Identify the factors in the transport of oxygen to the cells of the body and describe oxyhemoglobin association and disassociation; identify the factors in the transport of carbon dioxide from the cells.
   Review pages 741-747; refer to Figures 25-13 through 25-15 and 25-17.

6. Identify the normal values for arterial and venous blood gases.
   Refer to Figure 25-16.

7. Describe the factors controlling pulmonary vasodilation and vasoconstriction.
   Review page 747.

8. Note the pulmonary changes that occur with normal aging.
   Review page 748.

Practice Examination

1. Considering the sequence of structures through which air enters the pulmonary system, the pharynx is to the trachea as the:
   a. bronchioles are to the segmental bronchi.
   b. alveoli are to the alveolar ducts.
   c. alveolar ducts are to respiratory bronchioles.
   d. respiratory bronchioles are to the alveolar ducts.
   e. All of the above are correct.

2. The cilia of the bronchial wall:
   a. ingest bacteria.
   b. trigger the sneeze reflex.
   c. trap and remove bacteria.
   d. propel mucus and trapped bacteria toward the oropharynx.
   e. Both a and c are correct.

3. As the terminal bronchioles are approached:
   a. the epithelium becomes thicker.
   b. mucus-producing glands increase.
   c. the epithelium becomes thinner.
   d. cartilaginous support increases.
   e. the smooth muscle layer thickens.

4. The left bronchus:
   a. is shorter and wider than the right.
   b. is symmetrical to the right.
   c. has a course more vertical than the right's.
   d. is more angled than the right.
   e. has more bronchial wall layers.

5. The respiratory unit consists of:
   a. cilia.
   b. bronchiolar arteries and veins.
   c. goblet cells and alveoli.
   d. respiratory bronchioles and alveoli.
   e. All of the above are correct.

6. Alveoli are excellent gas exchange units because of:
   a. their large surface area.
   b. a very thin epithelial layer.
   c. extensive vascularization.
   d. Both b and c are correct.
   e. a, b, and c are correct.

7. Surfactant:
   a. facilitates O_2 exchange.
   b. produces nutrients for the alveoli.
   c. permits air exchange between alveolar ducts.
   d. facilitates alveolar expansion during inspiration.
   e. All of the above are correct.

8. During expiration, which relationship is true?
   a. As the lung volume decreases, the number of molecules of the gas increases.
   b. As the lung pressure increases, the number of molecules of the gas increases.
   c. As the lung volume decreases, the pressure increases.
   d. As the partial pressure increases, less gas will dissolve in a liquid.

9. When the diaphragm and external intercostal contract:
   a. the intrathoracic volume increases.
   b. the intrathoracic pressure increases.
   c. the intrathoracic volume decreases.
   d. None of the above is correct.

Match each term with its description or example.

_____10. inspiratory reserve volume

_____11. vital capacity

a. amount of air remaining in lungs after a forced expiration

b. taking an extra-deep breath of air just before diving

c. includes sum of tidal, expiratory reserve, and inspiratory reserve volumes

d. the extra air pushed out during a forced exhalation

12. Oxygen diffusion from the alveolus to the alveolar capillary occurs because:
    a. the pO_2 is less in the capillary than in the alveolus.
    b. the pO_2 is greater in the atmosphere than in the arterial blood.
    c. oxygen diffuses faster than CO_2.
    d. the pO_2 is higher in the capillary than in the alveolus.

13. A shift to the right in the oxyhemoglobin dissociation curve:
    a. prevents oxygen release at the cellular level.
    b. causes oxygen to bind tighter to hemoglobin.
    c. improves oxygen release and increases oxygen movement into the cells.
    d. Both a and b are correct.
    e. None of the above is correct.

14. In which sequence does pO_2 progressively decrease?
    a. blood in aorta, atmospheric air, body tissues
    b. body tissues, arterial blood, alveolar air
    c. body tissues, alveolar air, arterial blood
    d. atmospheric air, aortic blood, body tissues

15. Most O_2 is carried in the blood _____; most CO_2 is carried _____.
    a. dissolved in plasma; associated with salt or an acid
    b. bound to hemoglobin; associated with bicarbonate/carbonic acid
    c. combined with albumin; associated with carbonic acid and hemoglobin
    d. bound to hemoglobin; bound to albumin

16. Alveoli are well-suited for diffusion of respiratory gases because:
    a. they are small and thus have a small total surface area.
    b. vascularization is minimal, allowing greater air circulation.
    c. they contain four thick layers, preventing air leakage.
    d. they contain surfactant, which helps prevent alveolar collapse.

17. Which ordinarily brings about the greatest increase in the rate of respiration?
    a. excess carbon dioxide
    b. increased O_2
    c. increased arterial pH
    d. sudden rise in blood pressure

18. Given that the oxygen content of blood equals (1.34 ml of O_2 per gram of hemoglobin) times arterial oxygen saturation percentage, if hemoglobin concentration is 15 g/dl and arterial saturation is 98%, what is the arterial oxygen content?
    a. 13.2 ml/dl of blood
    b. 19.7 ml/dl of blood
    c. 14.7 ml/dl of blood
    d. None of the above is correct.

19. The major muscle(s) of inspiration is (are) the:
    a. diaphragm.
    b. sternocleidomastoid.
    c. external intercostals.
    d. internal intercostals.
    e. Both a and c are correct.

20. Stretch receptors:
    a. are sensitive to volume changes in the lung.
    b. are located in bronchial smooth muscles.
    c. decrease ventilatory rate when stimulated.
    d. prevent lung overinflation when stimulated.
    e. All of the above are correct.

21. Which of the following increases the respiratory rate?
    a. increased pCO_2, decreased pH, decreased pO_2
    b. increased pCO_2, increased pH, decreased pO_2
    c. decreased pCO_2, decreased pH, increased pO_2
    d. decreased pCO_2, decreased pH, decreased pO_2

22. The dorsal respiratory group (DRG) of neurons:
    a. sets the automatic rhythm of respiration.
    b. modifies the rhythm of respiration.
    c. is active when increased ventilation is required.
    d. None of the above is correct.

Match the normal range of blood gases with its arterial or venous state.

_____23. pCO_2 of 40 mm Hg

_____24. oxygen saturation of 70%

_____25. oxygen content of blood of 19 to 20 ml/dl

a. arterial blood

b. mixed venous blood

26

Alterations of Pulmonary Function

a. **Compare the structures of the lower airway as the generations of division move toward the alveoli.**
   Refer to Figures 25-1 and 25-3 through 25-6.

MEMORY CHECK!

- The trachea and mainstem bronchi are composed mainly of cartilage with a lining of mucous membrane. When the bronchi enter the lungs, they branch further. Instead of cartilaginous rings, smooth muscle encircles the bronchi with cartilage interspersed among the muscle bundles. By the time the bronchioles are reached, supportive cartilage is no longer present. The bronchioles are capable of constriction because of their layer of smooth muscle. Smooth muscle becomes thinner in the terminal bronchioles. The epithelium changes from pseudostratified and ciliated columnar in the bronchi to nonciliated cuboidal in the terminal bronchioles and finally to squamous in the alveoli. Macrophages must remove any debris that reaches the respiratory bronchioles and alveoli because of the absence of cilia.

b. **Identify the measurements of lung volume.**
Refer to Figure 25-9 and Table 25-2.

MEMORY CHECK!

- Tidal volume (TV) is the amount of gas inspired and expired during normal breathing. Inspiratory reserve volume (IRV) is the amount of gas that can be inspired in addition to the tidal volume. Expiratory reserve volume (ERV) is the amount of gas that can be expired after a passive or relaxed expiration. Residual volume (RV) is the volume of gas that cannot be expired and is always present in the lungs.

- Total lung capacity (TLC) is the total gas volume in the lung when the lung is maximally inflated. It includes RV, ERV, TV, and IRV. Vital capacity (VC) is the maximum amount of gas that can be expired from the lung. It includes IRV, TV, and ERV. Functional residual capacity (FRC) is the amount of gas remaining in the lung at the end of a passive expiration or RV and ERV. Inspiratory capacity (IC) is the amount of gas that can be inspired after a passive expiration from FRC. It includes TV and IRV. The lung capacities are always the sum of two or more volumes. Normal values for volumes and capacities are based on age, sex, and height.

- With each breath, a portion of the tidal volume remains in the conducting airways. This is the anatomic dead space. In certain disease conditions, some of the respiratory bronchioles and alveoli receive adequate ventilation but do not participate in gas exchange because they are not perfused by the pulmonary circulation. The volume of gas in unperfused alveoli is known as *alveolar dead space.*

c. **Describe the diaphragmatic movements in inspiration and expiration; indicate other factors involved in the mechanism of breathing.**

Review pages 738-741; refer to Figures 25-11 and 25-12.

MEMORY CHECK!

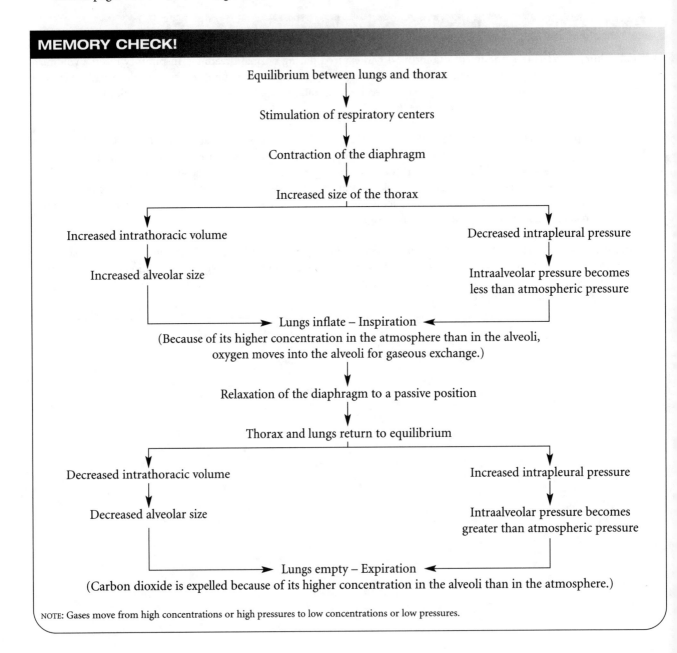

Equilibrium between lungs and thorax
↓
Stimulation of respiratory centers
↓
Contraction of the diaphragm
↓
Increased size of the thorax

Increased intrathoracic volume   Decreased intrapleural pressure
↓   ↓
Increased alveolar size   Intraalveolar pressure becomes
                                                  less than atmospheric pressure

→ Lungs inflate – Inspiration ←
(Because of its higher concentration in the atmosphere than in the alveoli,
oxygen moves into the alveoli for gaseous exchange.)
↓
Relaxation of the diaphragm to a passive position
↓
Thorax and lungs return to equilibrium

Decreased intrathoracic volume   Increased intrapleural pressure
↓   ↓
Decreased alveolar size   Intraalveolar pressure becomes
                                                  greater than atmospheric pressure

→ Lungs empty – Expiration ←
(Carbon dioxide is expelled because of its higher concentration in the alveoli than in the atmosphere.)

NOTE: Gases move from high concentrations or high pressures to low concentrations or low pressures.

MEMORY CHECK!—cont'd

- Other factors involved in the mechanics of breathing include alveolar surface tension, elasticity of the lungs and chest wall, and resistance to air flow through the conducting airways. Surface tension occurs at any gas-liquid interface and is the tendency for liquid molecules exposed to air to adhere to one another. This phenomenon decreases the surface area exposed to the air. According to the law of Laplace, the pressure (P) required to inflate a sphere is equal to 2 times the surface tension (T) divided by the radius (r) of the sphere, or $P = 2T/r$. As the surface tension increases and the radius of the sphere or alveolus becomes smaller, more pressure is required to inflate it.

- Surfactant in the alveoli has a detergent-like effect that separates the liquid molecules, thus decreasing alveolar surface tension. Surfactant reverses the law of Laplace. The alveoli are much easier to inflate at low lung volumes after expiration than at high volumes after inspiration. The decrease in the surface tension caused by surfactant also is responsible for keeping the alveoli free of fluid. In the absence of surfactant, the surface tension tends to attract fluid into the alveoli.

- The lung and chest wall have elastic properties that permit expansion during inspiration and relaxation to original dimension during expiration. During inspiration, the diaphragm and intercostal muscles contract, air flows into the lungs, and the chest wall expands. Muscular effort is needed to overcome the resistance of the lungs to expansion. During expiration, the muscles relax and the elastic recoil of the lungs causes the thorax to decrease in volume until balance between the chest wall and lung recoil forces is reached.

- Compliance is the measure of lung and chest wall distensibility. It represents the relative ease with which these structures can be stretched. Compliance is, therefore, the reciprocal of elasticity. An increase in compliance indicates that the lungs and/or chest wall are abnormally easy to inflate and have lost some elastic recoil. A decrease indicates that the lungs and/or chest wall are abnormally stiff or difficult to inflate.

- Airway resistance is determined by the length, radius, and cross-sectional area of the airways and density, viscosity, and velocity of the gas. Resistance (R) is computed by dividing change in pressure (P) by rate of flow (F), or $R = P/F$. Resistance is inversely proportional to the fourth power of the radius; thus anything decreasing the radius of the airways increases airway resistance.

Objectives

After studying this chapter, the learner will be able to do the following:

1. **Define the terms used in describing the signs and symptoms of pulmonary disease.**
   Study pages 752-753; refer to Figure 26-1.

Dyspnea is the subjective sensation of uncomfortable breathing. It is often described as breathlessness, air hunger, shortness of breath, or labored breathing. Dyspnea occurs if increased airway resistance or decreased compliance causes respiratory effort greater than appropriate for the ventilation achieved. The signs of dyspnea include anxiety, rapid labored breathing, and body position (usually leaning forward).

Orthopnea is experienced in the horizontal position. This position redistributes body water and causes the abdominal contents to exert pressure on the diaphragm, which decreases its efficiency of contraction and causes dyspnea.

Paroxysmal nocturnal dyspnea is seen in individuals with left ventricular failure who wake up at night gasping for air and have to sit up or stand to relieve the dyspnea. This dyspnea results from redistribution of body water into the lungs while the individual is recumbent.

Strenuous exercise or metabolic acidosis induces **Kussmaul respiration** or **hyperpnea**. Kussmaul respiration is characterized by a slightly increased ventilatory rate, effortless tidal volumes, and no expiratory pause.

Cheyne-Stokes respirations are characterized by alternating periods of deep and shallow breathing. Apnea, cessation of breathing lasting from 15 to 60 seconds, is followed by increased ventilation, after which ventilation decreases again to apnea. Cheyne-Stokes respirations occur in any condition that slows the blood flow to the brain stem or slows impulses to the respiratory centers of the brain stem.

Hypoventilation is inadequate alveolar ventilation in relation to metabolic demands. It is caused by alterations in pulmonary mechanics or in the neurologic control of breathing. With hypoventilation, CO_2 removal does not keep up with production and CO_2 rises in the blood, causing **hypercapnia**.

Hyperventilation is alveolar ventilation that exceeds metabolic demands. The lungs remove CO_2 at a faster rate than it is produced, which results in **hypocapnia** or low levels of CO_2 in the blood.

Coughing is a protective reflex that cleanses the lower airways by an explosive expiration that removes inhaled particles, accumulated mucus, or foreign bodies. Stimulation of the irritant receptors in the airway initiates the cough.

Hemoptysis is coughing up blood or bloody secretions. Hemoptysis indicates a localized infection or inflammation that has damaged the bronchi or the lung parenchyma.

Cyanosis is a bluish discoloration of the skin and mucous membranes caused by increasing amounts of desaturated or reduced hemoglobin in the blood. Cyanosis can result from decreased arterial oxygenation or decreased cardiac output.

Pain is caused by pulmonary disorders that originate in the pleurae, airways, or chest wall. Infection and inflammation of the parietal pleura cause pain when the pleura stretches during inspiration. Pain that is pronounced after coughing occurs in individuals with infection and inflammation of the trachea and/or bronchi. Pain in the chest wall occurs with excessive coughing, which makes the muscles sore.

Clubbing is the selective bulbous enlargement of the end of a finger or toe. Its pathogenesis is unknown, but it is associated with diseases that interfere with oxygenation and cause long-term hypoxia.

An **abnormal sputum** is seen with different pulmonary disorders. Changes in the amount and consistency of sputum provide information about the progression of disease and the effectiveness of therapy.

2. **Characterize lung conditions that are caused by pulmonary disease or injury.**
   Study pages 754-762; refer to Figures 26-2 through 26-6 and Table 26-1.

Conditions Caused by Pulmonary Disease or Injury

Condition	Pathology	Cause
Hypercapnia	Increased carbon dioxide in arterial blood	Drug depression of respiratory center; infections of CNS or trauma to medulla; spinal cord disruption or poliomyelitis; neuromuscular junction disease as in myasthenia gravis or muscular dystrophy affecting respiratory muscles; thorax cage abnormalities; airway obstruction; emphysema due to physiologic dead space
Hypoxemia	Reduced oxygenation of arterial blood	Decreased oxygen content of inspired gas, hypoventilation diffusion abnormalities in emphysema, abnormal ventilation/perfusion ratios in bronchitis, right-to-left shunts in RDS or atelectasis
Pulmonary edema	Excess water in lungs	Heart disease increases pulmonary capillary hydrostatic pressure, so fluid moves into interstitium; ARDS or inhalation of toxic gases injures capillaries and increases permeability; blockage of lymphatic vessels by CHF, edema, or tumors
Aspiration	Passage of fluid and solids into lungs, obstruction of airway, localized inflammation, noncompliance, edema, collapse	Decreased levels of consciousness, CNS abnormalities
Atelectasis	Collapse of lung tissue	External pressure from tumor or fluid or air in pleural space, abdominal distension, bronchi obstruction, inhalation of concentrated oxygen or anesthetics
Bronchiectasis	Persistent abnormal dilation of bronchi	Obstruction of airway, atelectasis, infection, cystic fibrosis, tuberculosis, weakness of bronchial wall
Bronchiolitis	Inflammatory obstruction of bronchioles	Chronic bronchitis, infection, inhalation of toxic gases
Pneumothorax	Air or gas in pleural space collapses the lung partially or totally	Rupture of pleura or chest wall
Pleural effusion	Fluid in the pleural space collapses the lung partially or totally	Fluid from blood or lymphatic vessels from CHF, hypoproteinemia, infections or malignancies cause mast cell release of capillary permeability mediators, trauma that damages blood vessels
Empyema	Pus in pleural space	Bacterial pneumonia
Pleurisy	Inflammation of the pleura, exudate of lymph, fibrin, and cells cause a friction rub	Respiratory infection
Abscess	Circumscribed area of suppuration of lung parenchyma	Aspiration pneumonia
Fibrosis	Fibrous or connective tissue in lung	Scar tissue following ARDS, tuberculosis, or inhalation of dust or asbestos
Chest wall restriction	Compromised ventilation	Grossly obese, lateral bending and rotation of spine, arthritis of spine, depression of the sternum, neuromuscular disease
Flail chest	Compromised ventilation	Fracture of ribs or sternum
Toxic gas exposure	Inflammation of airways, alveolar and capillary damage, pulmonary edema	Inhalation of smoke, ammonia, hydrogen chloride, sulfur dioxide, chlorine, phosgene, and nitrogen dioxide; prolonged levels of high concentrations of oxygen
Pneumoconiosis	Fibrous tissue or nodules in lungs	Silicosis—inhalation of silica, anthracosis—inhalation of coal dust, asbestosis—inhalation of asbestos
Allergic alveolitis	Lung inflammation or pneumonitis	Inhalation of allergens—grains, silage, bird droppings, feathers, cork dust, animal pelts, molds, mushroom compost

3. **In a diagrammatic scheme, interrelate the pathogenic factors in adult respiratory distress syndrome (ARDS).**
   Study pages 762-764; refer to Figure 26-7.

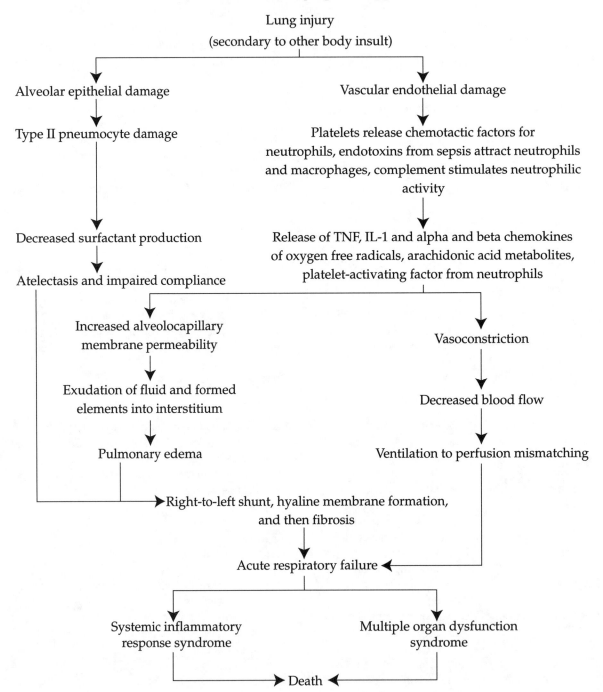

ARDS Pathophysiology

Lung injury
(secondary to other body insult)

Alveolar epithelial damage

Type II pneumocyte damage

Decreased surfactant production

Atelectasis and impaired compliance

Increased alveolocapillary
membrane permeability

Exudation of fluid and formed
elements into interstitium

Pulmonary edema

Vascular endothelial damage

Platelets release chemotactic factors for
neutrophils, endotoxins from sepsis attract neutrophils
and macrophages, complement stimulates neutrophilic
activity

Release of TNF, IL-1 and alpha and beta chemokines
of oxygen free radicals, arachidonic acid metabolites,
platelet-activating factor from neutrophils

Vasoconstriction

Decreased blood flow

Ventilation to perfusion mismatching

Right-to-left shunt, hyaline membrane formation,
and then fibrosis

Acute respiratory failure

Systemic inflammatory
response syndrome

Multiple organ dysfunction
syndrome

Death

4. Compare and contrast the obstructive pulmonary diseases.

Study pages 764-768 and 770; refer to Figures 26-8 through 26-12 and Tables 26-3 and 26-4.

Obstructive pulmonary disease is characterized by difficult expiration. More force or the use of accessory muscles of expiration is required to expire a given volume of air. The most common obstructive diseases are asthma, chronic bronchitis, and emphysema. Since many individuals have both chronic bronchitis and emphysema, these diseases are grouped together and are called chronic obstructive pulmonary disease (COPD). Asthma is more acute and intermittent than COPD, but it also can be chronic and is included as a type of COPD.

Obstructive Pulmonary Diseases

	Asthma*	Emphysema	Chronic Bronchitis
Cause of airway obstruction	Bronchial inflammation, bronchospasm, mucosal edema, and increased mucus production	Enlargement and destruction of alveoli, loss of elasticity, trapping of air during expiration	Bronchial smooth muscle hypertrophy and production of thick, tenacious mucus not cleared by ciliary function
Precipitating causes	Hyperresponsiveness to inflammatory mediators—histamine, prostaglandins and leukotrienes—leads to bronchoconstriction	Alpha$_1$-antitrypsin deficiency, cigarette smoke	Cigarette smoke, air pollutants, infections
Manifestations	Dyspnea, wheezing, nonproductive cough early but later mucoid, prolonged expiration, tachycardia, tachypnea, acidosis (varies over four distinct categories)	Marked dyspnea, no cough early but later, tachypnea with prolonged expiration, accessory muscles used for ventilation, barrel chest, normal or elevated hematocrit, late cor pulmonale	Exercise intolerance, late dyspnea, wheezing, productive cough, marked hypoxemia leading to polycythemia and cyanosis, early cor pulmonale, CHF
Treatment	Inhaled antiinflammatory agents, inhaled or oral bronchodilators	Prophylactic antibiotics for acute infections, bronchodilators, relief of dyspnea, cautious oxygen administration	Bronchodilators, expectorants, postural drainage, percussion, antiinflammatory agents

*Asthma classification is based on clinical severity with step 1 being mild intermittent and step 4 being severe persistent.
NOTE: Acute bronchitis is an acute infection or inflammation of the bronchi following a viral infection and is usually self-limiting.

5. Define pneumonia and describe its causes, manifestations, and treatment.
Study pages 771-773; refer to Figure 26-13.

Pneumonia is an acute infection of the lower respiratory tract or the lung caused by bacteria, bacterial-like microbes, fungi, viruses, protozoa, or parasites. The most common causal microbes are the following:

Gram-Positive Bacteria	Gram-Negative Bacteria	Nonbacterial Organisms
Streptococcus pneumoniae	Escherichia coli	Pneumocystis carinii
Staphylococcus aureus	Pseudomonas aeruginosa	Mycoplasma pneumoniae
Streptococcus pyogenes	Klebsiella pneumoniae	Fungi
	Proteus species	Viruses
	Bacteroides species	
	Haemophilus species	
	Legionella species	

Fungi infrequently cause pneumonia, but **fungal pneumonia** can be caused in immunosuppressed individuals by *Candida, Mucor,* and *Aspergillus* species. The most common cause of **community-acquired pneumonia** is *Streptococcus pneumoniae. Mycoplasma pneumoniae* is the next most common cause of community-acquired pneumonia. *Staphylococcus aureus* and *Klebsiella pneumoniae* cause some community-acquired disease, usually in individuals with other health problems such as COPD or alcoholism or in individuals with a primary viral illness.

Most **nosocomial** or **hospital-acquired pneumonias** are caused by gram-negative bacteria such as *Escherichia coli, Klebsiella pneumoniae,* and *Pseudomonas aeruginosa.* When the gram-positive organism *Staphylococcus aureus* infects hospitalized individuals, it causes a more serious infection. These staphylococcal infections also are more likely to result in lung necrosis, abscesses, or empyema.

The *Legionella* species are widely distributed in water environments and are present in cooling systems, condensers, shower heads, and water reservoirs. Infections may occur in outbreaks sporadically.

Pathogenic microorganisms can reach the lung by inspiration, by aspiration of oropharyngeal secretions, or via the circulation. This last source is usually by systemic infection, sepsis, or contaminated needles of intravenous drug users. The lungs' defense mechanisms, namely, the cough reflex, mucociliary clearance, and phagocytosis by alveolar macrophages, normally prevent infection by these pathogens. The body's immune system and various components of the inflammatory response further aid healthy individuals to prevent disease. In susceptible individuals, the invading pathogen is not contained. Instead, it multiplies and releases damaging toxins and stimulates full-scale inflammatory and immune responses. The immune response and the endotoxins released by some microorganisms damage bronchial mucous membranes and alveolocapillary membranes. Inflammation and edema cause the acinus and terminal bronchioles to fill with infectious debris and exudate; ventilation-perfusion abnormalities follow. If the pneumonia is caused by staphylococci or gram-negative bacteria, necrosis of lung parenchyma also may occur.

Streptococcus pneumoniae organisms cause most **bacterial pneumonias.** In this bacterial infection, the involved lobe undergoes consolidation or solidification of the tissue as it fills with exudate. A stage of red hepatization follows in which alveoli fill with blood cells, fibrin, edematous fluid, and pneumococci. This gives the lung tissue a red appearance. Next is a stage of gray hepatization in which affected tissues become gray because of fibrin deposition over the pleural surfaces and the presence of fibrin and leukocytes in the consolidated alveoli.

Viral pneumonia is usually mild and self-limiting, but it can set the stage for a secondary bacterial infection by providing an ideal environment for bacterial growth and by damaging ciliated epithelial cells. Viral pneumonia can be a primary infection or a complication of another viral illness such as chickenpox or measles. Viral pneumonia is usually caused by influenza viruses.

Most cases of pneumonia are preceded by an upper respiratory viral infection. Individuals then develop fever, chills, productive or dry cough, malaise, pleural pain, and sometimes dyspnea and hemoptysis. The white blood count is usually elevated, but it may be low if the individual is debilitated. Chest radiographs reveal infiltrates that may involve a single lobe of the lung (lobar pneumonia) or may be more diffuse (bronchopneumonia). Purulent sputum is expectorated by individuals with bacterial pneumonia, whereas viral pneumonia and pneumonia caused by *Mycoplasma pneumoniae* characteristically show scant sputum production.

Antibiotics are used to treat bacterial and mycoplasmal pneumonia. Viral pneumonia is treated with supportive therapy unless secondary bacterial infection is present. Adequate hydration, deep breathing, coughing, and chest physical therapy are important in treating all types of pneumonia.

6. Describe the pathogenesis of tuberculosis (TB).
Study pages 773-774.

Tuberculosis is an infection caused by *Mycobacterium tuberculosis,* which is an acid-fast bacillus that usually affects the lungs but may invade other body systems. Individuals with AIDS are highly susceptible to respiratory infections including tuberculosis. Recently, effective treatment of HIV infections has resulted in fewer cases of tuberculosis. Emigration of infected individuals from high-prevalence countries, transmission in crowded institutional settings, substance abuse, and lack of access to medical care also have contributed to the growing problem.

Tuberculosis is transmitted from person to person in airborne droplets. Once the bacilli are inspired into the lung, they multiply and cause nonspecific lung inflammation. Some bacilli migrate through the lymphatics and become lodged in the lymph nodes where they encounter lymphocytes and initiate an immune response.

Neutrophils and alveolar macrophages wall off the colonies of bacilli and form a granulomatous lesion called a *tubercle.* Infected tissues within the tubercle die and form a cheeselike material; this is called **caseation necrosis.** Collagenous scar tissue then grows around the tubercle, which prevents further multiplication of bacilli.

Once the bacilli are isolated in tubercles and immunity develops, tuberculosis may remain dormant for life. However, if the immune system is impaired or if live bacilli escape into the bronchi, active disease occurs and may spread through the blood and lymphatics to other organs. Endogenous reactivation of dormant bacilli in the elderly may be caused by poor nutritional status, insulin-dependent diabetes, long-term corticosteroid therapy, and other debilitating diseases.

In many infected individuals, tuberculosis is asymptomatic. In others, symptoms develop so gradually that they are not noticed until the disease is well advanced. Common clinical manifestations include fatigue, weight loss, lethargy, loss of appetite, and a low-grade fever that usually occurs in the afternoon. A cough with purulent sputum develops slowly and becomes more frequent after weeks or months. "Night sweats" and general anxiety are often present. A positive tuberculin skin test indicates that an individual has been infected and has produced antibodies against the bacillus. Chest radiographs and culturing the bacillus from the sputum aid in diagnosis of tuberculosis. Six grades of tuberculosis are possible: the grades aid in evaluation and the determination of appropriate therapy.

Treatment consists of antibiotic therapy to control active or dormant tuberculosis and prevent transmission. Today, with increased numbers of immunosuppressed and susceptible individuals and drug-resistant bacilli, the recommended treatment for those at high risk is a combination of drugs: isoniazid, rifampin, pyrazinamide, and ethambutol and streptomycin. Treatment is continued for at least 6 months until sputum cultures show that the active bacilli have been eliminated.

7. Compare and contrast pulmonary embolism, pulmonary hypertension, and cor pulmonale.
Study text pages 775-777; refer to Figures 26-14 and 26-15.

Blood flow through the lungs can be disrupted by a number of disorders that occlude the vessels, increase pulmonary vascular resistance, or destroy the vascular bed. Major disruptive disorders include pulmonary embolism, pulmonary hypertension, and cor pulmonale. (See the box on page 194.)

8. Describe laryngeal cancer.
Study page 778; refer to Figure 26-17.

The risk for **laryngeal cancer** is increased by and related to the amount of tobacco smoked; the risk is heightened when smoking is combined with alcohol consumption. Carcinoma of the glottis is more common than that of the epiglottis, aryepiglottic folds, arytenoids, and false cords. Squamous cell carcinoma is the most common cell type.

Progressive hoarseness is the most significant symptom and can result in voice loss. Dyspnea is rare with supraglottic tumors but can be severe in subglottic tumors. Laryngeal pain or a sore throat is likely with supraglottic lesions.

Radiation therapy has shown good results for early carcinoma of the vocal cords. Total laryngectomy is required when lesions are extensive and involve the cartilage.

Pulmonary Vascular Disease

	Embolism	Hypertension	Cor Pulmonale
Cause	Blood-borne substances from venous stasis, vessel injury, or hypercoagulation lodge in a branch of pulmonary artery and obstruct blood flow	Pulmonary arterial pressure is elevated by increased left atrial pressure, pulmonary blood flow, or vascular resistance secondary to lung disease	Right heart failure because of primary pulmonary disease and long-standing pulmonary hypertension
Manifestations	Earlier evidence of deep vein thrombosis of legs or pelvis, tachypnea, dyspnea, chest pain, hypotension, shock, possible radiographic wedge shape bordering the pleura	Fatigue, chest discomfort, tachypnea, dyspnea with exercise, a radiograph or electrocardiogram that shows right ventricle hypertrophy	Chest pain, second heart sound or closure of pulmonic valve is accentuated; tricuspid valve murmur; radiograph and electrocardiogram show right ventricular enlargement
Treatment	Avoid venous stasis; anticoagulant therapy; fibrinolytic agent if life-threatening	Supplemental oxygen, digitalis, and diuretics are palliative; lung transplantation is therapeutic	Same as pulmonary hypertension, success depends on reversal of underlying lung disease

9. Describe the major histologic types of lung cancer.
Study pages 779 and 781-782; refer to Figure 26-18 and Tables 26-5 and 26-6.

Lung cancers or **bronchogenic carcinomas** arise from the epithelium of the respiratory tract. Lung cancer and malignant melanoma are the only major cancers whose incidence is rapidly increasing in the United States.

The most common cause of lung cancer is cigarette smoking; heavy smokers have about 25 times greater chance of developing lung cancer than nonsmokers. Cigarette smoke contains several organ-specific carcinogens for organs or tissues other than lung tissue; smoking has been causally related to carcinogenesis of the larynx, oral cavity, esophagus, and urinary bladder. Genetic predisposition to developing lung cancer also plays a role in lung cancer pathophysiology.

Characteristics of Lung Cancer

Type/Frequency	Growth Rate	Metastasis	Manifestations/Treatment
Adenocarcinoma; 35%	Moderate	Early	Pleural effusion; surgical treatment
Squamous cell; 30%	Slow	Late	Cough, sputum production, airway obstruction; surgical treatment
Small cell (oat cell) carcinoma; 20%-25%	Very rapid	Very early and widespread	Airway obstruction, excessive ACTH secretion with its signs and symptoms; chemotherapy and radiation
Large cell carcinoma; 10%-15%	Rapid	Early and widespread	Pain, pleural effusion, cough, sputum production, hemoptysis, airway obstruction; surgical treatment to relieve pneumonitis or pleural effusion
Mesotheliomas; 80% of sarcomas of pleural membrane	Slow	Late	Dyspnea, pleuritive pain; surgical treatment

NOTE: The current accepted system for the staging of lung cancer is the TNM classification. In this system, *T* denotes the extent of the primary tumor, *N* indicates the nodal involvement, and *M* describes the extent of metastasis.

Practice Examination

Match the pulmonary condition with the characteristic or definition.

_____ 1. Kussmaul respiration

_____ 2. hemoptysis

_____ 3. cyanosis

_____ 4. Cheyne-Stokes respiration

_____ 5. pleural space atelectasis

_____ 6. bronchiectasis

_____ 7. pneumoconiosis

_____ 8. flail chest

_____ 9. pneumothorax

_____ 10. abscess

a. inadequate alveolar ventilation

b. ventilation exceeding metabolic demand

c. coughing blood or bloody secretions

d. abnormal dilation of bronchi

e. fibrous tissue or nodules in lungs

f. fractured ribs or sternum

g. increased ventilatory rate, effortless tidal volume, and no expiratory pause

h. decreased arterial oxygenation

i. alveolar collapse

j. pleural space air

k. pleural space pus

l. apnea, increased ventilations, then apnea again

m. aspiration pneumonia

---

11. High altitudes may produce hypoxemia by:
    a. right-to-left shunts.
    b. hypoventilation.
    c. decreased oxygen inspiration.
    d. diffusion abnormalities.
    e. All of the above are correct.

12. In ARDS, increased alveolocapillary membrane permeability is due to:
    a. PAF.
    b. oxygen-free radicals.
    c. TNF.
    d. Both a and c are correct.
    e. a, b, and c are correct.

13. Type II pneumocyte damage causes:
    a. increased alveolocapillary permeability.
    b. chemotaxis for neutrophils.
    c. exudation of fluid from capillaries into interstitium.
    d. decreased surfactant production.
    e. All of the above are correct.

14. Pulmonary edema may be caused by abnormal:
    a. capillary hydrostatic pressure.
    b. capillary oncotic pressure.
    c. capillary permeability.
    d. Both a and c are correct.
    e. a, b, and c are correct.

15. In bronchial asthma:
    a. bronchial muscles contract.
    b. bronchial muscles relax.
    c. mucous secretions decrease.
    d. imbalances within the CNS develop.

16. Asthma is precipitated by which of the following in-flammatory mediators? (More than one answer may be correct.)
    a. histamine
    b. prostaglandins
    c. leukotrienes
    d. neutrophilic infiltration

17. In emphysema:
    a. there is increased area for gaseous exchange.
    b. there are prolonged inspirations.
    c. the bronchioles are primarily involved.
    d. there is increased diaphragm movement.
    e. None of the above is correct.

18. Chronic bronchitis (more than one answer may be correct):
    a. is caused by lack of surfactant.
    b. is caused by air pollutants.
    c. exhibits a productive cough.
    d. causes collapsed alveoli.

19. Which is *inconsistent* with pneumonia?
    a. chest pain, cough, and rales
    b. involves only interstitial lung tissue
    c. may be caused by mycoplasmas
    d. can be lobar pneumonia or bronchopneumonia

20. Tuberculosis (more than one answer may be correct):
    a. is caused by an aerobic bacillus.
    b. may affect other organs.
    c. involves a type III hypersensitivity.
    d. antibodies may be detected by a skin test.

21. Pulmonary emboli usually (more than one answer may be correct):
    a. obstruct blood supply to lung parenchyma.
    b. originate from thrombi in the legs.
    c. occlude pulmonary vein branches.
    d. occlude pulmonary artery branches.

22. Pulmonary hypertension:
    a. is seen in elevated left arterial pressure.
    b. involves deep vein thrombosis.
    c. shows right ventricular hypertrophy.
    d. Both a and c are correct.
    e. a, b, and c are correct.

23. Cor pulmonale:
    a. occurs in response to long-standing pulmonary hypertension.
    b. is right heart failure.
    c. is manifested by altered tricuspid and pulmonic valve sounds.
    d. Both b and c are correct.
    e. a, b, and c are correct.

24. A lung cancer characterized by many anaplastic figures and the production of hormones is most likely:
    a. squamous cell carcinoma.
    b. small cell carcinoma.
    c. large cell carcinoma.
    d. adenocarcinoma.
    e. bronchial adenoma.

25. The metastasis of lung squamous cell carcinoma is:
    a. late.
    b. very early and widespread.
    c. early.
    d. early and widespread.
    e. never seen.

Case Study

Mr. S. is a retired 69-year-old county attorney who was on a buying trip with his wife looking for old, classic cars in the high, mountainous country of Colorado when he became extremely short of breath. His alarmed wife took him to a multispecialty medical clinic for evaluation.

On admission to the clinic, Mr. S. was restless and dyspneic. His chest had an increased anteroposterior dimension.

His past history revealed a habit of smoking two packs of cigarettes a day for 45 years (90 pack years). During the past few years, Mr. S. noticed a cough each morning on arising. Recently, while working in his flower garden, he had to stop at times to catch his breath. Even while watching television, he had experienced dyspnea.

A chest radiograph was taken, and pulmonary function tests were done. The chest radiograph revealed a flat, low diaphragm with lung hyperinflation but clear fields. Pulmonary function tests showed decreased tidal volume and vital capacity, increased total lung capacity, and prolonged forced expiratory volume.

Which pulmonary disease is exhibited by Mr. S.'s symptoms? Justify your answer.

27

Alterations of Pulmonary Function in Children

Foundational Objectives

a. Review Foundational Objectives *a*, *b*, and *c* of Chapter 26 and the following Memory Check box.

MEMORY CHECK!

Infants and young children have fewer alveoli than adults; their alveoli are much smaller and less complex than those of adults. The small diameter airways of infants and children produce increased resistance to airflow and are easily obstructed by mucosal edema or secretions. The airways and chest walls of the infant are much less rigid than those of the adult. The flexible and compliant infant chest wall may actually flex inward, and the airways may collapse somewhat during times of respiratory stress, thereby limiting functional respiratory capacity. The premature infant may not have attained adequate surfactant production by the time of birth and will be unable to maintain alveolar surface tension. Children have greater metabolic rates and oxygen consumption than adults; respiratory distress, acidosis, and dehydration develop more easily in children than in adults. By virtue of their immature immune systems, children have many more respiratory infections than do adults.

Objectives

After studying this chapter, the learner will be able to do the following:

1. **Identify two different forms of croup and differentiate between them by respective etiologies, anatomic involvement, and seriousness.**
   Study pages 788-790; refer to Figures 27-1 through 27-4 and Table 27-1.

Croup is a very generic term that refers to a number of primarily infectious processes of different etiologies affecting the structures of the upper airway. These vary from relatively benign to acutely life-threatening and are

usually easily differentiated by matching the symptoms with the probable anatomic site involved.

Inflammation above the epiglottis includes hoarseness or muffled voice. As respiration is compromised, accessory muscles retract, nasal flaring occurs, and agitation or fatigue may be seen. Inflammation of the glottis or below it often begins with a whispery, low-volume voice, and a barking cough.

Laryngotracheobronchitis or classic croup is generally a more common and a less severe form of croup than epiglottitis. The etiologic agent is usually parainfluenza virus, influenza A, or respiratory syncytial virus. The affected age range is usually 6 months to 5 years, and recurrences are common.

Classic symptoms are generally preceded by two to three days of "cold" symptoms such as rhinorrhea and low-grade fever that progress to a high-pitched cough, muffled voice, and inspiratory stridor that is variable in intensity. Obstruction is caused by swelling of the subglottic tissues, and spasm of the vocal cords occurs as the inflammation extends. Treatment is with air humidification or cool mist, and inhaled epinephrine to temporarily decrease airway edema.

Epiglottitis is an acutely life-threatening emergency. The etiologic agent is usually the bacteria Group A streptococci. Children aged 2 to 7 years are affected. The affected swollen structures are the epiglottis and the very small glottic space.

Onset is rapid, and respiratory distress tends to be severe and quickly progresses to respiratory arrest without appropriate intervention. The child will be quite restless and fearful because of air hunger and will generally have severe respiratory stridor and be unable to swallow, causing copious drooling. Symptoms are due to marked edema of the epiglottis secondary to infection.

Treatment consists of establishing an emergency airway by intubation. Appropriate antibiotics are necessary to treat the underlying bacterial infection. Administering oxygen, aerosolized epinephrine, and nebulized glucocorticoids will relieve inflammation and obstruction.

2. **Describe foreign body aspiration in infants and children.**
   Study page 790.

Foreign body aspiration is common and often life-threatening in children. Offending objects are often toys or bits of food. Cough, hoarseness, and dyspnea are common with any foreign body in the larynx. Similar symptoms with blood-streaked sputum are associated with bronchus obstruction. Complications include pneumonia, atelectasis, bronchiectasis, and lung abscesses if treatment is delayed. Lodged objects require endoscopic removal.

3. **Describe obstructive sleep apnea.**
   Study page 790.

Obstructive sleep apnea syndrome (OSAS) is partial or complete upper airway obstruction (UAO) during sleep with disruption of normal ventilation and normal sleep patterns. Childhood OSAS is quite common, with an estimated prevalence of 1% to 10%. OSAS is usually seen in children with adenotonsillar hypertrophy but also may occur in children who are obese or have craniofacial anomalies or neurologic disorders.

There usually is a history of snoring and labored breathing during sleep, which may be continuous or intermittent. There may be episodes of increased respiratory effort but no audible airflow, often terminated by snorting, gasping, repositioning, or arousal. Sleep is often described as restless. Daytime sleepiness is occasionally reported. Children are most often referred for tonsillectomy and adenoidectomy (T & A) on the basis of described symptoms and physical findings, such as enlarged tonsils, adenoidal facies, and mouth breathing.

4. **Describe the pathophysiologic processes involved in respiratory distress syndrome of the newborn.**
   Study pages 790-792; refer to Figure 27-5.

Respiratory distress syndrome (RDS) of the newborn is a lack of adequate surfactant to reduce alveolar surface tension and inadequate alveolar surface area for gas exchange due to prematurity. The small, underdeveloped alveoli of preterm infants require very high pressures to inflate. Absence of surfactant compounds this problem, and each breath the infant takes requires as much pressure as the first. Widespread atelectasis occurs, causing respiratory distress and increased pulmonary vascular resistance. Increased pulmonary vascular resistance causes shunting of the blood away from the lungs and results in a right-to-left shunt, which further compounds the problem of hypoxia and hypercapnia. Hypoxia and hypercapnia trigger vasoconstriction of the pulmonary vascular bed and exacerbate shunting. Prolonged anaerobic metabolism produces metabolic acidosis.

Tachypnea, expiratory grunting, intercostal and subcostal retractions, nasal flaring, and skin duskiness are clinical manifestations. Treatment is supportive with mechanical ventilation. Exogenous surfactant administration for low weight infants has contributed significantly to the treatment of RDS. Antenatal treatment with glucocorticoids for women in preterm labor (24 to 34 gestation weeks) induces a significant acceleration of lung maturation and reduces the incidence of RDS.

5. **Describe bronchopulmonary dysplasia.**
   Study pages 792-793; refer to Figure 27-6.

Bronchopulmonary dysplasia (BPD) is a severe form of lung damage associated with neonatal chronic lung disease. Risk factors include premature birth and immature lungs, oxygen toxicity, positive pressure ventilation, respiratory infection, antiprotease deficiency, genetic predisposition, and ductus arteriosus.

Clinically, the infants remain oxygen- and ventilator-dependent and have hypoxemia and hypercapnia. Intermittent bronchospasms, mucus plugging, and pulmonary hypertension characterize BPD. At one moment, the infant seems stable or improving and then suddenly deteriorates.

BPD can cause death within a few weeks or can continue for months or years. Treatment is designed to accelerate lung maturation, maintain normal oxygenation, prevent further lung damage and infections, and promote lung repair.

6. **Identify the most common etiologic agent in bronchiolitis; describe the pathophysiology and the usual clinical course of the disease.**
   Study page 794.

The most common cause of **bronchiolitis** is respiratory syncytial virus, followed by adenoviruses, influenza, parainfluenza, and mycoplasma in older children. Viral infection causes necrosis of the bronchial epithelium and destruction of ciliated epithelial cells. The submucosa of the bronchi becomes edematous and plugged with mucus and cellular debris, and bronchospasm narrows airways. Atelectasis occurs in some areas of the lungs and hyperinflation in others. The usual manifestation is an infant who develops mild cold symptoms. Symptoms progress to hypoxemia, overexpanded thoracic cage, and the diaphragm flattening causing downward displacement of the liver and spleen. Children younger than 1 year of age may require assisted ventilation. Bronchodilators and antiviral agents for RSV may be required.

Bronchiolitis obliterans is fibrotic obstruction of the respiratory bronchioles and alveolar ducts secondary to inflammation. Most cases are associated with pulmonary infections.

7. **Describe the most common etiologic agents of pneumonias in children.**
   Study pages 794 and 796; refer to Tables 27-2 and 27-3.

Pneumonia in young children is most often caused by *Streptococcus pneumoniae* followed by *Staphylococcus aureus* and group A streptococci. The milder viral pneumonias tend to occur in infancy and early childhood and are characterized by an antecedent "cold" followed by cough, fever, tachypnea, and mild systemic symptoms. Respiratory syncytial virus causes most viral pneumonia in infants. Mycoplasma and Chlamydia cause atypical pneumonia in young children and exhibit only upper respiratory tract involvement. Bacterial pneumonias tend to have more dramatic systemic features and exhibit high

fever, shaking, chills, restlessness, and malaise because they are more lobar in nature and require antibiotics therapy for resolution. Treatment for viral pneumonia is palliative.

Children at highest risk for **aspiration pneumonitis** are toddlers and children with poor airway reflexes or gastroesophageal reflux. The severity of lung injury after an aspiration incident is determined by the pH of the aspirated material, presence of pathogenic bacteria, and the volatility and viscosity of the substance. Very low or high pH and low-viscosity cause significant inflammatory response whereas high-viscosity substances are less likely to cause a pneumonitis.

8. **Describe the pathophysiologic processes, manifestations, and treatment of asthma.**
   Study pages 797-798 and 800; refer to Figures 27-7 and 27-8.

Asthma is a chronic illness of highly variable severity, which tends to be punctuated with more or less frequent episodes of acute exacerbation. The pathophysiologic basis of asthma involves hyperresponsive lower airways responding in an obstructive manner to various triggers. The triggers include allergens, exercise, viruses, and other infectious agents. Responses include spasm of the respiratory smooth muscle that encircles the airways, edema of the airway mucosa, mucus plugging of the airways, and cellular infiltration into the airways. Asthma attacks may have two phases. The early phase of the attack is caused by IgE mediation resulting from mast cell degranulation and histamine, leukotrienes, prostaglandins, platelet activating factor, and certain cytokines released in response to the triggering factors. The late phase follows in 4 to 8 hours and is caused by inflammatory mediators released from cells attracted to the airways. The typical abnormalities in acute asthma are hypoxemia, hypercapnia, and respiratory alkalosis; with severe airway obstruction, respiratory failure with acute CO_2 retention and respiratory acidosis occurs. Clinical manifestations may include persistent cough, expiratory wheeze, and signs of respiratory distress.

Treatment involves the administration of adrenergic and bronchodilator aerosols, and inhaled and systemic corticosteroids.

9. **Describe the pulmonary pathophysiology associated with cystic fibrosis and identify general modes of diagnostic testing and therapy.**
   Study pages 801-803; refer to Figures 27-10 and 27-11.

Cystic fibrosis (CF) is an autosomal recessive, genetically transmitted, multisystem disease in which exocrine or mucus-producing glands secrete abnormally thick mucus that obstructs the gastrointestinal system and lungs. Although CF is a multiorgan disease, respiratory failure is almost always the cause of death. An obstructed gastrointestinal system leads to malabsorption of nutrients related to pancreatic insufficiency. Thick secretions obstruct the bronchioles in the lung and predispose the lungs to recurrent or chronic infection. Chronic inflammation leads to destruction of the airway walls and hyperplasia of goblet cells. Bronchiectasis, pneumonia, and widespread pulmonary fibrosis follow in response to bacterial colonization with *Staphylococcus aureus* and *Pseudomonas aeruginosa*. End-stage disease is characterized by cor pulmonale, chronic hypoxia, and pulmonary hypertension.

Chronic cough, sputum production, and purulent mucus indicate lung involvement. Labored ventilation results in hypoxia, finger clubbing, and cyanosis. Pulmonary disorders are the most common causes of morbidity and mortality.

Genetic testing is available to detect carriers. Sweat chloride testing is a definitive diagnostic test because it measures defective epithelial chloride ion transport. Treatment includes aggressive chest physiotherapy and judicious use of antibiotics to control infection.

10. Describe SIDS.
Study pages 803-804.

Sudden infant death syndrome (SIDS) refers to the sudden, unexpected death of any infant or young child in whom a postmortem examination fails to demonstrate a cause for death. The highest incidence is between 3 and 4 months of age; it mostly occurs during sleep and with greater frequency during winter months.

The cause of SIDS in unknown; however, new information suggests that it involves an inflammatory response in the lungs to either bacterial pathogens from the nasopharynx or viral respiratory tract infections. The degranulation of eosinophil mediators could cause pulmonary edema, fatal respiratory obstruction, and hypoxia.

There is no treatment because the death is sudden and unexplained. There is evidence that infants should not be placed in the prone position during the first 6 months of life and should not be laid down to sleep on top of any soft surface.

Practice Examination

True/False

_____ 1. Inflammation above the epiglottis causes a "barking" cough.

_____ 2. Laryngotracheobronchitis is more severe than epiglottis.

_____ 3. Surfactant production accelerates airway lumenal growth.

_____ 4. Failure to produce surfactant at birth results in severe atelectasis and RDS.

_____ 5. Cystic fibrosis is a disease process due primarily to hyperresponsive airways that are sensitive to certain environmental triggers.

_____ 6. Bronchiolitis and asthma produce similar symptoms.

7. Epiglottitis is characterized by:
a. gradual onset.
b. severe stridor.
c. drooling.
d. All of the above are correct.
e. Both b and c are correct.

8. Laryngotracheobronchitis (croup) is characterized by:
a. mild to moderate stridor, often worse at night.
b. antecedent "cold" symptoms.
c. swelling of subglottic tissues.
d. a "barking" cough.
e. All of the above are correct.

9. The most common cause of bronchiolitis is:
a. *H. influenzae.*
b. exposure to allergens.
c. parainfluenza virus.
d. respiratory syncytial virus.

10. Streptococcal pneumonia in children is acute and tends to occur in:
a. the winter.
b. the early spring.
c. the fall months.
d. the summer.
e. any season.

11. Staphylococcal pneumonia in children has its highest incidence at:
a. 2 to 3 years.
b. 1 to 4 years.
c. 1 week to 2 years.
d. 1 to 12 years.

12. Bronchiolitis:
    a. causes destruction of ciliated cells.
    b. can cause atelectasis.
    c. can cause hyperinflation.
    d. All of the above are correct.

13. All of the following statements about foreign body aspiration are true *except:*
    a. it is a relatively common occurrence in childhood.
    b. the offending objects include food and toys.
    c. can cause pneumonia and atelectasis.
    d. it may cause pneumonias and lung abscess.
    e. Both b and c are correct.

14. Which statement is true concerning cystic fibrosis?
    a. It is a multisystem disease.
    b. Defect results in overproduction of viscous mucus.
    c. It is difficult to detect carriers through genetic testing.
    d. Infectious complications are common.
    e. a, b, and d are correct.

15. Which statement is true concerning asthma?
    a. Its triggers include allergy, viruses, and exercise.
    b. Once asymptomatic for a number of years, affected individuals may be assumed to be cured.
    c. It is characterized by hyperresponsive airways.
    d. Both a and c are correct.
    e. a, b, and c are correct.

16. Which statement is true concerning childhood obstructive sleep apnea syndrome?
    a. Its estimated prevalence is 1% to 10%.
    b. It is usually seen when accompanied by adeno-tonsillar hypertrophy.
    c. There may be episodic increased respiratory effort but no audible airflow.
    d. All of the above are correct.

Match the characteristic or cause with the alteration.

_____17. expiratory wheezing

_____18. autosomal recessive disease

_____19. a right-to-left shunt

_____20. may be an outcome of prematurity

_____21. acute life-threatening infection

_____22. parainfluenza virus

_____23. prone position increases incidence

_____24. spasm of vocal cords occurs as inflammation intensifies

_____25. inflammatory basis with hyperresponsive airways

a. asthma

b. cystic fibrosis

c. laryngotracheobronchitis (croup)

d. SIDS

e. epiglottitis

f. respiratory distress syndrome

Case Study

Tyler C. is a 2-month-old boy who saw his physician 3 days ago with a history of mild nasal congestion without fever, cough, vomiting, or other complaints. His parents stated, however, that they were just getting over "terrible winter colds" and hoped they had not given it to Tyler.

Tyler has returned today because his mother is concerned that he is coughing severely, not feeding well at all, and "breathes funny." He still has no significant fever but is somewhat lethargic with a high respiratory rate, moderate intercostal retractions, nasal flaring, and light expiratory wheeze. Tyler is admitted to the hospital for further treatment.

A chest radiograph was taken, and pulmonary function tests were done. The chest radiograph revealed a flat, low diaphragm with lung hyperinflation but clear fields. Pulmonary function tests showed decreased tidal volume and vital capacity, increased total lung capacity, and prolonged forced expiratory volume.

What do Tyler's signs and symptoms suggest, and what is causing his signs? Why is hospitalization necessary?

28

Structure and Function of the Renal and Urologic Systems

Objectives

After reviewing this chapter, the learner will be able to do the following:

1. **Describe or identify the organs of the urinary system and the gross anatomic features of the kidneys.**
   Review pages 808 and 811-812; refer to Figures 28-1, 28-2, and 28-7.

2. **Describe the microscopic structure of the nephron.**
   Review pages 808-812; refer to Figures 28-3 through 28-6.

3. **Identify the determinants of renal blood flow.**
   Review pages 813-815; refer to Figures 28-8 and 28-9.

4. **Describe the process of glomerular filtration.**
   Review pages 815-817; refer to Figures 28-10 and 28-11 and Table 28-1.

5. **Describe the process of tubular reabsorption and tubular secretion.**
   Review pages 817-818; refer to Figure 28-12.

6. **Differentiate the substances reabsorbed and secreted by different segments of the nephron tubules.**
   Refer to Figure 28-10.

7. **Describe the purposes of the countercurrent exchange system; note the actions of diuretics.**
   Review pages 818-820; refer to Figure 28-13 and Table 28-2.

8. **Identify the effects of hormones activated or synthesized by the kidney.**
   Review pages 820-821.

9. **Identify the changes that occur in renal function with advancing age.**
   Review page 822.

Practice Examination

1. Which sequence of structures does urine pass through as it leaves the body?
   a. 2, 4, 6, 1, 3, 5   1. ureter
   b. 4, 2, 6, 1, 3, 5   2. renal pelvis
   c. 6, 4, 2, 1, 3, 5   3. urinary bladder
   d. 2, 6, 4, 5, 3, 1   4. major calyx
   e. 6, 4, 2, 5, 3, 1   5. urethra
                        6. minor calyx

2. The functional unit of the human kidney is the:
   a. nephron.
   b. collecting tubule (duct).
   c. major calyx.
   d. minor calyx.
   e. pyramid.

3. One feature of the renal blood circulation that makes it unique is that:
   a. blood flows from arterioles into venules.
   b. blood flows from venules into arterioles.
   c. there is a double set of venules.
   d. there are two sets of capillaries.

4. Which has the opposite effect on urine production from the others?
   a. decreased solutes in blood
   b. decreased blood pressure
   c. increased ambient temperature
   d. dehydration
   e. reduced water consumption

5. The glomerular filtration rate is regulated by:
   a. the autonomic nervous system.
   b. the renin-angiotensin system.
   c. atrial natriuretic factor.
   d. All of the above are correct.
   e. Both a and b are correct.

6. If the following hypothetical conditions exist in the nephron, what would be the net (effective) filtration pressure?
   Glomerular blood hydrostatic = 80 mm Hg
   Glomerular blood osmotic = 20 mm Hg
   Capsular hydrostatic = 30 mm Hg
   a. 40 mm Hg
   b. 30 mm Hg
   c. 20 mm Hg
   d. 10 mm Hg

7. The capillaries of the glomerulus differ from other capillary networks in the body because they:
   a. have a larger area of anastomosis.
   b. branch from and drain into arterioles.
   c. lack endothelium.
   d. force filtrate from the blood.

8. Which is *not* a function of the kidney?
   a. Water volume control
   b. Blood pressure control
   c. Urine storage
   d. Converts vitamin D to an active form

9. Potassium is secreted by the _____ and reabsorbed by the _____.
   a. Bowman capsule; loop of Henle
   b. proximal convoluted tubule; distal convoluted tubule
   c. loop of Henle; collecting ducts
   d. distal convoluted tubule; proximal convoluted tubule
   e. collecting ducts; loop of Henle

10. ADH causes water to:
    a. diffuse into the ascending limb of the vasa recta.
    b. return to the systemic circulation.
    c. be reabsorbed at the proximal tubule.
    d. Both a and b are correct.
    e. a, b, and c are correct.

11. Water reabsorbed from the glomerular filtrate initially enters the:
    a. afferent arterioles.
    b. efferent arterioles.
    c. Bowman's capsule.
    d. glomerulus.
    e. vasa recta.

12. Plasma contains a much greater concentration of _____ than the glomerular filtrate.
    a. sodium
    b. protein
    c. urea
    d. creatinine

13. An increase in water permeability of the distal convoluted tubules and collection duct is due to:
    a. a decrease in the production of antidiuretic hormone (ADH).
    b. an increase in production of ADH.
    c. a decrease in blood plasma osmolality.
    d. an increase in water content within tubular cells.
    e. None of the above is correct.

14. The descending loop of the nephron allows:
    a. sodium secretion.
    b. potassium secretion.
    c. hydrogen ion secretion.
    d. water reabsorption.

15. Which most accurately describes the pressures affecting net glomerular filtration?
    a. Blood osmotic opposes capsular hydrostatic and blood hydrostatic.
    b. Blood hydrostatic opposes capsular hydrostatic and blood oncotic.
    c. Capsular hydrostatic opposes blood osmotic and blood hydrostatic.
    d. None of the above is correct.

16. Tubular secretion of urea is accomplished in the:
    a. glomerulus.
    b. urethra.
    c. renal pelvis.
    d. distal convoluted tubule.
    e. None of the above is correct.

17. Tubular reabsorption and tubular secretion differ in that:
    a. secretion adds material to the filtrate; reabsorption removes materials from the filtrate.
    b. secretion is a passive process; reabsorption is an active transport process.
    c. reabsorption tends to increase urine volume; secretion tends to decrease urine volume.
    d. secretion adds materials to the blood; reabsorption removes materials from the blood.

18. The kidneys (more than one answer may be correct):
    a. conserve H^+.
    b. conserve NH_4^+.
    c. eliminate H^+.
    d. eliminate NH_4^+.
    e. conserve HCO_3^-.

19. If a small person excretes about 1 liter of urine during a 24-hour period, estimate the total amount of glomerular filtrate formed.
    a. 4 liters
    b. 10 liters
    c. 18 liters
    d. 100 liters

20. Which should *not* appear in the glomerular filtrate (in any significant quantity) just after the process of glomerular filtration has been accomplished?
    a. protein
    b. urea
    c. glucose
    d. Both a and b are correct

21. Loop of Henle is to vasa recta as convoluted tubules are to:
    a. afferent arterioles.
    b. peritubular capillaries.
    c. efferent arterioles.
    d. renal arteries.

22. The two "currents" used in the countercurrent exchange system are the:
    a. afferent and efferent arterioles.
    b. glomerulus and glomerular (Bowman) capsule.
    c. ascending and descending limbs.
    d. proximal and distal tubules.
    e. All of the above are correct.

23. The countercurrent exchange system:
    a. prevents water reabsorption from the collecting duct.
    b. concentrates sodium in the renal cortex.
    c. facilitates osmosis.
    d. concentrates chloride in the renal cortex.
    e. None of the above is correct.

24. Atrial natriuretic factor (ANF):
    a. increases ADH secretion.
    b. is produced by the kidney.
    c. increases urine output.
    d. decreases urine output.

25. A waste product of protein metabolism is:
    a. pepsinogen.
    b. trypsin.
    c. amino acid.
    d. urea.
    e. urine.

29

Alterations of Renal and Urinary Tract Function

a. **Define the renal processes of filtration, reabsorption, and secretion.**
   Review pages 815-818; refer to Figure 28-10.

MEMORY CHECK!

- Glomerular filtration is the first step in urine formation in which permeable substances from the blood are filtered at the endothelial-capsular membrane into the Bowman capsule; the filtrate there enters the proximal convoluted tubule.

- Tubular reabsorption retains substances needed by the body, including water, glucose, sodium, potassium, and bicarbonate. This process removes materials from the filtrate and returns them to the blood.

- Tubular secretion excretes chemicals not needed by the body, including hydrogen and some amino acids, urea, creatinine, and some drugs. Secretion adds material to the filtrate from the blood.

b. **Identify the forces and factors determining net filtration pressure; explain cause and effect of decreased filtration pressure.**
   Refer to Figure 28-11 and Table 28-1.

MEMORY CHECK!

- Net filtration pressure (NFP) is equal to glomerular blood hydrostatic pressure (GBHP) minus capsular hydrostatic pressure (CHP) plus blood oncotic pressure. Stated mathematically, the formula is NFP = GBHP − (CHP + BOP). The pressure promoting filtration into the Bowman space is 47 mm Hg due to GBHP, whereas the pressure resisting flow to the Bowman space is 35 mm Hg due to 10 mm Hg of pressure from the Bowman capsule CHP and 25 mm Hg from BOP. This provides a small net filtration pressure of 12 mm Hg. This net filtration pressure can be reduced by renal vasoconstriction, hypotension, hypovolemia, or low cardiac output. Any of these circumstances will reduce glomerular filtration rate (GFR). The GFR is directly related to renal blood flow (RBF), which is regulated by intrinsic neural and hormonal autoregulation. The blood flow is determined by arteriovenous pressure differences across the vascular bed divided by the vascular resistance or, stated mathematically, RBF = PA − PV/R. As pressure increases and resistance decreases, renal blood flow increases. Sympathetic nerve activity stimulates renal arteriolar vasoconstriction and decreases both RBF and GFR.

MEMORY CHECK!—cont'd

EFFECTS OF RENIN-ANGIOTENSIN SYSTEM

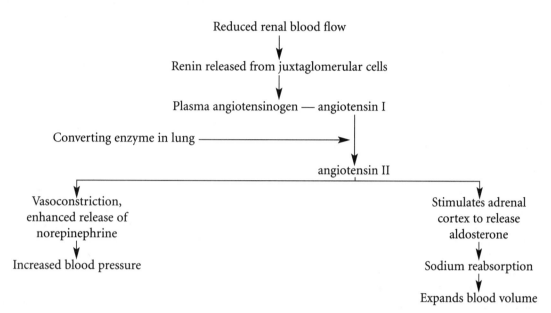

NOTE: The increase in circulating blood volume increases venous return and arterial pressure. The renin-angiotensin system affects both the renal and cardiovascular systems.

c. **Explain the basis of serum and urinalysis examinations to evaluate renal function.**
   Review pages 821-822; refer to Table 28-3.

MEMORY CHECK!

LABORATORY TESTS FOR KIDNEY FUNCTION
- Blood urea nitrogen (BUN) measures the concentration of urea in the blood. Urea is formed from protein metabolism and is elevated in reduced glomerular filtration. Normal BUN is 10 to 20 mg/dl. The BUN rises in states of dehydration and acute and chronic renal failure because passage of fluid through the tubules is slowed.

- The serum creatinine level should have a stable value because creatinine is a byproduct of muscle metabolism and its levels of production are constant and are proportional to muscle mass. Normally, it is not reabsorbed. If normal serum levels of 0.7 to 1.2 mg/dl exist, it indicates normal renal function. When creatinine rises and accumulates in the plasma, it represents decreasing GFR. If doubled, renal function is probably half of normal. If tripled, about 75% of renal function is lost.

- Creatinine clearance is the amount of blood theoretically "cleared" of creatinine by the kidney in 1 minute of filtration; 90 to 130 ml/min is normal. Creatinine clearance provides a good measure of renal blood flow and GFR because serum levels are related to a 24-hour urine volume. Inulin, a substance with a stable plasma concentration, can be used to assess clearance. The amount of inulin filtered is equal to the volume of plasma filtered multiplied by the plasma concentration of insulin.

- The urinalysis is an essential part of the examination of all individuals who may have renal disease because materials in the urine can be diagnostic for many disorders. It is normal to have inorganic material such as Na^+, Cl^-, and K^+ and organic materials such as urea and creatinine in the urine. It is abnormal to find RBCs, more than a few WBCs, bacteria, protein, glucose, or ketones in the urine.

Objectives

After studying this chapter, the learner will be able to do the following:

1. **Describe the general features of urinary tract obstruction.**
   Study pages 826-827; refer to Figures 29-1 and 29-2.

Urinary tract obstruction is an interference with the flow of urine at any site along the urinary tract. The obstruction may be anatomic or functional; it impedes flow proximal to the blockage, dilates the urinary system, increases the risk for infection, and compromises renal function. Common causes of upper urinary tract obstruction include stricture or congenital compression of a calyx or the ureteropelvic or ureterovesical junction, stones (calculi), compression from an aberrant vessel, tumor or abdominal inflammation and scarring (retroperitoneal fibrosis), or ureteral blockage from a malignancy of the renal pelvis, ureter, bladder, or prostate. Obstruction of the lower urinary tract is often caused by benign or malignant prostate enlargement in men, urethral stricture, incoordination between the detrusor muscle and urethral sphincter (vesicosphincter dyssynergia) or severe pelvic organ prolapse in women.

The most serious complications are hydronephrosis, hydroureter, ureterohydronephrosis, and infection caused by accumulation of urine behind the obstruction. Another complication is hypertension.

2. **Describe kidney stones.**
   Study pages 827-829; refer to Figure 29-2.

Calcium is a common constituent of renal stones; about 80% of stones, or **renal calculi,** are composed of calcium oxalate, calcium phosphate, or a combination of both. Another stone, the struvite stone (makes up 15% of stones), is composed of magnesium ammonium phosphate. Uric acid stones, about 7% of stones, may be seen with gout. Rarely, cystine stones are seen in individuals with a genetic defect in transporting cystine.

A colicky pain occurs as the rhythmic contractions of the ureter attempt to dislodge and advance the sharp-edged stone. The accumulation of urine behind the stone causes infection or damage to organs. This consequence of obstruction depends on the location of the obstruction. If high and complete, glomerular filtration may be affected. The pain may be in the flank or between the last rib and the lumbar vertebrae, or it may radiate into the groin, depending on the stone's location.

Treatment involves dilution of stone-forming substances by a high fluid and fiber intake, extraction of larger stones by instrumentation and fragmentation of stones by ultrasonic lithotripsy, and laser treatment. Some smaller stones may pass spontaneously.

3. **Characterize neurogenic bladder dysfunction.**
   Study pages 829-831; refer to Figure 29-3.

Neurogenic bladder is a functional urinary tract obstruction caused by an interruption of the nerve supply to the bladder. The neurologic disruption can occur in the central nervous system or at the level of the spinal cord. Resulting bladder paralysis interferes with the normal flow of urine. Lesions occurring in the cortex or below the cortex but above the sacral level of the spinal cord cause loss of voluntary control of voiding. Lesions occurring at the sacral level of the spinal cord cause loss of both voluntary and involuntary control of urination.

Because of disordered sensation, symptoms are difficult to assess. Management involves use of a pessary to compensate for reversal of pelvic organ prolapse, catheterization, drugs, or surgery to relieve obstruction. Any infection must be treated with appropriate antibiotics.

4. **Describe renal and bladder tumors.**
   Study pages 831-832; refer to Figure 29-4 and Tables 29-1 and 29-2.

Renal adenomas are uncommon, but they may become malignant and are therefore usually surgically removed. **Renal carcinoma** is the most common renal neoplasm and usually occurs in men between the ages of 50 and 60 years. An association between tobacco use and renal cell carcinoma exists. The tumors usually occur unilaterally and spread through the lymph nodes and blood vessels to the lungs, liver, and bones.

The manifestations are hematuria, flank pain, palpable flank mass, and weight loss. These signs and symptoms are infrequent; when they occur, they indicate an advanced stage of disease.

Treatment is usually surgical removal of the affected kidney combined with use of chemotherapy. Radiation therapy and biologic response modifiers may be useful.

Bladder tumors represent about 2% of all malignant tumors and are the fifth most common malignancy. The development of bladder cancer is most common in men older than 60 years of age.

The risk of primary bladder cancer is greater among individuals who smoke or work in the chemical, rubber, and textile industry and among women who take large amounts of phenacetin (an analgesic). Bladder cancer re-

Cystitis and Pyelonephritis

	Cystitis (bladder)	Pyelonephritis* (kidney tubules, pelvis, and interstitium)
	Lower Tract Infection	Upper Tract Infection
Signs/Symptoms	Low back or suprapubic pain, painful burning on urination, frequent voiding/urgency, hematuria, cloudy urine	Fever, chills, backache, abdominal pain, nausea, vomiting, urinary urgency and frequency, costovertebral tenderness
Etiology	Urinary obstruction, prostatitis, ascending infection with gram-negative rods ("honeymoon cystitis"), irritable bladder from sphincter dysfunction, interstitial "nonbacterial" cystitis caused by an inflammatory autoimmune response	Inflammation or scarring of the interstitial tissue and tubules; causative organism is usually an ascending gram-negative rod but can be fungi or viruses; a risk factor is any urinary obstruction or condition that causes urine reflux or residual urine

*Acute pyelonephritis involves an infection that exhibits inflammation of the pelvis, calyce, and medulla. Chronic pyelonephritis is persistent or recurrent autoimmune infection usually associated with an obstructive pathologic condition. It can lead to renal failure.

sults from a genetic alteration in normal bladder epithelium. Metastasis is usually to lymph nodes, liver, bones, and lungs. Secondary bladder cancer develops by invasion of cancer from bordering organs such as cervical carcinoma in women and prostatic carcinoma in men.

Bladder tumors may be asymptomatic or accompanied by hematuria. Advanced cancers are associated with pelvic pain and frequent urination. Treatment depends on the type and size of the lesion and involves resection, chemotherapy, or immunotherapy.

5. **Identify the predisposing risk factor, and the most likely pathogens responsible for urinary tract infections (UTIs).**
   Study pages 832-833.

In these infections, predisposing factors are very important. Factors include fecal contamination of the urethra, particularly in the female; sexual activity; catheterization or instrumentation of the urinary tract; urinary obstruction, which causes the flushing effects of urination to be reduced; and diaphragm spermatocidal usage.

The most common route in the development of acute urinary tract infection is by an ascending infection. Common pathogens in these infections are the gram-negative rods, namely *E. coli*, Klebsiella, *Staphylococcus saprophyticus*, Proteus, and Pseudomonas. Other possible infectious agents are gram-positive cocci, mycobacteria, and fungi.

6. **Compare and contrast the signs, symptoms, and etiology of cystitis and pyelonephritis.**
   Study pages 834-835; refer to Figure 29-5 and Table 29-3.

7. **Describe the types of glomerulonephritis, its features, manifestations, and treatment.**
   Study pages 835-838; refer to Figure 29-6 and Tables 29-4 through 29-6.

Glomerular damage generally occurs from activation of biochemical mediators of inflammation, namely complement, leukocytes, and fibrin. Damage begins after antibodies against glomerular basement membrane or antigen-antibody complexes have localized in the glomerular capillary wall. Complement activation attracts neutrophils and monocytes. The neutrophils and monocytes further the inflammatory reaction by releasing lysosomal enzymes, which damage glomerular walls and increase glomerular capillary wall permeability. Membrane damage can lead to platelet aggregation and degranulation, wherein platelets release vasoactive amines. Changes in membrane permeability permit the passage of protein molecules and red blood cells into the urine, causing proteinuria and hematuria. The coagulation system also may be activated and may lead to fibrin deposition in the Bowman space; this reduces renal blood flow and depresses glomerular filtration.

Mild proteinuria and hematuria occur during the early years of the disease. After 10 or 20 years, renal insufficiency will develop followed by nephrotic syndrome and an accelerated progression to end-stage renal failure.

The diagnosis of glomerular disease is confirmed by a urinalysis that shows proteinuria, red blood cells, white blood cells, and casts. The basic principles for treating glomerulonephritis are related to treating the primary disease, preventing or minimizing immune responses, and correcting accompanying problems such as edema, hypertension, and hyperlipidemia. Antibiotic therapy is essential for management of underlying infections. Dialysis or kidney transplantation ultimately may be necessary. (See the box on this page.)

8. Identify and explain key features of nephrotic syndrome.
Study pages 838-839; refer to Table 29-7.

In **nephrotic syndrome,** there is increased glomerular permeability and protein leakage of 3.5 g or more in the urine per day.

The key features of nephrotic syndrome include proteinuria, edema, hypoalbuminemia, hyperlipidemia, and lipiduria. Proteinuria occurs with protein leakage from the serum into the urine; this process reduces blood oncotic pressure. Thus water leaves the capillaries more easily and tissue edema follows. The edema is soft, pitting, and generalized. Hypoalbuminemia develops as albumin leaks through the capillaries and depletes its serum level. Hyperlipidemia occurs as the liver responds to the hypoalbuminemia by synthesizing replacement albumin. While synthesizing albumin, the liver also synthesizes lipoproteins in large amounts; therefore, hyperlipidemia develops. As tubular cells containing fat are sloughed into the urine, lipiduria can be seen. Also, free fat from the hyperlipidemia leaks across the glomerulus. Loss of protein immunoglobulins increases susceptibility to infection in nephrotic syndrome.

Treatment is with a normal protein, low-fat diet; salt restriction; diuretics; steroids; and occasionally, albumin replacement.

Common Types of Glomerulonephritis

Type and Cause	Pathophysiology
Poststreptococcal Group A beta-hemolytic streptococci	Diffuse, subepithelial deposits of immune and complement complexes, phagocytic infiltration, and occlusion of glomerular capillary blood flow decreasing glomerular filtration
Rapidly progressive (RPGN)* or crescentic Nonspecific response to glomerular injury	Diffuse accumulation of immune deposits and macrophages or epithelial cell proliferation into Bowman space, which form crescents and occlude glomerular filtration; antiglomerular basement membrane antibodies lead to damaged tissue and renal failure
Membranoproliferative Usually idiopathic, associated with activation of complement pathways	Thickened basement membrane reduces glomerular capillary blood flow and decreases glomerular filtration
IgA nephropathy Usually idiopathic, no systemic immunologic disease	Focal, some diffuse lesions, IgA deposits, and mediators decrease GFR
Minimal change disease or lipoid nephrosis Usually idiopathic	Diffuse fusion of epithelial processes, loss of negative charge in basement membrane, and increased permeability lead to proteinuria and nephrotic syndrome
Focal glomerulosclerosis Usually idiopathic	Similar pathology to minimal change disease
Membranous nephropathy Usually idiopathic, can be associated with systemic disease	Diffuse thickening of glomerular capillary wall increases permeability with proteinuria and nephrotic syndrome

*Goodpasture syndrome is a type of RPGN associated with antibody formation against both pulmonary capillary and glomerular basement membranes.

9. Define and identify the common etiologies for prerenal, intrarenal, and postrenal disease.

Study pages 839-842; refer to Figure 29-7 and Tables 29-8 and 29-9.

Acute renal failure is the rapid deterioration of renal function with accompanying elevation of BUN and plasma creatinine; oliguria also develops. The etiology may be either prerenal (before kidney) because of renal hypoperfusion, intrarenal (within kidney) from renal functional impairment, or postrenal (after kidney) following obstruction of urinary flow.

The clinical progression has three phases: oliguria, diuresis, and recovery of renal function. BUN and plasma creatinine concentrations increase. The primary goal is to maintain life until renal function returns. Management involves correcting fluid and electrolyte imbalances, treating infections, and providing nutrients.

10. Describe chronic renal failure; identify the systemic manifestations of uremia.

Study page 842; refer to Tables 29-10 and 29-11.

Chronic renal failure symptoms and signs usually do not develop until GFR declines to 25% of normal. The chronic alteration is primarily because of loss of nephron mass. The clinical manifestations of chronic renal failure are described as **uremia.** The uremic state is characterized by a decline in renal function and the accumulation of toxins in the blood. If the lesions are tubular, electrolyte imbalances, volume depletions, and metabolic acidosis occur. In glomerular lesions, hematuria and nephrotic syndrome develop.

Uremia is a toxic condition associated with widespread effects on all body systems.

Causes of Acute Renal Failure

Prerenal	Intrarenal	Postrenal
Hypovolemia	Prolonged renal ischemia	Ureteral obstructions
Hemorrhage	Nephrotoxins	Edema, tumors, stones, clots
Hypotension	Glomerulonephritis	Bladder outlet obstruction
Cardiac failure	Intratubular obstructions or necrosis	Prostatic hyperplasia, urethral strictures
Interruption of renal artery flow		

Uremia

Skeletal	Cardiopulmonary	Integumentary	Hematologic
Bone demineralization	Hypertension	Pruritus	Anemia
	Pericarditis	Pigmentation	Bleeding
	Pulmonary edema		Infection
			Suppressed immunity

Metabolic	Gastrointestinal	Neurologic	Reproductive
Acidosis	Diarrhea	Fatigue	Infertility
Hyperuricemia	Nausea	Attention deficit	Decreased libido
Hypocalcemia	Vomiting	Irritability	Impotence
Hyperkalemia	Anorexia	Peripheral neuropathy	Amenorrhea
	Urinous breath	Stupor	
		Coma	

NOTE: If chronic renal failure cannot be managed with diet, diuretics, and fluid restriction, then dialysis or transplantation becomes necessary.

Practice Examination

1. Renal function tests include:
   a. the urinalysis.
   b. BUN and serum creatinine.
   c. SGOT/SGPT.
   d. Both a and b are correct.
   e. a, b, and c are correct.

2. Which substance is an abnormal constituent of urine?
   a. urea
   b. glucose
   c. sodium chloride
   d. creatinine

3. The presence of albumin in the urine would indicate probable damage to:
   a. glomeruli.
   b. renal columns.
   c. collecting tubules.
   d. pyramids.
   e. None of the above is correct.

4. Which statement is *not* true concerning urinary tract infections?
   a. Once cystitis develops, pyelonephritis will certainly occur.
   b. They are usually due to coliforms, especially *E. coli.*
   c. Organisms probably enter the bladder by way of the urethra.
   d. The patient may be asymptomatic.

5. Renal calculi may be composed of:
   a. calcium oxalate.
   b. uric acid.
   c. cholesterol.
   d. All of the above are correct.
   e. Both a and b are correct.

6. Which can be characteristic of ureteral stones?
   a. severe pain in back
   b. severe pain in abdomen
   c. nausea and vomiting
   d. All of the above are correct.
   e. Both a and c are correct.

7. Which are predisposing factors for acute urinary tract infections? (More than one answer may be correct.)
   a. congenital deformities of urinary tract
   b. the sex of the patient
   c. decreased urine flow
   d. increased urine flow
   e. increased fluid intake

8. A common cause of both pyelonephritis and cystitis is:
   a. urinary calculi.
   b. invading microorganisms, such as *E. coli.*
   c. allergy reactions.
   d. heavy metals.

9. Uremia exhibits:
   a. polycythemia.
   b. retention of metabolic acids.
   c. low plasma calcium levels.
   d. increased erythropoiesis.
   e. Both a and d are correct.

10. Pyelonephritis is (more than one answer may be correct):
    a. an inflammation and infection of the urinary bladder.
    b. characterized by fever, chills, and flank pain.
    c. characterized by pyuria, bacteriuria, and hematuria.
    d. more common in young women than in young men.

11. Which renal condition usually has a history of recent infection with beta-hemolytic streptococci?
    a. pyelonephritis
    b. chronic renal failure
    c. nephrosis
    d. glomerulonephritis
    e. calculi

12. Which statement is *not* true concerning glomerulonephritis?
    a. Significant damage to kidneys occurs during the body's response to an infection.
    b. Fever and flank pain occur.
    c. Complement activation attracts neutrophils.
    d. It is characterized by hematuria, proteinuria, and the presence of casts.
    e. Approximately 90% of individuals develop chronic disease.

13. Nephrotic syndrome is associated with _____ to
    plasma _____.
    a. increased glomerular permeability; urea
    b. decreased glomerular permeability; proteins
    c. decreased glomerular permeability; tubular fil-
       trate
    d. increased glomerular permeability; proteins

14. Causes of acute renal failure include:
    a. cholecystitis.
    b. stones and strictures in kidneys or ureters.
    c. heart failure leading to poor renal perfusion.
    d. Both b and c are correct.
    e. a, b, and c are correct.

15. Which describe a patient in acute renal failure?
    (More than one answer may be correct.)
    a. elevated serum creatinine
    b. leukocytosis
    c. low BUN
    d. fever
    e. oliguria

16. Which is *not* a characteristic of chronic renal fail-
    ure?
    a. hyperkalemia
    b. anuria
    c. anemia
    d. pruritus
    e. acidosis

17. Chronic renal failure:
    a. may result from hypertension.
    b. is usually the result of chronic inflammation of
       the kidney.
    c. may be treated with dialysis or transplants.
    d. All of the above are correct.
    e. Both a and c are correct.

18. An individual has an elevated blood level of urea
    and creatinine because of complete calculi blockage
    of one ureter. This is referred to as:
    a. prerenal disease.
    b. intrarenal disease.
    c. postrenal disease.
    d. preeclampsia.
    e. hypercalcemia.

19. Nephrotoxins, such as antibiotics, may be responsi-
    ble for:
    a. acute tubular necrosis.
    b. acute glomerulonephritis.
    c. pyelonephritis.
    d. cystitis.

20. Uremia, as seen in chronic renal failure, would in-
    clude:
    a. metabolic acidosis.
    b. elevated BUN and creatinine.
    c. cardiovascular disturbances.
    d. All of the above are correct.

21. The earliest symptom of chronic renal failure is:
    a. pruritus.
    b. oliguria.
    c. polyuria.
    d. decreased BUN.

22. In chronic renal failure, tubulointerstitial disease
    leads to:
    a. sodium retention.
    b. sodium wasting.
    c. no significant changes in sodium levels.
    d. increased phosphate excretion.

Match the condition with its characteristic.

_____23. Goodpasture syndrome

_____24. hypovolemia

_____25. uremia

a. prerenal failure

b. postrenal failure

c. chronic glomerulonephritis

d. pulmonary capillary and glomerular basement membrane antibodies

e. pruritus

Case Study

Mr. and Mrs. C. returned from a weekend of downhill skiing to find their 9-year-old son, Eddie, with bloody urine. About 6 weeks earlier, they had spent a week skiing, during which Eddie had a severe sore throat that was not treated because his teenage sitter did not take him to a physician.

Eddie was taken to his pediatrician where it was established that he had been lethargic and without appetite for the past 10 days and had complained of back pain. His physical examination showed a temperature of 101° F and a blood pressure of 140/102. The remainder of the physical was noncontributory. Eddie's urinalysis showed blood, protein, and RBC casts with an elevated specific gravity. BUN and serum creatinine were elevated.

What do you think is the likely cause of Eddie's symptoms and signs? What do you think the pediatrician will do?

Alterations of Renal and Urinary Tract Function in Children

Foundational Objective

a. **Describe fluid balance in children; explain the implications of imbalances.**
   Review page 822.

MEMORY CHECK!

- Infants and young children have a larger ratio of body water to body weight than adults. Children exchange half of their extracellular water each day. When children become ill, they tend to retain fluid because of lowered osmotic pressure. Children have limited ability to concentrate urine because of higher renal blood flow and shorter tubular length. Fluid and electrolyte balance is very sensitive to the slightest changes in any of these factors.

Objectives

After studying this chapter, the learner will be able to do the following:

1. **Describe the common congenital/structural anomalies that occur within the renal and urologic system.**
   Study pages 850-852; refer to Figures 30-1 through 30-3.

   Structural defects range from minor, easily correctable anomalies to those incompatible with life. **Hypospadias,** with or without **chordae** and its band of fibrous tissue that deviates the penis ventrally, has the urethral meatus located ventrally. **Epispadias** has the urethra opening dor-

sally. Hypospadias is the more common penile defect, with an incidence of 1 in 300 infant boys, and is usually easily corrected with surgery. Epispadias is a more complex problem because it extends into the bladder, but it has a lower incidence rate, approximately 1 in 200,000 boys and 1 in 400,000 girls. This also can be surgically corrected but requires a more involved intervention.

   Exstrophy of the bladder is a defect wherein the bladder and associated urinary tract structures are exposed to the surface of the body. This defect involves the abdominal wall and the pubic bone. Incidence is 1 in

40,000, of which three-fourths are boys. This defect allows urine to leak from the ureters onto the abdominal wall, leading to excoriation of the skin and the persistent odor of urine. The exposed bladder mucosa becomes edematous, bleeds easily, and is painful. Surgical repair requires several stages, the first during the first few days of life and the last at about age 3. Neoplastic changes have been associated with exstrophy of the bladder.

Congenital urethral valves consist of thin membranes of tissue that occlude the urethral lumen and obstruct urinary flow in males. Another bladder outlet obstruction can be a polyp that arises from the prostatic urethra and may cause severe obstruction and impair renal embryogenesis. Both must be resected early.

Ureteropelvic junction (UPI) obstruction is a blockage at the point where the renal pelvis transitions into the ureter. It is the most common cause of hydronephrosis in the neonate. Any infection must be treated and recurrent infections may require surgical repair.

Structural changes of the kidney may be categorized as those that affect renal function and those that do not; they may occur unilaterally or bilaterally. **Unilateral agenesis** occurs in approximately 1 in 1000 births and has little or no effect on function if one of the kidneys is normal. **Bilateral agenesis,** or Potter syndrome, occurs in approximately 1 in 3000 births and is usually associated with other anomalies including facial defects; affected infants rarely live more than a few hours. A **hypoplastic kidney** may be small but functionally normal, or underdeveloped and functionally abnormal. The bilateral form is a common cause of chronic renal failure. **Renal dysplasia** is associated with obstructions of the renal collecting system. **Polycystic kidney disease** is an autosomal dominant inherited disorder. The affected kidney has large fluid-filled cysts of the tubules and collecting ducts.

2. **Note glomerular disorders in children; describe the pathophysiology and clinical manifestations of hemolytic uremic syndrome and immunoglobulin A nephropathy and their treatment.**
   Study pages 852-854.

Nephrotic syndrome and **glomerulonephritis** in children express pathophysiologic mechanisms similar to those observed in adults. **Hemolytic uremic syndrome** is associated with a viral or bacterial illness and is preceded 1 or 2 weeks by an upper respiratory or gastrointestinal infection. The antecedent infection causes endothelial injury to the glomerular arterioles. This event triggers the inflammatory cascade, resulting in platelet aggregation and fibrin clot formation that narrows the arterioles. Anemia results when erythrocytes and platelets are damaged while passing through narrowed and inflamed glomerular arterioles and are later removed by the spleen. This same thrombocyte and fibrin clot mechanism activates the fibrinolytic cascade that prompts the release of damaged platelets from the arterioles. These damaged platelets are also removed by the spleen. Thrombocytosis eventually results.

Classic symptoms of hemolytic uremic syndrome are pallor, bruising or purpura, and oliguria that may be accompanied by fever, vomiting, bloody diarrhea, abdominal pain, and jaundice. Central nervous system involvement, seizures, and lethargy may be features of severe disease.

Treatment is supportive and includes transfusions of red blood cells and platelets to treat the anemia and thrombocytopenia. Peritoneal dialysis may be required to regulate fluids and electrolytes until renal function returns to normal.

Immunoglobulin A (IgA) nephropathy is the most common form of glomerulonephritis worldwide. It is characterized by deposition mainly of the immunoglobulin IgA in glomerular capillaries and mesangium. No systemic immunologic disease is evident. Deposits of IgA cause immune injury to the glomerulus, which is usually reversible.

Children with the disease have recurrent gross hematuria, often after a respiratory infection. Most continue to have microscopic hematuria between the attacks of gross hematuria and have a mild proteinuria as well. Treatment is supportive because kidney damage is generally insignificant. Approximately 20% of affected children develop the progressive form of the disease with hypertension and decreasing renal function. These children eventually require dialysis and transplantation.

3. **Identify the structural cause of vesicoureteral reflux and explain the potential effects on renal function.**
   Study pages 855-856; refer to Figures 30-4 and 30-5.

Primary vesicoureteral reflux is caused by the congenital malpositioning of a ureter or ureters into the bladder that allows retrograde urine to flow up the ureters. If the urine contains microorganisms and can reach the renal parenchyma, chronic infection and scarring may result. The combination of reflux and infection can cause pyelonephritis. This condition is classified by a grading system, with grade I the most mild and grade V the most severe. **Secondary vesicoureteral reflux** occurs because an infection causes mucosal edema and interferes with the antireflux mechanisms of the urinary tract. It is also associated with malformations of the ureterovesical (UV) junction, increased intravesical pressures, or surgery of the UV junction.

Symptoms associated with vesicoureteral reflux include fever, recurrent urinary tract infections, and poor feeding. Diagnosis is confirmed by a radiologic procedure that allows visualization of reflux during voiding. Treatment goals are to prevent infection and to protect and preserve renal function. Recurrent infection and grade V status are indications for surgical repair.

4. Characterize nephroblastoma (Wilms tumor).
Study page 856; refer to Table 30-1.

Nephroblastoma, or Wilms tumors, is an embryonic tumor. The peak age of diagnosis is 2 to 3 years of age, with an incidence of approximately 400 cases yearly in the United States. Nephroblastoma may occur as a sporadic phenomenon, or it may be inherited. The inherited form is an autosomal dominant disorder but is rare. The occurrence has been found to be caused by the deletion or inactivation of genes on the short arm of chromosome 11. This finding tends to support the theory of tumor-suppressor genes. Other congenital genitourinary anomalies have been associated with nephroblastoma in 18% of children.

Children with nephroblastoma may be asymptomatic or may present with vague abdominal pain, hematuria, fever, or hypertension. The tumor is smooth, firm, and usually encapsulated and separated from the renal parenchyma. Diagnosis is made by locating the tumor and assessing its site by radiologic procedures such as ultrasound, computerized tomography (CT scan), or magnetic resonance imaging (MRI). Treatment is surgical excision with a heminephrectomy or total nephrectomy. Depending on the stage of the tumor, resection, chemotherapy, radiation therapy, or a combination of these modalities may be required.

5. Define primary and secondary enuresis; discuss their likely causes and common approaches to management.
Study pages 856-857; refer to Table 30-2.

Enuresis, or involuntary urination after voluntary bladder control should exist, can be classified in two categories; **primary enuresis** occurs when a child has never obtained continence and **secondary enuresis** occurs when a child has had and then loses bladder control. Secondary enuresis is also termed *acquired enuresis.* The origin may be neurologic, anatomic, or functional. Diabetes that increases the normal urinary output and renal failure that impairs the kidney's concentrating ability may cause this disorder. Enuresis shows a familial tendency. Psychologic problems have been related to enuresis in some cases and must be considered a legitimate cause in the absence of organic findings. Enuresis may be associated with sleep apnea.

Management depends on cause and may include a combination of interventions such as medication, limited fluid intake, behavior modification, alarms, or periodic awakening during sleep. Psychological counseling also may benefit the child and family.

Practice Examination

True/False

_____ 1. Exstrophy of the bladder occurs because of birth trauma.

_____ 2. Vesicoureteral reflux is caused by a congenitally malpositioned entry of the ureter or ureters into the bladder.

_____ 3. Children are at no greater risk for fluid and electrolyte imbalances than adults.

_____ 4. Grade V vesicoureteral reflux can be medically managed.

_____ 5. Polycystic kidney disease is an autosomal dominant disorder.

_____ 6. Secondary enuresis occurs when the child has never been continent.

7. Nephrotic syndrome in children manifests as:
   a. proteinuria.
   b. hyperlipidemia.
   c. lipiduria.
   d. All of the above are correct.
   e. None of the above is correct.

8. Poststreptococcal glomerulonephritis in children:
   a. is a noninfectious renal disease.
   b. causes hypotension.
   c. causes dehydration.
   d. Both b and c are correct.

9. Infants cannot concentrate urine because of:
   a. shorter tubular length.
   b. increased tubular weight.
   c. increased blood flow to the kidneys.
   d. Both a and c are correct.
   e. a, b, and c are correct.

10. Vesicoureteral reflux causes urine to _____ up the ureters and places the young child at risk for _____.
    a. retrograde; glomerulonephritis
    b. regrade; nephrotic syndrome
    c. retrograde; pyelonephritis
    d. regrade; cystitis

11. Which manifestation may be associated with vesicoureteral reflux?
    a. recurrent urinary tract infections
    b. poor growth
    c. irritability
    d. Both a and b are correct.
    e. a, b, and c are correct.

12. Children are at risk for hemolytic uremic syndrome after:
    a. upper respiratory tract infection.
    b. vomiting and/or diarrhea.
    c. viral infections.
    d. All of the above are correct.

13. Organic causes of enuresis may include:
    a. congenital abnormalities of the urinary tract.
    b. a neurologic origin.
    c. diabetes insipidus.
    d. All of the above are correct.

14. Children with enuresis may be managed by:
    a. sleep interruption.
    b. psychotherapy.
    c. diet.
    d. All of the above are correct.

15. Which characterizes IgA nephropathy?
    a. no systemic immunologic disease
    b. Injury to the glomerulus is usually reversible.
    c. gross hematuria
    d. All of the above are correct.
    e. Both a and b are correct.

16. Identify the sequence of events in hemolytic uremic syndrome that cause anemia.
    1. The damaged cells are removed from the circulation by the spleen.
    2. The endothelial lining of the glomerular arterioles becomes swollen.
    3. Narrowed vessels damage erythrocytes.
    4. Fibrin split-products appears in the urine and serum.
    a. 1, 3, 4
    b. 2, 4, 1
    c. 3, 1, 2
    d. 2, 3, 1

17. Which factor influences the prognosis of a child with nephroblastoma?
    a. the child's height
    b. genetics
    c. stage
    d. congenital anomalies
    e. b, c, and d are correct.

18. What causes neonate bladder outlet obstruction?
    a. polyps arising from the prostatic urethra
    b. congenital urethral valves
    c. impaired renal embryogenesis
    d. Both b and c are correct.
    e. a, b, and c are correct.

Match the description with the structural abnormality.

_____19. small, normally developed kidney

_____20. facial anomalies

_____21. urethral opening on the dorsal surface of the penis; a cleft along the ventral urethra in girls

_____22. results from abnormal differentiation of renal tissue

_____23. exposed bladder mucosa through a fissure in the abdominal wall

_____24. urethral meatus opening on the ventral side of the penis

_____25. obstruction of the renal collection system

a. hypospadias

b. epispadias

c. bladder exstrophy

d. hypoplastic kidney

e. renal dysplasia

f. bilateral agenesi

g. renal dysplasia

Case Study

A 3-year-old girl is brought to the emergency room of a local hospital because she has bloody stools. Her parents reveal a history of gastrointestinal illness 2 weeks ago after a weekend of camping. The girl has been well since the GI illness until yesterday when the bloody stools began. At that time, they noticed how pale she was; they believe she has not voided at all today. Her assessment reveals pallor and bruising. A urine collection bag is placed on the child; however, she does not void while in the emergency room. A complete blood count reveals low Hgb, Hct, and platelets.

From the laboratory values, what diagnosis is likely? What treatment will she require?

31

Structure and Function of the Reproductive Systems

1. **Describe the hormonal stimulation of the reproductive systems; note secondary sex characteristics.**
   Review pages 862-865; refer to Figures 31-1 through 31-3.

2. **Identify female external and internal genitalia and female sex hormones.**
   Review pages 865-871; refer to Figures 31-4 through 31-9 and Table 31-1.

3. **Describe the menstrual cycle, noting its differential hormonal effects, levels, and cellular events.**
   Review pages 871-875; refer to Figures 31-10 and 31-11 and Table 31-2.

4. **Identify male external and internal genitalia.**
   Review pages 875-876 and 878-879; refer to Figures 31-12 through 31-16.

5. **Describe spermatogenesis and male sex hormones.**
   Review pages 879-880; refer to Figures 31-17 and 31-18.

6. **Identify the structure of and cyclical hormones associated with female breast tissue; describe the lymphatic drainage.**
   Review pages 880-882; refer to Figures 31-19 and 31-20.

7. **Identify changes in the female and male reproductive systems that occur with advancing age; describe the perimenopause.**
   Review pages 882-884; refer to Figure 31-21.

Practice Examination

1. GnRh reaches the anterior pituitary gland and causes the release of which of the following? (More than one answer may be correct.)
   a. growth hormone
   b. FSH
   c. ADH
   d. LH
   e. oxytocin

2. Which is *not* a structure of the female external genitalia?
   a. vagina
   b. clitoris
   c. vestibule
   d. labia minora
   e. labia majora

3. A new menstrual cycle has a rise in the levels of:
   a. LH.
   b. GH.
   c. estrogen.
   d. progesterone.
   e. FSH.

4. Progesterone:
    a. stimulates lactation.
    b. increases uterine tube motility.
    c. thins the endometrium.
    d. maintains the thickened endometrium.
    e. causes ovulation.

5. The ovaries produce:
    a. ova, estrogen, and oxytocin.
    b. ova only.
    c. ova and estrogen.
    d. testosterone and semen.
    e. None of the above is correct.

6. During which days of the menstrual cycle does the endometrium achieve maximum development?
    a. 2-6
    b. 7-12
    c. 14
    d. 20-24
    e. 26-28

7. Hormones necessary for the growth and development of female breasts are:
    a. estrogens and progesterone.
    b. oxytocin and ADH.
    c. androgens and steroids.
    d. gonadocorticoids.
    e. relaxin.

8. The structure that releases a mature ovum is the:
    a. corpus albicans.
    b. graafian follicle.
    c. primary follicle.
    d. corpus luteum.
    e. infundibulum.

9. A major duct of the female reproductive system is the:
    a. suspensory tube.
    b. uterosacral duct.
    c. broad duct.
    d. mesovarian duct.
    e. uterine tube.

10. Prostate is to the accessory gland as gonad is to the:
    a. ejaculatory duct.
    b. ovary.
    c. bulbourethral gland.
    d. accessory gland.
    e. urethra.

11. Cells that produce testosterone are called:
    a. interstitial endocrinocytes.
    b. testicular endocrine cells.
    c. sustentacular cells.
    d. spermatogonia.
    e. None of the above is correct.

12. The function of testosterone includes:
    a. development of male gonads.
    b. bone and muscle growth.
    c. influencing sexual behavior.
    d. growth of testes.
    e. All of the above are correct.

13. Immediately after the sperm cells leave the ductus epididymis, they enter the:
    a. ejaculatory duct.
    b. ductus deferens.
    c. urethra.
    d. seminiferous tubules.
    e. None of the above is correct.

14. A substance produced in the reproductive system mainly by the bulbourethral glands is:
    a. fructose.
    b. HCl.
    c. mucus.
    d. an alkaline, viscous fluid.

15. Which produce(s) a secretion that helps maintain the motility of spermatozoa?
    a. prostate
    b. penis
    c. greater vestibular glands
    d. interstitial tissues
    e. All of the above are correct.

16. Semen is:
    a. vaginal secretions needed to activate sperm.
    b. the product of the testes.
    c. the sperm and secretions of the seminal vesicles, prostate, and bulbourethral gland.
    d. responsible for engorgement of the erectile tissue in the penis.
    e. the secretion that causes ovulation in the female.

17. The vulva consists of the:
    a. labia majora and labia minora.
    b. clitoris.
    c. vaginal orifice.
    d. Both a and b are correct.
    e. a, b, and c are correct.

18. The major difference between female and male hormone production is:
    a. LH is without effect in the male.
    b. GnRH doesn't cause the release of FSH in the male.
    c. hormonal production is relatively constant in the male.
    d. Both a and b are correct.
    e. None of the above is correct.

19. The primary spermatocyte has:
    a. 46 chromosomes.
    b. the same number of chromosomes as a sperm.
    c. 23 chromosomes.
    d. a diploid number of chromosomes.
    e. Both a and d are correct.

20. During the follicular/proliferative phase of the menstrual cycle:
    a. vascularity of breast tissue increases.
    b. vascularity of breast tissue decreases.
    c. progesterone constricts the ducts.
    d. Both b and c are correct.

21. Most of the lymphatic drainage of the female breast occurs through the:
    a. axillary nodes.
    b. internal mammary nodes.
    c. subclavian nodes.
    d. brachial nodes.
    e. anterior pectoral nodes.

Match the aging reproductive changes with the term or response.

_____22. primary follicles resist gonadotropin stimulation

_____23. corpus luteum fails to develop

_____24. less effective erection

_____25. first menstruation

a. menarche

b. premenopause

c. menopause

d. vasomotor flush

e. vasocongestive response

f. luteal/secretory phase

g. follicular/proliferative phase

32

Alterations of the Reproductive Systems Including Sexually Transmitted Infections

Foundational Objectives

a. **Identify the female and male reproductive structures.**
   Review pages 865-870, 875-876 and 878-879.

MEMORY CHECK!

- The female external genitalia collectively are called the *vulva* and comprise the structures externally visible: the mons pubis, the labia majora, the labia minora, the clitoris, and the vestibule. The urethral meatus, the vaginal opening, and two sets of glands—Skene glands and Bartholin glands—open onto the vestibule. The internal organs of the female reproductive system are two ovaries, two fallopian tubes or uterine tubes, the uterus, and the vagina. The ovaries are the primary female reproductive organs. They are located on both sides of the uterus and are suspended and supported by ligaments.

- The fallopian tubes extend from the ovaries to the uterus and open into the uterine cavity, thus providing a direct communication between the peritoneal cavity and the uterine cavity. The uterus lies centrally in the pelvis and is divided structurally into the body, or corpus, and the cervix. The inner layer, the endometrium, consists of surface epithelium, glands, and connective tissue. The endometrium is shed during menstruation. At the lowest portion of the corpus is the internal os of the cervix. The external os is at the lower end of the cervix. The canal of the cervix provides a direct communication from the cavity of the uterine body through the internal os and the external os to the vagina.

- The vagina extends from the cervix of the uterus to the vaginal opening. Thus there is continuous communication from outside the body to the peritoneal cavity through the reproductive system structures.

Continued

MEMORY CHECK!—cont'd

- The male reproductive structures are the penis; the testes in the scrotal sac; the duct system, which includes the epididymis, the vas deferens, the ejaculatory ducts, and the urethra; and the accessory glands, which include the seminal vesicles, the prostate, and the bulbourethral glands.

- The testes are divided internally into lobules that contain the seminiferous tubules and Leydig cells. Sperm production takes place in the seminiferous tubules; Leydig cells secrete testosterone. On the posterior portion of each testis is a coiled duct, the epididymis. The head of the epididymis is connected with the seminiferous tubule of the testis, and its tail is continuous with the vas deferens. The vas deferens is the excretory duct of the testis. It extends to the duct of the seminal vesicle and joins with it to form the ejaculatory duct. The ejaculatory duct joins the urethra, which is the common passageway to outside the body for both sperm and urine. The accessory glands communicate with the duct system. The prostate surrounds the neck of the bladder and the upper urethra. Its glandular ducts open into the urethra. The bulbourethral glands, or Cowper's glands, are located near the urethral meatus. The penis is composed of three elongated cylindrical masses of erectile tissue, which comprise the shaft of the penis. The inner, ventral mass is the corpus spongiosum, which contains the urethra. The two outer, dorsal, parallel masses are the corpus cavernosa. The distal end of the penis or the glans is covered by the prepuce, or foreskin.

b. **Describe the relationships of hormones to the normal menstrual cycle.**
   Review pages 871-875; refer to Figures 31-10 and 31-11 and Table 32-2.

MEMORY CHECK!

- The three phases of the menstrual cycle are the follicular/proliferative phase, the luteal/secretory phase, and menstruation. During menstruation, the functional layer of the endometrium disintegrates and is discharged through the vagina. Menstruation is followed by the follicular/proliferative phase. During this phase, the anterior pituitary gland secretes FSH, which causes cells of the endometrium to proliferate. By the time the ovarian follicle is mature, the endometrial lining is restored. At this point, ovulation occurs.

- Ovulation marks the beginning of the luteal/secretory phase of the menstrual cycle. The ovarian follicle begins its transformation into a corpus luteum. LH from the anterior pituitary stimulates the corpus luteum to secrete progesterone, which initiates the secretory phase of endometrial development. If conception occurs, the nutrient-laden endometrium is ready for implantation. If conception and implantation do not occur, the corpus luteum degenerates and ceases its production of progesterone and estrogen. Without progesterone or estrogen to maintain it, the endometrium enters the ischemic phase and disintegrates. Then, menstruation occurs, marking the beginning of another cycle.

c. **Characterize the structure and development of the female breast.**
   Review pages 880-882; refer to Figures 31-19 and 31-20.

MEMORY CHECK!

- The female breast is composed of 15 to 20 pyramid-shaped lobes, which are separated and supported by Cooper ligaments. Each lobe contains 20 to 40 lobules, which subdivide into many functional units called *acini*. Each acinus is lined with a layer of epithelial cells capable of secreting milk and a layer of subepithelial cells capable of contracting to squeeze milk from the acinus. The acini empty into a network of lobular collecting ducts that reach the skin through openings in the nipple. The lobes and lobules are surrounded and separated by muscle strands and fatty connective tissue. An extensive capillary network surrounds the acini. Lymphatic draining of the breast occurs largely through the axillary nodes.

MEMORY CHECK!—cont'd

- The nipple is a pigmented, cylindrical structure that has multiple openings. The areola is the pigmented, circular area around the nipple. A number of sebaceous glands are located within the areola and aid in lubrication of the nipple during lactation. The nipple's smooth muscle is innervated by the sympathetic nervous system.

- During childhood, breast growth is latent and growth of the nipple and areola keeps pace with body surface. At the onset of puberty in the female, estrogen secretion stimulates mammary growth. Full differentiation and development of breast tissue are mediated by a variety of hormones, including estrogen, progesterone, prolactin, growth hormone, thyroid hormone, insulin, and cortisol.

- During the reproductive years, the breast undergoes cyclic changes in response to changes in the levels of estrogen and progesterone associated with the menstrual cycle. Because the length of the menstrual cycle does not allow for complete regression of new cell growth, breast growth continues at a slow rate until approximately age 35. The number of acini increase with each cycle, so epithelial tissue proliferation is under the influence of hormones as long as secretion occurs.

Objectives

After studying this chapter, the learner will be able to do the following:

1. **Distinguish between various menstrual disorders and their hormonal alterations or causes; identify manifestations of premenstrual syndrome.**
   Study pages 890-896; refer to Figures 32-1 through 32-3 and Tables 32-1 and 32-2.

Premenstrual syndrome (PMS) is the cyclic recurrence in the luteal phase of the menstrual cycle of physical, psychologic, or behavioral changes distressing enough to impair interpersonal relationships or usual activities. It has been estimated that 5% to 10% of menstruating women have severe to disabling premenstrual symptoms and 3% to 8% of these women have exaggerated feelings of depression known as **premenstrual dysphoric disorder (PMDD)** warranting treatment. Currently, it is believed that PMS is the end result of abnormal tissue response of nervous, immunologic, vascular, and gastrointestinal systems to the normal hormone changes of the menstrual cycle. This biologic response may be triggered by fluctuating estrogen and progesterone levels. Serotonin levels likely play a role in type and severity of symptoms.

A predisposition to PMS runs in families and is likely due to genetics and/or environmental factors. There is some evidence that supports a relationship between the severity and frequency of premenstrual symptoms and perfectionism, increased stress, poor nutrition, lack of exercise, low self-esteem, and history of sexual abuse or family conflict. Depression, anger, irritability, and fatigue have been reported as the most prominent and the most distressing symptoms; physical symptoms seem less prevalent and problematic.

Treatment for PMS is symptomatic. After a trial of nonpharmacologic therapies including dietary changes, various medications may be added to the treatment plan even if their efficacy in the treatment of PMS is questionable in the hopes of relieving symptoms.

Menstrual Disorders

Disorder	Alteration
Primary dysmenorrhea	Excessive endometrial prostaglandin production
Secondary dysmenorrhea	Endometriosis, pelvic adhesions, uterine fibroids, adenosis, myosis
Painful menstruation	Increases myometrial contractions and constricts blood vessels
Amenorrhea	Amenorrhea is divided into compartments that reflect the underlying disorder: Compartment I—disorders of outflow tract or uterine target organ; Compartment II—disorders of the ovary; Compartment III—disorders of the anterior pituitary; and Compartment IV—central nervous system disorders or altered hypothalamic factors. Galactorrhea (lactation not associated with childbirth or nursing) might be observed in any of the compartment types.
Primary: menarche failure Absence of menstruation	No ovulation occurs; no menstruation or secondary sex characteristics
Secondary: menstruation absence following menarche	Anovulation
Dysfunctional uterine bleeding (DUB)	Progesterone deficiency or estrogen excess; an imbalance between progesterone and estrogen
Heavy or irregular bleeding caused by disturbance of menstrual cycle	Estrogen proliferates endometrium, whereas progesterone limits it; large mass of tissue available for heavy, irregular bleeding
Polycystic ovarian syndrome (PCO) Anovulation causes enlarged, polycystic ovaries	Related to hypertension, hyperinsulinemia, and dyslipidemia; leads to infertility, hirsutism, acne, endometrial hyperplasia, cardiovascular disease, and diabetes mellitus

2. **Describe pelvic inflammatory disease.**
Study pages 896 and 898; refer to Figures 32-4 through 32-6.

Pelvic inflammatory disease (PID) is an acute inflammatory process caused by infection. PID involves organs of the upper genital tract, the uterus, fallopian tubes or uterine tubes, or ovaries. In its most severe form, the entire peritoneal cavity may be involved. Infection of the fallopian tubes is **salpingitis;** infection of the ovaries is **oophoritis.** Most cases of PID are caused by sexually transmitted microorganisms that ascend from the vagina to the uterus, fallopian tubes, and ovaries.

PID is considered a polymicrobial infection with the majority of cases being caused by gonorrheal or chlamydial microbes, such as anaerobes and facultative organisms. These organisms may induce a response that causes necrosis with repeated infections and may predispose a woman to PID. After one episode of pelvic infection, 15% to 25% of women develop long-term sequelae such as infertility, ectopic pregnancy, chronic pelvic pain, and pelvic adhesions. The incidence of complications increases markedly with repeated infections.

The clinical manifestations of PID are variable. Subclinical infections occur in 67% to 75% of women with salpingitis. The first sign of the ascending infection may be the gradual onset of low bilateral abdominal pain often characterized as dull and steady. Symptoms are more likely to develop during or immediately after menstruation. The pain of PID may worsen with walking, jumping, or intercourse. Other manifestations of PID are difficult or painful urination and irregular bleeding. Other conditions causing pelvic pain must be excluded, such as ectopic pregnancy, threatened abortion, or appendicitis before treatment.

Treatment involves bed rest, avoidance of intercourse, and combined antibiotic therapy. Hospitalization is required for 25% to 40% of women for intravenous administration of antibiotics and treatment of peritonitis or tubo-ovarian abscess.

3. **Define and cite causes of vaginitis, cervicitis, vulvitis, and bartholinitis.**
Study pages 899-900; refer to Figure 32-7.

Vaginitis is an infection of the vagina most often caused by sexually transmitted pathogens and *Candida albicans.* Because the acidic nature of vaginal secretions during the reproductive years provides protection against a variety of sexually transmitted pathogens, variables that alter the vaginal pH may predispose a woman to infection. The use of antibiotics may destroy *Lactobacillus acidophilus,* which helps maintain an acidic vaginal pH.

Thus there may be an overgrowth of *C. albicans,* which could cause a yeast vaginitis.

Cervicitis is an inflammation of the cervix usually caused by one or more sexually transmitted pathogens. A mucopurulent exudate drains from the external os.

Vulvitis is an inflammation of the skin of the vulva and often of the perianal area. Vulvitis can be caused by contact with soaps, detergents, lotions, hygienic sprays, menstrual pads, perfumed toilet paper, or nonabsorbent or tight-fitting clothes.

Bartholinitis is an inflammation of one or both of the ducts that lead from the vaginal opening to the Bartholin glands. The causes of bartholinitis are microorganisms that infect the lower female reproductive tract; this disorder is usually preceded by cervicitis, vaginitis, or urethritis. Infection or trauma causes inflammatory changes that narrow the distal portion of the duct, leading to obstruction and stasis of glandular secretions and causing further inflammation.

4. **Describe pelvic relaxation disorders.**
    Study pages 900-902; refer to Figures 32-8 and 32-9 and Table 32-3.

The bladder, urethra, and rectum are supported by the endopelvic fascia and perineal muscles. This muscular and fascial tissue loses tone and strength with aging and may fail to maintain the pelvic organ in the proper position. Trauma such as childbirth or pelvic surgery damages or weakens the supporting structures.

Cystocele is descent of the bladder and the anterior vaginal wall into the vaginal canal. A cystocele may cause the woman to lose urine when she laughs, sneezes, coughs, or does anything that strains the abdominal muscles. Cystocele is usually accompanied by **urethrocele,** or sagging of the urethra. Urethrocele is usually caused by the shearing effect of the fetal head on the urethra during childbirth. A **rectocele** is the bulging of the rectum and posterior vaginal wall into the vaginal canal. An **enterocele** is herniation of the rectouterine pouch into the rectovaginal septum. **Uterine prolapse** is descent of the cervix or entire uterus into the vaginal canal.

Treatment includes isometric exercises to strengthen muscles, estrogens to improve tone and vascularity of fascial support, a pessary device to hold the uterus in position, stool softeners, and surgery.

5. **Characterize the benign growth and proliferative conditions of the female reproductive system.**
    Study pages 902-905; refer to Figures 32-10 through 32-13. (See table below.)

Benign Lesions of the Female Reproductive System

Lesion	Cause	Manifestations
Ovarian cysts		
Follicular cyst	Ovarian follicle fails to release ovum; fluid not reabsorbed from degenerating follicle	Pelvic and abdominal pain, menstrual irregularities
Corpus luteum cyst	A persistent corpus luteum secretes progesterone	Pelvic pain, amenorrhea with subsequent heavy bleeding
Endometrial polyps	Estrogen stimulation	Premenstrual or intermenstrual bleeding
Leiomyomas (smooth muscle tumors)	Unknown, hormonal fluctuations alter size	Abnormal or increased uterine bleeding, pain, pressure
Adenomyosis (endometrial tissue in the myometrium)	Repeated pregnancies	Dysmenorrhea, uterine enlargement and tenderness
Endometriosis (ectopic endometrial tissue)	Depressed T_c cells tolerate ectopic tissue, genetics	Ectopic tissues respond to hormonal stimulation, bleeding causes pelvic adhesions and pain

NOTE: Dermoid cysts are ovarian teratomas having malignant potential and should be removed. Ovarian torsion may occur as a complication of ovarian cysts.

6. **Characterize the malignant tumors of the female reproductive system.**

Study pages 905-910; refer to Figures 32-14 through 32-17 and Tables 32-4 through 32-6.

Malignant Tumors of the Female Reproductive System

Tumor	Causes	Manifestations
Cervical cancer*	STD, human papilloma virus (HPV), early sexual activity, multiple sex partners, smoking, poor nutrition	Asymptomatic; vaginal bleeding or discharge; grade of epithelial thickness enables precursor lesion diagnosis
Vaginal cancer	Previous cervical cancer, nonsteroidal estrogen exposure in utero	Asymptomatic; vaginal bleeding or discharge
Vulvar cancer	HPV in younger women, chronic inflammation in older women	Visible appearance
Endometrial cancer	Obesity, high-fat diet, no pregnancies, late menopause, hypertension	Vaginal bleeding
Ovarian cancer	Unknown; risk factors are similar to those for endometrial cancer	Systemic manifestations, pain and abdominal swelling, postmenopausal bleeding

*Preceding invasive cervical carcinoma are the progressively serious alterations of cervical intraepithelial neoplasia (cervical dysplasia) and cervical carcinoma in situ.

NOTE: Treatments for these malignancies depend on the clinical staging, the extent of metastasis, and the age of the individual. Each lesion can be managed by surgery, radiation, and/or chemotherapy; a combination of all these modalities may be necessary as well as lymphadenectomy.

7. **Define terms used in female sexual dysfunction.**

Study pages 910-911; refer to Table 32-7.

Inhibited sexual desire may be a biologic manifestation of depression, alcohol or other substance abuse, prolactin-secretin pituitary tumors, or testosterone deficiency. Beta-adrenergic blockers used for heart disease also may inhibit sexual desire.

Vaginismus is an involuntary muscle spasm in response to attempted penetration. Common causes include prior sexual trauma, fear of sex, or organic disorders.

Anorgasmia is the inability of the woman to reach or achieve orgasm. Drugs such as narcotics, tranquilizers, antidepressants, and antihypertensive medications can inhibit orgasm.

Dyspareunia, or painful intercourse, is common. Inadequate lubrication may make penetration or intercourse unpleasant. Drugs with a drying effect—such as antihistamines, certain tranquilizers, and marijuana—and disorders such as diabetes, vaginal infections, and estrogen deficiency can decrease lubrication. Other causes of dyspareunia include infections and anatomic constraints around the introitus or the vulva.

Infertility is the inability to conceive after 1 year of unprotected intercourse and affects approxmately 15% of all couples. Important causes of infertility in the female are malfunctions of the fallopian tubes, the ovaries, or the reproductive hormones. Endometriosis also may contribute to infertility.

8. **By site, describe common disorders of the male reproductive system; distinguish between benign prostatic hyperplasia, prostatitis, and prostatic cancer.**

Study pages 912 and 914-926; refer to Figures 32-18 through 32-34.

Urethritis is an inflammatory process usually caused by sexually transmitted microorganisms. Nonsexual origins of urethritis are inflammation or infection as a result of urologic procedures, insertion of foreign bodies into the urethra, anatomic abnormalities, or trauma.

Symptoms of urethritis include urethral tingling or itching or a burning sensation when urinating. Frequency, urgency, and purulent or clear mucus-like discharge from the urethra may occur. Treatment is appropriate antibiotic therapy for infectious urethritis and avoidance of mechanical irritation.

Urethral stricture is a narrowing of the urethra because of scarring. The scars may be congenital but are more likely to result from trauma or untreated or severe urethral infections.

Symptoms include urinary frequency and hesitancy, diminished force and size of the urinary stream, dribbling after voiding, and nocturia. Treatment is usually surgical and may involve urethral dilation, urethrotomy, or a variety of other surgical techniques.

Phimosis and **paraphimosis** are both disorders in which the penile foreskin, or prepuce, is "too tight" to be moved easily over the glans penis. In phimosis, the foreskin cannot be retracted back over the glans; in paraphimosis, the foreskin is retracted and cannot be moved forward to cover the glans. Phimosis can occur at any age and is most commonly caused by poor hygiene and chronic infection. Circumcision, if needed, is performed after infection has been eradicated. In paraphimosis, surgery must be performed to prevent necrosis of the glans caused by constricted blood vessels.

Peyronie disease is a fibrotic condition that causes lateral curvature of the penis during erection. The problem usually affects middle-aged men and is associated with painful erection, painful intercourse for both partners, and poor erection distal to the involved area. There is no definitive treatment for Peyronie disease. Spontaneous remissions occur about 50% of the time. Pharmacologic therapies that increase oxygenation may hasten resolution. Surgical resection of the fibrous plaque followed by grafting has been successful.

Balanitis is an inflammation of the glans penis and usually occurs in conjunction with an inflammation of the prepuce. It is associated with poor hygiene and phimosis. The accumulation under the foreskin of glandular secretions, sloughed epithelial cells, and *Mycobacterium smegmatis* can irritate the glans directly or lead to infection. Balanitis is most commonly seen in men with poorly controlled diabetes mellitus and candidiasis. Antimicrobials are used to treat infection, and circumcision can prevent recurrences.

Penile cancer is rare in the United States. Although the exact etiology is unknown, cancer of the penis is likely a result of chronic irritation caused by smegma beneath a phimotic foreskin.

Varicocele, hydrocele, and spermatocele are common intrascrotal disorders. **Varicocele** is an abnormal dilation of a vein within the spermatic cord, and most occur on the left side. They may be painful or tender. They occur in 10% to 15% of males, frequently after puberty. The cause of varicocele is incompetent or congenitally absent valves in the spermatic veins that normally prevent backflow of blood. Thus blood pools in the veins rather than flowing into the venous system. Decreased blood flow through the testis interferes with spermatogenesis and can cause infertility.

A **hydrocele** is a collection of fluid within the tunica vaginalis and is the most common cause of scrotal swelling. Hydroceles in infants are congenital malformations that often resolve spontaneously by 1 year of age. Hydroceles in adults may be caused by an imbalance between the secreting and absorptive capacities of scrotal tissues.

The **spermatocele** is a cyst located between the head of the epididymis and the testis that usually is asymptomatic or produces mild discomfort that is relieved by scrotal support. Neither hydroceles nor spermatoceles are associated with infertility.

Cryptorchidism is a condition in which one or both testes fail to descend into the scrotum. It is the most common congenital condition involving the testes. In approximately 75% to 90% of infants with cryptorchidism, the testes descend into the scrotum by 1 year of age. The cause of cryptorchidism is not clear, but it may result from a developmental delay, a defect of the testis, deficient maternal gonadotropin stimulation, or some mechanical factor that prevents descent through the inguinal canal.

Untreated cryptorchidism is associated with lowered sperm count and impaired fertility. Undescended testes are susceptible to neoplastic processes. Treatment often begins with administration of human chorionic gonadotropin. If hormonal therapy is not successful, the testis is located and moved into the scrotum surgically.

Torsion of the testis is a condition wherein the testis rotates on its vascular pedicle; this interrupts its blood supply. Onset may be spontaneous, or it may follow physical exertion or trauma. If the torsion cannot be reduced manually, surgery must be performed within 6 hours after the onset of symptoms to preserve normal testicular function.

Orchitis is an acute inflammation of the testes and is uncommon except as a complication of systemic infection or as an extension of an associated epididymitis. Mumps is the most common infectious cause of orchitis and usually affects postpubertal males. The onset is sudden and occurs 3 to 4 days after the onset of parotitis. Irreversible damage to spermatogenesis results in about 30% of affected testes.

Treatment is supportive and includes bed rest, scrotal support, elevation of the scrotum, hot or cold compresses, and analgesic agents for relief of pain. Appropriate antimicrobial drugs should be used for bacterial orchitis. Corticosteroids are indicated in proved cases of nonspecific granulomatous orchitis.

Testicular cancers are rare, accounting for approximately 1% of all male cancers; yet they are the most common solid tumor of young adult men. The cure rate is greater than 95%.

The etiology of testicular neoplasms is unknown. Because young men are affected most often, it is believed that high levels of androgens may contribute to carcinogenesis. A genetic predisposition exists. Cryptorchidism also is statistically associated with the development of testicular cancer. Apparently, the undescended testis has a developmental defect or undergoes gradual involution and degeneration over time, which may contribute to neoplastic changes.

Painless testicular enlargement usually is the first sign of testicular cancer. Enlargement is gradual and may be accompanied by a sensation of testicular heaviness or a dull ache in the lower abdomen. Occasionally, acute pain occurs because of rapid growth; then, there may be hemorrhage and necrosis. Besides surgery, treatment involves radiation and chemotherapy singly or in combination. Orchiectomy does not affect sexual function.

Epididymitis, inflammation of the epididymis, generally occurs in sexually active young males. In young men, the usual cause is a sexually transmitted microorganism. In men over 35 years of age, intestinal bacteria and *Pseudomonas aeruginosa* found in urinary tract infections and prostatitis also may cause epididymitis. The pathogenic microorganism reaches the epididymis by ascending the vas deferens from an infected urethra or bladder. **Chemical epididymitis** may result from inflammation caused by urine reflux into ejaculatory ducts; it is usually self limiting.

Acute and severe scrotal or inguinal pain is caused by inflammation of the epididymis and surrounding tissues. The individual may have pyuria and bacteriuria and a history of urinary symptoms including urethral discharge. Complications of epididymitis include abscess formation, infarction of the testis, recurrent infection, scarring of epididymal endothelium, and infertility. Treatment includes antibiotic therapy for the infection and various measures to provide symptomatic relief. The individual's sexual partner should be treated with antibiotics if the causative microorganism is a sexually transmitted pathogen.

Benign prostatic hyperplasia (BPH) was formerly called *benign prostatic hypertrophy* and causes problems as enlarged prostatic tissue compresses the prostatic urethra. More than half of all men between 60 and 69 years of age have prostatic enlargement. During the third decade of life, the prostate reaches adult size. Between 40 and 45 years of age, benign hyperplasia begins and continues slowly until death. Current etiologic theories of BPH implicate estrogen/androgen synergism or prostatic growth factors such as insulin-like growth factors (IGFs) with possible additional hormonal involvement.

BPH begins in the periurethral glands, which are the inner glands or layers of the prostate. As nodular hyperplasia and cellular hypertrophy progress, the compressed prostatic urethra usually, but not always, causes bladder outflow obstruction. The urge to urinate frequently, some delay in starting urination, and decreased force of the urinary stream develop. Over a period of several years, the bladder is unable to empty all of the urine, and urine retention becomes chronic.

Progressive bladder distention causes sacculations or diverticular outpouchings of the bladder wall. The ureters may be obstructed as they pass through the hypertrophied detrusor muscle. Bladder or kidney infection then develops. Hyperplastic tissue may be removed surgically.

Prostatitis is an inflammation of the prostate usually limited to a few of the gland's excretory ducts. Prostatitis is categorized as acute bacterial prostatitis, chronic bacterial prostatitis, or nonbacterial prostatitis.

Acute bacterial prostatitis is an ascending infection of the urinary tract that tends to occur in men between the ages of 30 and 50 but also is associated with BPH in older men. Urinary tract bacteria are common causes of acute bacterial prostatitis.

Symptoms include dysuria and urinary frequency and lower abdominal and suprapubic discomfort. The individual also may have a slow, small urinary stream, inability to empty the bladder, and the need to urinate frequently during the night. Systemic signs of infection include sudden onset of a high fever, fatigue, joint pain, and muscle pain. Long-term, broad-spectrum antibiotics may be required to resolve the infection and control its spread. Pain relievers, antipyretics, bed rest, and adequate hydration also are used therapeutically.

Chronic bacterial prostatitis is characterized by recurrent urinary tract infections and the persistence of pathogenic bacteria. This prostatitis is the most common recurrent urinary tract infection in men.

Symptoms are variable and may be similar to those of acute bacterial prostatitis. The prostate may be only slightly enlarged, but fibrosis causes it to be firm and irregular in shape. Treatment of chronic bacterial prostatitis is difficult mainly because fibrosis blocks passage of antibiotics into prostatic tissues. Therefore, therapeutic levels are hard to achieve. If chronic bacterial prostatitis is not cured medically, a radical transurethral prostatectomy may be required.

Nonbacterial prostatitis is the most common prostatitis syndrome and consists of prostatic inflammation without evidence of bacterial infection. Its etiology is unclear.

Men with nonbacterial prostatitis may complain of continuous or spasmodic pain in the suprapubic, infrapubic, scrotal, penile, or inguinal areas. The prostate gland generally feels normal upon palpation. Nonbacterial prostatitis is diagnosed by exclusion. There is no generally accepted treatment for nonbacterial prostatitis. A course of antibiotics for both affected individuals and sexual partners may minimize symptoms.

Prostatic cancer accounts for more than 14% of all cancer deaths and more than 29% of all cancers in men in the United States; only lung cancer accounts for more male deaths. Incidence increases with advancing age; over 80% of all prostate cancers are diagnosed in men over 65. More than 95% of prostatic neoplasms are adenocarcinomas, and most occur in the periphery of the prostate. Aggressiveness appears related to the degree of differentiation rather than the size of the tumor.

Possible causes include genetic predisposition, environmental and dietary factors, alterations in testosterone, dihydrotestosterone, estradiol, and insulin growth factor (IGF-1), which is a powerful mitogen and inhibitor of apoptosis. Dietary risk reduction factors for prostate cancer include reduction of fats; avoiding refined sugars; decreasing total caloric intake; increasing antioxidants, lycopenes, soy, and fiber; and maintaining calcium intake.

Local extension is usually posterior, although late in the disease the tumor may invade the rectum or encroach on the prostatic urethra and cause bladder outlet obstruction. Sites of distant metastasis occur via lymph and blood vessels and include the lymph nodes, bones, lungs, liver, and adrenals. The pelvis, lumbar spine, femur, thoracic spine, and ribs are the most common sites of bone metastasis.

Prostatic cancer often causes no symptoms until it is far advanced. The first manifestations of disease are slow urinary stream, hesitancy, incomplete emptying, frequency, nocturia, and dysuria. Unlike the symptoms of obstruction caused by BPH, the symptoms of obstruction caused by prostatic cancer are progressive and do not temporarily remit. Symptoms of late disease include bone pain at sites of bone metastasis, edema of the lower extremities, enlarged lymph nodes, liver enlargement, pathologic bone fractures, and mental confusion associated with brain metastases.

Transrectal ultrasound (TRUS), prostatic-specific antigen (PSA) blood tests, and digital examination can assist in the diagnosis of prostatic cancer. PSA density (PSAD) can differentiate BPH from prostatic cancer. PSAD is calculated by dividing PSA serum levels by the volume of prostate tissue, which is determined by TRUS. Tissue biopsy can confirm the presence of prostatic cancer. Treatment options include hormonal therapy, chemotherapy, radiation therapy, surgery, or any combination of these. Symptomatic relief of urinary obstruction, bladder outlet obstruction, colon obstruction, and spinal cord compression may be required.

9. **Describe sexual dysfunction in the male.**
   Study pages 926-927.

Male sexual dysfunction is the impairment of erection, emission, and ejaculation. In men over 40 years of age, organic factors are involved in more than 50% of dysfunctional cases. Vascular disorders cause erectile dysfunction. Neurologic disorders can interfere with the important sympathetic, parasympathetic, and central nervous system mechanisms of erection, emission, and ejaculation. Men who are taking antihypertensives, antidepressants, antihistamines, antispasmodics, sedatives or tranquilizers, barbiturates, diuretics, sex hormone preparations, narcotics, or psychoactive drugs or who consume ethyl alcohol experience sexual dysfunction. Treatments for organic sexual dysfunction include both medical and surgical approaches. Viagra (sildenafil) has the ability to maintain erections.

10. **Differentiate between benign and malignant female breast disease.**
    Study pages 927-930 and 932-937; refer to Figures 32-35 through 32-43 and Tables 32-8 through 32-12.

Many terms have been used to describe benign breast lesions of epithelial origin. **Fibrocystic disease** or physiologic nodularity is one description, and it is manifested by palpable lumps in the breast. These lumps fluctuate with the menstrual cycle and may become progressively worse until menopause. This terminology is not altogether accurate because physiologic nodularity is present in approximately 50% of menstruating women. Also, some of the lesions attributed to fibrocystic disease are associated with an increased risk of breast cancer.

Breast cancer is the most common cancer in American women and the most common killer after lung cancer. Lifetime risk for breast cancer is approximately 1 in every 8 women. About 77% of these cancers will occur in women older than 50 years. The risk factors and possible etiologies of breast cancer can be classified as reproductive, hormonal, environmental, and familial.

Benign/Malignant Female Breast Disorders

Disorder	Risks	Pathophysiology	Manifestations	Treatment
Fibrocystic disease (FCC) • Microcysts • Macrocysts • Adenosis • Apocrine change • Fibrosis • Fibroadenomas • Ductal hyperplasia *Other lesions	Puberty to lifetime; nonproliferative lesions demonstrate no added risk for cancer; proliferative lesions with atypia hyperplasia have increased risk for cancer development	Increased estrogen levels, alterations in estrogen-to-progesterone ratio	Fluctuating pain; pain increases as menstruation approaches; fluctuating lesion size; multiple lesions; may be nipple discharge	Cyst drainage; surgical excision; pain relief by synthetic androgens
Breast cancer	Increase with age: Lifetime, 1 in 8. No term pregnancies, long reproductive life; ionizing radiation, high-fat diet, alcohol ingestion, first-degree relatives	Estrogens have a proliferative effect on mammary gland epithelium; estrogens may increase susceptibility to environmental carcinogens, transforming growth factor (TGF), insulin-like growth factor (IGF), epidermal growth factor (EGF), platelet-derived growth factor (PGF); mutations of $BRCA_1$ on chromosome 17 and $BRCA_2$ on chromosome 13	Painless or painful lumps, skin retraction over lesion, nipple puckering and discharge; hemorrhage *After* metastasis: palpable axillary lymph nodes, bone pain, site-specific signs and symptoms	Surgery to remove lesion, radiation to prevent metastasis, chemotherapy, hormones for hormone-dependent tumors; Herceptin to block growth-promoting signal for HER_2 (in some cases); bone marrow transplantation

*Other benign lesions include comedomastitis, solitary and multiple intraductal papillomas, and fat necrosis caused by breast trauma.
NOTE: Ductal carcinoma in situ (DCIS) refers to a heterogenous group of lesions. These lesions are presumed to be malignant epithelial cells of the ductal system. The increase in the incidence of DCIS may reflect an increase in cancer or increased detection by mammography.

11. **Describe male gynecomastia and breast cancer.**
    Study pages 940-941.

Gynecomastia is the overdevelopment of breast tissue in a male. Gynecomastia accounts for approximately 85% of all masses that develop in the male breast and affects approximately 35% of the male population. Incidence is greatest among adolescents and men older than age 50.

Gynecomastia usually involves an imbalance of the estrogen-testosterone ratio. The ratio can be altered by tumor- and drug-induced hyperestrogenism that elevates the estrogen levels while testosterone levels remain nor-mal. Gynecomastia also can be caused by increased breast tissue responsiveness to estrogen or decreased responsiveness to androgen. Estrogen-testosterone imbalances are associated with hypogonadism, Klinefelter syndrome, testicular neoplasms, cirrhosis of the liver, infectious hepatitis, chronic renal failure, chronic obstructive lung disease, hyperthyroidism, tuberculosis, and chronic malnutrition.

Hyperplasia results in a firm, palpable mass at least 2 cm in diameter located beneath the areola. Identification and treatment of the cause likely will resolve the gynecomastia.

Breast cancer in males is uncommon. Incidence is greatest in men in their 60s. Most male breast cancers are estrogen receptor positive. It has a poor prognosis be-cause men tend to delay seeking treatment.

12. Discuss the current status of sexually transmitted infections (STIs).
Study pages 941-942; refer to Table 32-13.

The study and categorization of **STIs** has broadened to include bacterial, viral, and other agents as causes of STIs. The viral-induced STIs are generally considered incurable. It is estimated that more than 15 million cases of STIs are contracted by Americans each year. The

incidence and increase in STIs is due to increased pre-marital sex, an increase in the divorce rate, non-monogamy among married people, and bisexuality. These factors contribute to the increase in numbers of sexual partners and an increased exposure to STIs. The number of individuals who fail to take protective mea-sures when engaging in sexual activities also contributes to the problem.

13. Characterize the bacterial and bacterial-like STIs, focusing on infectious agents and manifestations.
Refer to Table 32-15 and color plates 1 through 25.

Bacterial and Bacterial-Like STIs

Disease/Infectious Agent	Manifestations
Gonorrhea *Neisseria gonorrhoeae*	Possibly asymptomatic, urethritis, cervicitis, mucopurulent discharge, anorec-tal infection, pharyngitis, conjunctivitis, ophthalmia
Syphilis *Treponema pallidum*	Primary: nonpainful chancre at site of invasion Secondary: systemic involvement with skin rash and lymphadenopathy Tertiary: gummas
Chancroid *Haemophilus ducreyi*	Papule erodes into painful ulcer, superficial exudate, painful lymphadenopathy
Bacterial vaginosis *Gardnerella vaginitis*	Thin and scant malodorous vaginal discharge

Urogenital infections
  Lymphogranuloma venereum
  Chlamydia trachomatis
	Commonly associated with other STIs, purulent discharge, cervicitis, urethri-tis, proctitis, newborn conjunctivitis and pneumonia, tender lymph nodes, and inguinal buboes

NOTE: Treatment of bacterial and bacterial-like STIs is with appropriate antibiotics.

14. Characterize the viral STIs, focusing on infectious agents and manifestations.
Refer to Table 32-15 and color plates 1 through 25.

Viral STIs

Disease/Infectious Agent	Manifestations

Genital herpes
  Herpes simplex virus
  (HSV-1 or HSV-2)
  (latent virus)
	Painful blister-like lesions on external genitalia and genital tract

Condylomata acuminata (warts) Human papillomavirus (HPV)	Soft, skin-colored single or clustered growths, asymptomatic

NOTE: Treatment for HSV is not curative, but oral and topical antiviral agents (acyclovir) are used to lower recurrence; HPV lesions are treated with topical agents and cosmetic surgery because there is no cure.

15. Characterize the parasitic STIs by infectious agents and manifestations.
Refer to Table 32-15 and color plates 1 through 25.

Parasitic STIs

Disease/Infectious Agent	Manifestations
Trichomoniasis *Trichomonas vaginalis*	Pain during intercourse, dysuria, spotting
Scabies *Sarcoptes scabiei*	Intense pruritus
Pediculosis pubic (crabs) *Phthirus pubis*	Pruritus

NOTE: Treatment is by antitrichosomal agents, scabicides, and prescription creams.

Practice Examination

1. Secondary amenorrhea is:
   a. failure to begin menstruation by age 20.
   b. menarche failure.
   c. increased myometrial vasculature constriction.
   d. the absence of menstruation following menarche.

2. What is the likely pathophysiology of PMS?
   a. Elevated prolactin levels cause salt and water retention.
   b. Elevated aldosterone levels cause salt and water retention.
   c. An abnormal nervous, immunologic, vascular, and gastrointestinal response to hormone fluctuations of the menstrual cycle likely occurs.
   d. Both a and b are correct.

3. Acute pelvic inflammatory disease (PID):
   a. primarily affects males.
   b. is usually caused by viruses.
   c. never causes peritonitis.
   d. involves the epididymis.
   e. may cause infertility or tubular pregnancy.

4. Anovulatory cycles having prolonged estrogen levels and absent progesterone production are found in:
   a. cervical cancer.
   b. corpus luteum cysts.
   c. adenomyosis.
   d. endometrial hyperplasia.
   e. Both b and c are correct.

5. Depressed T cell function is associated with:
   a. follicular cysts.
   b. endometrial polyps.
   c. leiomyomas.
   d. adenomyosis.
   e. endometriosis.

6. A 42-year-old retired prostitute who became sexually active at age 14 is at risk to develop:
   a. endometriosis.
   b. cervical carcinoma.
   c. breast cancer.
   d. uterine carcinoma.

7. Polycystic ovary syndrome is:
   a. the most common cause of infertility in the United States.
   b. associated with hyperinsulinemia.
   c. sometimes a precursor of endometrial carcinoma.
   d. a, b, and c are correct.

8. Endometriosis:
   a. has the ectopic endometrium responding to hormonal fluctuations of the menstrual cycle.
   b. occurs primarily in the pleural cavity.
   c. causes infertility in most women having the disorder.
   d. does not reoccur after treatment.

9. Phimosis is:
   a. thickening of the fascia in the erectile tissue of the corpora cavernosa.
   b. the condition of a retracted foreskin that cannot be moved forward.
   c. a condition in which the foreskin cannot be retracted.
   d. caused by poor hygiene and chronic infection.
   e. Both c and d are correct.

10. A varicocele is an intrascrotal disorder:
    a. that results in a collection of fluid within the tunica vaginalis.
    b. occurring because of independent or congenitally absent valves in the spermatic veins.
    c. located between the head of the epididymis and the testis.
    d. that does not interfere with spermatogenesis.

11. Cryptorchidism is:
    a. underdevelopment of the testes.
    b. the absence of scrotal tissue.
    c. relieved by scrotal support.
    d. failure of testes to descend into the scrotum.
    e. an imbalance between secreting and absorptive capacities of scrotal tissues.

12. The infectious cause of orchitis is:
    a. streptococci.
    b. gonococci.
    c. chlamydial organisms.
    d. mumps virus.

13. Which organisms can cause epididymitis?
    a. Enterobacteriaceae
    b. *Neisseria gonorrhoeae*
    c. *Chlamydia trachomatis*
    d. All of the above are correct.
    e. None of the above is correct.

14. In benign prostatic hyperplasia, enlargement of periurethral tissue of the prostate causes:
    a. obstruction of the urethra.
    b. inflammation of the testis.
    c. decreased urinary outflow from the bladder.
    d. abnormal dilation of a vein within the spermatic cord.
    e. tension of the spermatic cord and testis.

15. Recurrent urinary tract infections in the male cause:
    a. orchitis.
    b. balanitis.
    c. epididymitis.
    d. chronic bacterial prostatitis.
    e. nonbacterial prostatitis.

16. A symptom or sign of late-stage, metastatic prostatic cancer is:
    a. a slow urinary stream.
    b. frequency of urination.
    c. incomplete emptying.
    d. mental confusion associated with brain metastases.
    e. a, b, and c are correct.

17. Male sexual dysfunction may be caused by:
    a. infection around the introitus.
    b. diabetes mellitus.
    c. infected hymenal remnants.
    d. None of the above is correct.

Match the characteristic with the benign or malignant female breast disorder.

_____18. fluctuating lesion size

_____19. palpable axillary lymph node

_____20. mutated gene on chromosome 13 or 17

a. fibrocystic disease

b. breast cancer

Match the STI with its causative agent.

_____21. gonorrhea   a. *Haemophilus ducreyi*

_____22. syphilis   b. *Mycoplasma hominis*

_____23. condylomata acuminata   c. *Neisseria gonorrhoeae*

_____24. pediculosis pubis   d. *Gardnerella vaginalis*

_____25. lymphogranuloma   e. *Treponema pallidum*

                                                 f. human papillomavirus

                                                 g. *Sarcoptes scabiei*

                                                 h. *Phthirus pubis*

                                                 i. *Chlamydia trachomatis*

                                                 j. *Trichomonas vaginalis*

Case Study

Mrs. B., a 46-year-old female, consults her physician about the nature of a lump in one breast. About 3 months ago, her spouse noticed a small lump in her left breast; however, she was unconcerned because she had experienced small lumps in her breast around the times of her menses in the past. Yet, this lump seemed to be growing and did not seem to fluctuate in size as had other lumps. Three small lumps that did fluctuate in size were noticed by Mrs. B. in her right breast. She states she is in excellent health, exercises daily, and neither smokes nor drinks alcohol.

Mrs. B. is the mother of two preteen children. After the birth of her last child, she took birth control pills for 8 years and then selected an alternative method of birth control. Her onset of menses occurred at age 10. Her family history reveals that her mother and one of three aunts died of breast cancer; otherwise, the history is noncontributing.

On examination, a 2- to 3-cm mass is palpated in the upper quadrant of her left breast. This mass is firm, fixed to the chest wall, and slightly tender to touch. The skin and nipple appear normal. Under the left axilla, a node about the size of a pea is palpable. Three 1- to 2-cm soft, movable masses are palpated in Mrs. B.'s right breast.

Mammography confirms the presence of a 3-cm mass in the left breast and four 1.5-cm masses in the right breast. All other diagnostic procedures are negative.

What thoughts do you have concerning Mrs. B.'s examination and her risk factors?

33

Structure and Function of the Digestive System

Objectives

After reviewing this chapter, the learner will be able to do the following:

1. List sequentially the parts of the alimentary canal from mouth to anus.
   Refer to Figure 33-1.

2. Describe the structural layers of the gastrointestinal tract.
   Review page 956; refer to Figure 33-2.

3. Describe the mouth and esophagus, noting specific structure and function.
   Review pages 957-958; refer to Figures 33-3 and 33-4.

4. Describe the stomach, noting specific structure, function, and secretions.
   Review pages 958-961; refer to Figures 33-5 through 33-8 and Table 33-1.

5. Describe the small intestine, noting specific structure, function, and secretions.
   Review pages 961 and 963-964; refer to Figures 33-9 through 33-11 and Table 33-1.

6. Describe the structure and function of the large intestine and identify normal intestinal flora and their activities.
   Review pages 964 and 966-968; refer to Figure 33-12.

7. Note the significance of splanchnic blood flow.
   Review page 968; refer to Figure 33-13.

8. Describe the structure, function, and secretions of the liver and characterize the gallbladder.
   Review pages 968-974; refer to Figures 33-14 through 33-18 and Table 33-3.

9. Explain the relationship between cell types and function of the exocrine pancreas.
   Review pages 974-976; refer to Figure 33-19 and Table 33-4.

10. Describe the alterations in the digestive system associated with normal aging.
    Review page 977.

Practice Examination

1. The muscularis of the gastrointestinal tract is:
   a. skeletal muscle throughout the tract, particularly in the esophagus and large intestine.
   b. the layer that contains the blood capillaries for the entire wall of the tract.
   c. composed principally of keratinized epithelium.
   d. composed of circular fibers and longitudinal fibers.

2. The digestive functions performed by the saliva and salivary amylase, respectively, are:
   a. moistening and protein digestion.
   b. deglutition and fat digestion.
   c. peristalsis and polysaccharide digestion.
   d. lubrication and carbohydrate digestion.

3. The nervous pathway involved in salivary secretion requires stimulation of:
   a. receptors in the taste buds and somatic motor impulses to salivary glands.
   b. receptors in the mouth, sensory impulses, and parasympathetic impulses to salivary glands.
   c. taste receptors, sensory impulses, and somatic motor impulses to salivary glands.
   d. pressoreceptors in blood vessels and autonomic impulses to salivary glands.

4. Food would pass rapidly from the stomach into the duodenum if it were not for the:
   a. fundus.
   b. epiglottis.
   c. rugae.
   d. cardiac sphincter.
   e. pyloric sphincter.

5. The secretion of gastric juice:
   a. occurs only when swallowed food comes in contact with the stomach.
   b. is entirely under the control of the hormone gastrin.
   c. is entirely under the control of the hormone enterogastrone.
   d. is stimulated by the presence of saliva in the stomach.
   e. occurs in three phases: cephalic, gastric, and intestinal.

6. During nervous control of gastric secretion, the gastric glands secrete before food enters the stomach. This stimulus to the glands comes from:
   a. gastrin.
   b. impulses over somatic nerves from the hypothalamus.
   c. motor impulses from the cerebral cortex and cerebellum.
   d. parasympathetic impulses over the vagus nerve.

7. Pepsinogen:
   a. must be activated by HCl.
   b. is secreted by the chief cells.
   c. is a precursor to pepsin.
   d. All of the above are correct.

8. Beginning at the lumen of the tube, the sequence of layers of the gastrointestinal tract is:
   a. mucosa, submucosa, muscularis, serosa.
   b. submucosa, mucosa, serosa, muscularis.
   c. submucosa, mucosa, muscularis, skeletal muscle.
   d. serosa, muscularis, mucosa, submucosa.

9. Normally, when chyme leaves the stomach:
   a. the nutrients are ready for absorption into the blood.
   b. the amount of inorganic salts have been increased by the action of hydrochloric acid.
   c. its pH is neutral.
   d. the proteins have been partly digested into polypeptides.
   e. All of the above are correct.

10. Which layer of the small intestine includes microvilli?
    a. submucosa
    b. mucosa
    c. muscularis
    d. serosa

11. Which is *not* an example of mechanical digestion?
    a. chewing
    b. churning and mixing of food in the stomach
    c. peristalsis and mastication
    d. conversion of protein molecules into amino acids

12. Pancreatic juice is to trypsin as gastric juice is to:
    a. salivary amylase.
    b. pepsin.
    c. mucin.
    d. intrinsic factor.

13. Which part of the small intestine is most distal from the pylorus?
    a. jejunum
    b. pyloric sphincter
    c. duodenum
    d. cardiac sphincter
    e. common bile duct

14. The pancreas:
    a. lies mostly on the left side of the abdominal cavity, anterior to the stomach and the spleen.
    b. secretes all of its products directly into the bloodstream.
    c. is a gland with its duct ultimately opening into the duodenum.
    d. contains cells with endocrine function for the determination of secondary sex characteristics.
    e. is classified as a digestive exocrine gland, not having endocrine functions.

15. The chief role played by the pancreas in digestion is to:
    a. secrete insulin and glucagon.
    b. churn the food and bring it into contact with digestive enzymes.
    c. secrete enzymes, which digest food in the small intestine.
    d. assist in absorbing the digested foods.

16. Among the structural features of the small intestine are villi, microvilli, and circular folds. Their function is to:
    a. liberate hormones.
    b. promote peristalsis.
    c. liberate digestive enzymes.
    d. increase the surface area for absorption.

17. The fate of carbohydrates in the small intestine is:
    a. digestion to monosaccharides.
    b. conversion to simple sugars by the activity of trypsin.
    c. hydrolysis to amino acids.
    d. conversion to glycerol and fatty acids.

18. The absorptive fate of the end products of digestion may be summarized as:
    a. most fatty acids are absorbed into the blood; glucose and amino acids are absorbed into the lymphatic system.
    b. amino acids and monosaccharides are absorbed into blood capillaries; most fatty acids are absorbed into lymph.
    c. amino acids and fatty acids are absorbed into the lymph capillaries; glycerol and glucose are absorbed into the blood capillaries.
    d. fatty acids are absorbed into blood capillaries; glycerol, glucose, and amino acids are absorbed into lymph.

19. A lobule of the liver contains a centrally located:
    a. vein with radiating hepatocytes and sinusoids.
    b. arteriole with radiating capillaries and Kupffer cells.
    c. hepatic sinus with radiating sinusoids.
    d. hepatic duct with radiating Kupffer cells and cords of hepatic cells.

20. An obstruction of the common bile duct would cause blockage of bile coming from:
    a. the gallbladder.
    b. the liver but not from the gallbladder.
    c. both the liver and the gallbladder.
    d. the pancreatic duct but not from the gallbladder.

21. The human adult liver does not:
    a. store glycogen.
    b. produce erythrocytes.
    c. convert ammonia to urea.
    d. produce blood coagulation proteins.

22. The chyme that enters the large intestine is converted to feces by activity of:
    a. specific mucosal enzymes.
    b. gastric and duodenal hormones.
    c. bacteria and water reabsorption.
    d. the microvilli, villi, and circular muscles.

Match the substance/structures with its function.

_____23. splanchnic organs

_____24. Kupffer cells

_____25. cholecystokinin

a. stimulates gallbladder to eject bile

b. activates pepsinogen

c. trap bacteria

d. increases gastrointestinal mobility

e. act as blood reservoir for heart and lungs

f. stimulates liver to secrete bile

34

Alterations of Digestive Function

Foundational Objectives

a. **Describe the structure and function of the gastrointestinal tract and accessory organs of digestion.**
   Review pages 956-961 and 968-976; refer to Figure 33-1.

MEMORY CHECK!

- The gastrointestinal system includes the oral structures (mouth, salivary glands, pharynx), the alimentary tract (esophagus, stomach, small intestine, large intestine, appendix, anus), and the accessory organs of digestion (liver, gallbladder, bile ducts, pancreas). The function of the alimentary tract is to digest masticated food, to absorb digestive products, and to excrete the digestive residue and certain waste products excreted by the liver through the bile duct.

- The esophagus is a straight tube that carries food from the pharynx to the stomach. The stomach is a distensible organ. The stomach's mucosal cells secrete hydrochloric acid and proteolytic enzymes, which aid in digestion. The mucosa of the lower part of the stomach is lined by mucous cells. The distal end of the stomach is called the *pylorus.* The small intestine is divided into the duodenum, jejunum, and ileum. The large intestine or colon consists of the cecum, ascending colon, transverse colon, descending colon, sigmoid colon, and rectum. The vermiform appendix is a nonfunctional vestigial structure attached to the cecum. The colon is a storage reservoir for undigested food and a site for water absorption.

- The alimentary tract has four layers: mucosa, submucosa, muscularis, and serosa. The mucosal layer consists of epithelial cells lining the lumen's surface, supporting connective tissue called the *lamina propria,* and a unique thin, muscular layer called the *muscularis mucosae.* The structure of the inner mucosal layer varies to provide specialized function at each part of the tract. The esophagus is lined by stratified squamous epithelium, which enables rapid gliding of masticated food from the mouth to the stomach. The stomach has a thick glandular mucosa, which provides mucus, acid, and proteolytic enzymes to help digest food. The small intestinal mucosa has a villous structure to provide a large surface of cells for active absorption. The large intestinal mucosa is lined by abundant mucus-secreting cells that facilitate storage and evacuation of the residue. Beneath the mucosa is the submucosa, which gives structural support to the tract because of its abundant collagenous tissue. The muscle layer contracts rhythmically to move materials through the alimentary tract. The serosal layer is a thin, smooth membrane present on the outer surface of the alimentary tract. It keeps the tortuous loops of bowel from becoming tangled and is continuous with the mesentery. The mesentery is a connective tissue attachment of the bowel to the abdominal wall; it contains blood vessels, lymphatics, and nerves.

Continued

MEMORY CHECK!—cont'd

- A wave of muscle contraction carries a bolus of swallowed food down the esophagus, where a sphincter at the lower end of the esophagus prevents regurgitation. Contractions in the stomach mix the food and push the partially digested contents into the duodenum. The muscle of the pylorus only partially closes the outlet to the stomach, so intestinal contents can regurgitate into the stomach if the small intestine is not emptying properly. Normally, movement of luminal contents in the small intestine is more rapid in the upper small intestine and slows as chyme moves distally. Contents pass from the ileum into the colon, where reverse proximal movement is partially prevented by the ileocecal valve. Water is absorbed in the colon, and the contents become solid; the solid residue is moved to the left side of the colon and rectum. When the rectum becomes distended, an urge for defecation develops.

- The liver and the pancreas are glandular organs with excretory ducts emptying into the duodenum at a site called the *ampulla of Vater.* The excretory ducts of the liver are called *bile ducts.* The gallbladder is a storage reservoir connected to the bile ducts by the cystic duct.

- Most of the blood from the abdominal organs is carried to the liver via the portal vein. Therefore, blood is filtered by the glandular cells of the liver before it returns to the heart via the hepatic vein and vena cava. Because portal blood has little oxygen left after passing through the abdominal organs, the liver has the hepatic artery to provide oxygenated blood. The bulk of the liver is composed of hepatocytes, which are aligned in cords with sinusoids between the cords to diffuse the blood from the portal areas to the central vein. Between adjacent hepatocytes are tiny canaliculi that carry bile produced by the hepatocytes to the portal area, where they empty into epithelial lined bile ducts. In the sinusoids, waste products and nutrients are removed and metabolized by the hepatocytes. The metabolites may be returned to the blood, stored in the hepatocytes, or excreted into bile canaliculi. The liver also contains many mononuclear cells or Kupffer cells that line the sinusoids. They phagocytize particulate material from the blood. Metabolically, the liver (1) produces bile salts, (2) excretes bilirubin, (3) metabolizes nitrogenous substances, (4) produces serum proteins, and (5) detoxifies drugs and poisons.

- The gallbladder is a distension of the common bile duct that becomes a storage reservoir for bile. The gallbladder empties its contents into the duodenum after meals when bile salts are needed for fat absorption. This reservoir function is not essential, because the gallbladder can be removed without loss of digestive function.

- The pancreas is a long, narrow glandular organ lying horizontally and retroperitoneally in the midabdomen region. The pancreatic duct runs the length of the pancreas and empties into the duodenum after joining the bile duct. The bulk of the pancreas is made up of glands that secrete digestive enzymes into the pancreatic duct. When activated by intestinal juices, these enzymes digest carbohydrate, fat, and protein. Pancreatic enzymes are essential for life. Scattered among the pancreatic glands are clusters of endocrine cells known as the *islets of Langerhans,* which produce insulin and other hormones.

- The digestive process begins in the mouth, where a carbohydrate-splitting enzyme or amylase from the salivary glands mixes with food during mastication. In the stomach, proteolytic pepsin and hydrochloric acid are added to speed the digestive process. The greatest volume of digestive enzymes originates from the pancreas and is added to the digesting mixture of food in the duodenum. In addition, bile salts secreted by the liver and stored in the gallbladder are added to emulsify lipids into small water-soluble micelles. The final phase of the digestive process occurs at the surface of small intestinal epithelial cells. Complex endocrine and nervous mechanisms coordinate the timing of the secretion of digestive enzymes, hydrochloric acid, and bile salts. The sight of food may cause salivation and gastric secretions because of nervous stimulation. Distention of the stomach causes release of gastrin, which stimulates acid production and gastric emptying. Movement of food into the duodenum causes the pancreas to secrete more fluid and enzymes and the gallbladder to release bile. The products of both enter the duodenum.

Objectives

After studying this chapter, the learner will be able to do the following:

1. **Describe the common terms used in identifying the manifestations of gastrointestinal dysfunction.** Study pages 982-984; refer to Figure 34-1 and Table 34-1.

Anorexia is the absence of a desire to eat despite physiologic stimuli that would normally produce hunger. Anorexia is a nonspecific symptom often associated with nausea, abdominal pain, and diarrhea. Disorders of other systems besides the digestive system are accompanied by anorexia. These include cancer, heart disease, and renal disease.

Vomiting is the forceful emptying of stomach and intestinal contents, referred to as chyme, through the mouth. The vomiting reflex is stimulated by the presence of ipecac or copper salts in the duodenum, severe pain, or distention of the stomach or duodenum. Torsion or trauma affecting the ovaries, testes, uterus, bladder, or kidney also elicit vomiting.

Nausea and retching usually precede vomiting. **Nausea** is a subjective experience associated with many different conditions. **Retching** is a strong involuntary effort to vomit. In retching, the lower esophageal sphincter and body of the stomach relax, but the duodenum and antrum of the stomach go into spasm. The reverse peristalsis forces chyme from the stomach and duodenum up into the esophagus. Because the upper esophageal sphincter is closed, chyme does not enter the mouth. As the abdominal muscles relax, the contents of the esophagus drop back into the stomach. This process may be repeated several times before vomiting occurs.

Vomiting occurs when the stomach is full of gastric contents and the diaphragm is forced high into the thoracic cavity by strong abdominal muscle contractions. The higher intrathoracic pressure forces the upper esophageal sphincter to open and chyme is discharged from the mouth. Spontaneous vomiting not preceded by nausea or retching is called **projectile vomiting.** This vomiting is caused by direct stimulation of the vomiting center because of neurologic lesions involving the brain stem. The metabolic consequences of vomiting are fluid, electrolyte, and acid-base disturbances.

Constipation is difficult or infrequent defecation involving decreased numbers of bowel movements per week, hard stools, and difficult evacuation. Constipation is often caused by unhealthy dietary and bowel habits combined with inadequate exercise and low fluid intake. It also can occur as a result of intestinal immobility or obstruction disorders.

Constipation resulting from life-style or bowel habits usually has a long duration. Dysfunctional constipation is more likely to be sudden and can accompany the development of organic lesions.

Diarrhea is increased frequency of defecation accompanied by changes in fecal fluidity and volume. In **osmotic diarrhea,** the presence of nonabsorbable substances in the intestine causes water to be drawn into the lumen by osmosis. The excess water and the nonabsorbable substances increase stool weight and volume. This causes large-volume diarrhea. **Secretory diarrhea** is a form of large-volume diarrhea caused by excessive mucosal secretion of fluid and electrolytes. Excessive intestinal secretion is caused mostly by bacterial enterotoxins released by cholera or strains of *Escherichia coli.* A lesion that impairs autonomic control of motility such as diabetic neuropathy can cause large-volume diarrhea. Excessive motility decreases transit time, mucosal surface contact, and opportunities for fluid absorption. **Motility diarrhea** can be caused by resection of the small intestine, surgical bypass of an area of the intestine, or fistula formation between loops of the intestine.

Small-volume diarrhea is usually caused by inflammatory disorders of the intestine or by fecal impaction from severe constipation. In the latter case, the diarrhea consists of mucus and fluid produced by the colon to lubricate the impacted feces and move it toward the anal canal.

Abdominal pain is observed in a number of gastrointestinal diseases. Abdominal organs are sensitive to stretching and distention, which can activate nerve endings in both hollow and solid structures. Histamine, bradykinin, and serotonin, when released during inflammation, stimulate organic nerve endings and produce abdominal pain. The edema and vascular congestion that accompany inflammation also cause painful stretching. Any obstruction of blood flow because of distention of bowel obstruction or mesenteric vessel thrombosis produces ischemic pain. **Parietal pain** arises from the parietal peritoneum and is more localized and intense than **visceral pain,** which arises from the organs themselves. **Referred pain** is visceral pain felt at some distance from a diseased or affected organ. Referred pain is usually well localized and is felt in the skin or deeper tissues, which share a central, common afferent pathway with the affected organ.

Numerous disorders cause gastrointestinal tract bleeding. Acute **gastrointestinal bleeding** is usually characterized by hematemesis, or the presence of blood in the vomitus; **hematochezia,** or frank bleeding from the rectum; or **melena,** which is dark, tarry stools. **Occult bleeding** is slow, chronic blood loss that results in iron deficiency anemia as iron stores in the bone marrow are slowly depleted.

2. **Compare and contrast the various disorders of digestive motility.**
   Study pages 984-990; refer to Figures 34-2 and 34-3 and Tables 34-2 and 34-3.

Motility Disorders

Disorder	Causes	Manifestations

Dysphagia (swallowing difficulty)	Esophageal obstruction
	  Tumors, strictured, or diverticula
	Impaired esophageal motility
	  Neural dysfunction, muscular disease, CVA
	Achalasia (decreased ganglion cells in myenteric plexus, muscle cell atrophy)
		Distention and spasm of esophagus after swallowing, regurgitation of undigested food

Gastroesophageal reflux (chyme reflux into esophagus)	Increased abdominal pressure, ulcers, pyloric edema and strictures, hiatal hernia	Regurgitation of chyme within 1 hour of eating
Hiatal hernia (protrusion of upper stomach through diaphragm into thorax)	Congenitally short esophagus, trauma, weak diaphragmatic muscles at gastroesophageal junction, increased abdominal pressure	Gastroesophageal reflux, dysphagia, epigastric pain
Pyloric obstruction (narrow pylorus)	Peptic ulcer or carcinoma near pylorus	Epigastric fullness, nausea and pain, vomitus without bile
Intestinal obstruction (impaired chyme flow through intestinal lumen)	Hernia, telescoping of one part of intestine into another, twisting, inflamed diverticula, tumor growth, loss of peristaltic activity	Colicky pain to severe and constant pain, vomiting, diarrhea, constipation, dehydration and hypovolemia, and acidosis with their complications

3. **Describe the pathogenesis of acute and chronic gastritis.**
   Study page 990, refer to Figure 34-4.

Gastritis is a common inflammatory disorder of the gastric mucosa that may be acute or chronic affecting the fundus or antrum or both. Antiinflammatory drugs are known to cause **acute gastritis,** which erodes the epithelium, probably because they inhibit prostaglandins that normally stimulate the secretion of protective mucus. Alcohol, histamine, digitalis, and metabolic disorders such as uremia are contributing factors for gastritis.

The clinical manifestations of acute gastritis can include vague abdominal discomfort, epigastric tenderness, and bleeding. Healing usually occurs spontaneously within a few days. Discontinuing injurious drugs, using antacids, or decreasing acid secretion with drugs facilitates healing.

Chronic gastritis is a progressive disease that tends to occur in elderly individuals. This gastritis causes thinning and degeneration of the stomach wall.

Chronic fundal gastritis is the most severe type, because the gastric mucosa degenerates extensively. The loss of chief cells and parietal cells diminishes secretion of pepsinogen, hydrochloric acid, and intrinsic factor. Pernicious anemia develops because intrinsic factor is unavailable to facilitate vitamin B_{12} absorption. Chronic fundal gastritis becomes a risk factor for gastric carcinoma, particularly in individuals who develop pernicious anemia. A significant number of individuals with chronic fundal gastritis have antibodies to parietal cells, intrinsic factor, and gastric cells in their sera, thus suggesting an autoimmune mechanism in the pathogenesis of the disease.

Chronic antral gastritis is more common than fundal gastritis. It is not associated with decreased hydrochloric acid secretion, pernicious anemia, or the presence of parietal cell antibodies. *Helicobacter pylori* is a major etiologic factor associated with the inflammation seen in chronic gastritis. The longstanding inflammatory process and gastric atrophy may develop without a history of abdominal distress. Individuals may report vague symptoms including anorexia, fullness, nausea, vomiting, and epigastric pain. Gastric bleeding may be the only clinical manifestation of gastritis.

4. **Compare duodenal, gastric, and stress ulcers; identify the complications of surgical management of ulcers.**
   Study pages 990-991 and 993-996; refer to Figures 34-4 through 34-6 and Tables 34-4 and 34-5.

A **peptic ulcer** is a break or ulceration in the protective mucosal lining of the lower esophagus, stomach, or duodenum. Such breaks expose submucosal areas to gastric secretions and autodigestion.

Risk factors for peptic ulcer disease are smoking and habitual use of NSAIDs or alcohol. NSAIDs inhibit prostaglandins and decrease mucous production. Some chronic diseases such as emphysema, rheumatoid arthritis, and cirrhosis are associated with the development of peptic ulcers. Infection of the gastric and duodenal mucosa with *H. pylori* causes peptic ulcers. Studies of life stress and ulcer disease are inconclusive regarding causation of peptic ulcers.

Postgastrectomy syndromes are a group of signs and symptoms that occur after gastric resection. They are caused by alterations in motor and control functions of the stomach and upper small intestine. **Dumping syndrome** is the rapid emptying of hypertonic chyme from the surgically reduced and smaller stomach into the small intestine 10 to 20 minutes after eating.

Alkaline reflux gastritis is stomach inflammation caused by reflux of bile and alkaline pancreas secretions that contain proteolytic enzymes that disrupt the mucosal barrier. Clinical manifestations include nausea, vomiting in which the vomitus contains bile, and sustained epigastric pain that worsens after eating and is not relieved by antacids.

Afferent loop obstruction is a problem caused by volvulus, hernia, adhesion, or stenosis in the duodenal stump on the proximal side of the surgery. The symptoms of afferent loop obstruction include intermittent severe pain and epigastric fullness after eating.

Postgastrectomy **diarrhea** appears to be related to rapid gastric emptying of large amounts of high carbohydrate liquids. **Weight loss** often follows gastric resection because the stomach is less able to mix, churn, and break down food.

Anemia after gastrectomy results from iron, vitamin B_{12}, or folate deficiency.

Bone disorders are related to altered calcium levels, which increase the risk for fractures and bone deformity.

Features of Ulcers

Feature	Duodenal	Gastric	Stress
Age incidence	25-50 years	50-70 years	Related to severe stress, trauma, sepsis, head injuries
Sex prevalence	Men	No sex difference	
Stress factors	Average	Increased	Increased
Acid production	Increased	Normal to low	Increased
Ulcerogenic drugs	Heavy use of alcohol and tobacco	Moderate use of alcohol and tobacco	
Associated gastritis	Seldom	Common	
Helicobacter pylori	Usually present	May be present	
Pain	Pain-food-relief; common nocturnal pain; remission and exacerbations	Pain-food-relief; uncommon nocturnal pain; chronic; no remission and exacerbations	Asymptomatic until hemorrhage or perforation
Hemorrhage	Common	Less common	Very common (most frequent complication)
Malignancy	Almost never	Possible	

H. pylori's urease lead to ammonia formation, which is toxic to mucosal cells, and the phospholipases of these organisms damage mucosa. Also, *H. pylori* infection stimulates gastrin production, which increases acid secretion.

NOTE: Medical treatment is directed toward inhibiting or buffering acid secretions to relieve symptoms and promote healing. Antacids, dietary management, anticholinergic histamine blockers, and physical and emotional rest are used to accomplish relief and promote healing. *H. pylori* is treated with a combination of antibiotics and bismuth.

5. **Define malabsorption syndrome and maldigestion; characterize pancreatic insufficiency and lactase and bile salt deficiency.**
    Study page 996.

Malabsorption syndromes interfere with nutrient absorption in the small intestine; the intestinal mucosa fails to absorb or transport the digested nutrients into the blood. **Malabsorption** is the result of mucosal disruption caused by gastric or intestinal resection, vascular disorders, or intestinal disease. **Maldigestion** is failed or faulty digestion because of deficiencies of chemical enzymes.

Pancreatic insufficiency occurs because of deficient production of lipase, amylase, trypsin, or chymotrypsin by the pancreas. Causes of pancreatic insufficiency include chronic pancreatitis, pancreatic carcinoma, pancreatic resection, and cystic fibrosis. Fat maldigestion is the chief problem. A large amount of fat in the stool is the most common sign of pancreatic insufficiency.

Lactase deficiency inhibits the breakdown of lactose or milk sugar into monosaccharides and therefore prevents lactose digestion and absorption across the intestinal wall. Lactase deficiency is most common in blacks. The undigested lactose remains in the intestine, where bacterial fermentation causes gases to form. The osmotic gradient in the intestine also increases, which causes irritation and osmotic diarrhea.

Conjugated bile acids or bile salts are necessary for the digestion and absorption of fats. When bile from the liver enters the duodenum, the bile salts aggregate with fatty acids and monoglycerides to form micelles. Micelle formation solubilizes fat molecules and allows them to pass through the unstirred layer at the brush border. Advanced liver disease that causes **bile salt deficiency,** obstruction of the common bile duct, intestinal immotility, and diseases of the ileum all lead to poor intestinal absorption of fat and fat-soluble vitamins A, D, E, and K. Increased fat in the stool leads to diarrhea and decreased plasma proteins. The loss of fat-soluble vitamins causes night blindness, bone demineralization, and bleeding abnormalities.

6. **Compare ulcerative colitis and Crohn disease.**
    Study pages 996-997; refer to Table 34-6. (See box on next page.)

7. **Distinguish between diverticular disease and appendicitis.**
    Study pages 998-999; refer to Figure 34-7.

Diverticula are herniations or saclike outpouchings of mucosa through the muscle layers of the colon wall. **Diverticulosis** is asymptomatic diverticular disease. **Diverticulitis** represents symptomatic inflammation. The most common site of diverticula is the sigmoid colon at weak points in the colon wall where arteries penetrate the muscularis. Habitual consumption of a low-residue diet reduces fecal bulk and reduces the diameter of the colon. According to the law of Laplace, wall pressure increases as the diameter of the lumen decreases. Pressure within the narrow lumen can increase enough to rupture the diverticula and cause abscess formation or peritonitis. An increase of dietary fiber intake often relieves symptoms. Surgical resection may be required if there are severe complications.

Appendicitis is an inflammation of the vermiform appendix. Obstruction of the lumen with feces, tumors, or foreign bodies followed by bacterial infection is the most likely cause of appendicitis. The obstructed lumen does not allow drainage of the appendix, and as mucosal secretion continues, intraluminal pressure increases. The increased pressure decreases mucosal blood flow, and the appendix becomes hypoxic. The mucosa ulcerates, which promotes bacterial inflammation and edema. Gangrene develops from thrombosis of the luminal blood vessels followed by perforation.

Epigastric or periumbilical pain is the typical symptom of an inflamed appendix. Right lower quadrant pain that exhibits rebound tenderness is associated with extension of the inflammation to the surrounding tissues. Nausea, vomiting, and anorexia follow the onset of pain. Leukocytosis and a low-grade fever are common. Perforation, peritonitis, and abscess formation are the most serious complications of appendicitis.

Appendectomy is the treatment for simple or perforated appendicitis.

Ulcerative Colitis and Crohn Disease

Feature	Ulcerative colitis	Crohn disease
Family history	Less common	More common
Location of lesions	Large intestine; no "skip" lesions; mucosal layer involved	Large or small intestine; "skip" lesions common; entire intestinal wall involved
Granulomas	Rare	Common
Anal and perianal fistulas and abscesses	Rare	Common
Narrowed lumen and possible obstruction	Rare	Common
Abdominal pain	Common, mild to severe	Common, mild to severe
Diarrhea	Common	Common
Bloody stools	Common	Less common
Abdominal mass	Rare	Common
Small intestinal malabsorption	Rare	Common
Steatorrhea	Rare	Common
Cancer risk	Increased	Not increased

8. **Characterize the disorders of overnutrition and undernutrition.**

Study pages 1000-1002.

Overnutrition, or excessive caloric intake, leads to **obesity,** or excessive body fat, which is associated with three leading causes of death: cardiovascular disease, cancer, and diabetes mellitus. Obesity also is a risk factor for breast, cervical, endometrial, and liver cancer in women. Obese men are at greater risk for prostatic, colon, and rectal cancer than nonobese men.

Obesity is classified by cause as either exogenous, resulting from an excess of ingested calories, or endogenous, resulting from inherent metabolic problems. Physiologically, obesity can be (1) hyperplastic, caused by a greater-than-normal number of fat cells; or (2) hypertrophic, caused by a greater-than-normal size of fat cells. In children the adipose tissue is dispersed over the entire body and is both hyperplastic and hypertrophic with few metabolic abnormalities. Adult-onset obesity is hypertrophic, with the adipose tissue centrally located, and metabolic abnormalities are more common. Genotype is an important predisposing factor.

A number of theories have been postulated to explain the physiology of obesity. In the genetic theory, an elevated obese gene product, leptin, may control fat stores by regulating food intake. A fat-cell theory suggests that an excessive number and size of fat cells increases whenever a positive energy balance exists. In the lipoprotein-lipase (LPL) theory, lipase hydrolyzes fats into their components, which then reenter the fat cells and are converted back into fats; LPL promotes fat storage and hypertrophic

cells. The lipostatic theory states that obese individuals have a higher set-point, which makes it difficult to maintain weight loss.

Another theory of obesity is based on the thermogenesis of brown fat cells that are responsible for heat production. Subcutaneous brown fat cells release excess energy through heat production instead of converting the energy to fat stores; obese people are believed to have very few brown fat cells.

The sodium-potassium-adenosine triphosphatase (ATPase) pump transports sodium out of the cell and potassium into the cell and splits adenosine triphosphate, thus releasing energy. Obese people have fewer ATPase pumps, which could lead to less energy release and obesity.

One psychologic theory proposes that obese people are directed more by the sight, smell, and taste of food than by hunger and satiety. Another psychologic theory is that eating creates the desire to eat more.

Diabetes mellitus is often associated with obesity. The excess serum glucose is stored as glycogen in the liver or as triglycerides in adipose cells, thus enhancing hypertrophy and hyperplasia of fat cells.

Treatment of obesity caused by excessive nutrient intake is a regimen of reduced nutrient intake and increased energy expenditure. Individuals with adult-onset obesity can reduce the size of the adipose cells and achieve a standard weight. Those with child-onset obesity may never achieve standard weight. Additional treatments such as psychotherapy, behavioral modification, medication, and surgery may be needed.

Many young adults and adolescents in the United States are affected by two complex and related eating disorders, anorexia nervosa and bulimia. **Anorexia nervosa** is characterized by refusal to eat because of distorted body image perceptions that one is too fat. As the disease progresses, fat and muscle depletion give the individual a skeleton-like appearance. The loss of 25% to 30% of ideal body weight can eventually lead to death caused by starvation-induced cardiac failure. Treatment objectives for anorexia nervosa include reversing the compromised physical state, promoting insights and knowledge about the disorder, and modifying food habits.

Bulimia is characterized by binging or the consumption of normal to large amounts of food followed by self-induced vomiting or purging of the intestines with laxatives. Although individuals with bulimia are afraid of gaining weight, their weight usually remains within normal range. Because of negative connotations associated with vomiting and purging, individuals who have bulimia often binge and purge secretly. Bulimics may binge and purge as often as 20 times a day. Continual vomiting of acidic chyme can cause pitted teeth, pharyngeal and esophageal inflammation, and tracheoesophageal fistulas. Overuse of laxatives can cause rectal bleeding.

Starvation can be either short-term or long-term. Therapeutic short-term starvation is part of many weight-reduction programs, whereas therapeutic long-term starvation is used in medically controlled environments to facilitate rapid weight loss in morbidly obese individuals. Pathologic long-term starvation can be caused by poverty or chronic diseases such as cardiovascular, pulmonary, hepatic, and digestive disorders, malabsorption syndromes, and cancer.

Short-term starvation consists of several days of total dietary abstinence or deprivation. Glucose is the preferred energy source for cells. Once all available energy has been absorbed from the intestine, glycogen in the liver is converted to glucose through glycogenolysis, or the splitting of glycogen into glucose. This process peaks within 4 to 8 hours after glycogenolysis, and gluconeogenesis in the liver begins by the formation of glucose from noncarbohydrate molecules. Both of these processes deplete stored nutrients and thus cannot meet the body's energy needs indefinitely. Proteins continue to be catabolized in gluconeogenesis to a minimal degree to provide carbon for the synthesis of glucose.

The main characteristics of **long-term starvation** are decreased dependence on gluconeogenesis and increased use of products of lipid and pyruvate metabolism for cellular energy sources. Once the supply of adipose tissue is depleted, proteolysis begins. The breakdown of muscle protein is the last process to supply energy for life. Death results from severe alteration in electrolyte balance and loss of renal, pulmonary, and cardiac function.

Adequate ingestion of appropriate nutrients is the obvious treatment for starvation. Starvation caused by chronic disease, long-term illness, or malabsorption is treated by enteral or parenteral nutrition.

9. **Describe the complications of liver dysfunction.**
   Study pages 1002-1006; refer to Figures 34-8 through 34-10 and Table 34-7.

The complications of liver disease include portal hypertension, ascites, hepatic encephalopathy, jaundice, and hepatorenal syndrome. (See box on next page.)

10. **Compare the viral hepatitis types.**
    Study pages 1006-1008; refer to Table 34-8.

The clinical manifestations of the different types of hepatitis are very similar and usually consist of three phases: the prodromal, icteric, and recovery phases. The **prodromal phase** of hepatitis begins about 2 weeks after exposure and ends with appearance of jaundice. Fatigue, anorexia, malaise, nausea, vomiting, headache, hyperalgia, cough, and low-grade fever precede the onset of jaundice. The infection is highly transmissible during this phase.

The **icteric phase** begins about 1 to 2 weeks after the prodromal phase and lasts 2 to 6 weeks. The icteric phase is the actual phase of illness. The liver is enlarged, smooth, and tender, and percussion over the liver causes pain.

The posticteric or **recovery phase** begins with resolution of jaundice at about 6 to 8 weeks after exposure. In most cases, liver function returns to normal within 2 to 12 weeks after the onset of jaundice.

Liver Disease Complications

Complication	Causes	Manifestations
Portal hypertension	Obstruction or impeded blood flow in portal venous system or vena cava, cirrhosis, viral hepatitis, parasitic infection, hepatic vein thrombosis, right heart failure	Esophageal and stomach varices with vomiting of blood, splenomegaly, ascites
Ascites	Portal hypertension and reduced serum albumin levels increase capillary hydrostatic pressure that pushes water into the peritoneal cavity, cirrhosis, heart failure, constrictive pericarditis, abdominal malignancies, nephrotic syndrome, malnutrition	Abdominal distension, displaced diaphragm, dyspnea, peritonitis
Hepatic encephalopathy	Blood that contains toxins such as ammonia is shunted from gastrointestinal tract to systemic circulation, toxins reach brain	Subtle changes in cerebral function, confusion, tremor of hands, stupor, convulsions, coma
Jaundice		Dark urine, light-colored stools, anorexia, malaise, fatigue, pruritus
Hemolytic (unconjugated bilirubin)	Excessive hemolysis of red blood cells because of immune reactions, infections, toxic substances, or transfusions of incompatible blood	
Obstructive (conjugated bilirubin)	Obstruction of bile flow by gallstones or tumor prevents flow into duodenum, drugs	
Hepatocellular (conjugated and unconjugated bilirubin)	Intrahepatic disease, obstruction by bile calculi, genetic enzyme defects, infections	
Hepatorenal syndrome	Decrease in blood volume; intrarenal vasoconstriction because the liver may fail to remove excessive vasoactive substances from the blood	Oliguria, sodium and water retention, hypotension, BUN and creatinine increases

Fulminant hepatitis is a clinical syndrome resulting in severe impairment or necrosis of liver cells and potential liver failure. It may occur as a complication of hepatitis C or hepatitis B and is compounded by infection with the delta virus. The hepatic necrosis is irreversible.

Treatment of fulminant hepatitis is supportive, and many individuals die. Liver transplantation may be lifesaving. Survivors usually do not develop cirrhosis or chronic liver disease. (See box on page 250.)

Characteristics of Viral Hepatitis

	Hepatitis A	Hepatitis B	Hepatitis D	Hepatitis C	Hepatitis E	Hepatitis G
Transmission route	Fecal-oral, parenteral, sexual	Parenteral, sexual	Parenteral, fecal-oral, sexual	Parenteral	Fecal-oral	Parenteral, sexual
Incubation period	30 days	60-180 days	30-180 days	35-60 days	15-60 days	
Carrier state	No	Yes	Yes	Yes	No	
Severity	Mild	Severe, may be pro- longed	Severe	Unknown	Severe in preg- nant women	
Chronic hepatitis	No	Yes	Yes	Yes	No	
Prophylaxis	Hygiene, im- mune serum globulin	Hygiene, HBV vaccine	Hygiene, HBV vaccine	Hygiene, screening blood	Hygiene, safe water	

Transfusion transmission virus (TTV) was recently discovered but its pathogenesis is uncertain.

NOTE: Treatment is supportive, physical activity is restricted, low-fat and high-carbohydrate diet is recommended, and interferon is useful in chronic B and C types.

11. **Describe cirrhosis and contrast various types.**
    Study pages 1008-1010; refer to Figure 34-11 and Table 34-9.

    Cirrhosis is an irreversible inflammatory disease that disrupts liver structure and function. Structural changes result from fibrosis, which is a consequence of inflammation. (See box below.)

12. **Compare cholelithiasis to cholecystitis.**
    Study pages 1010-1011; refer to Figure 34-12.

Obstruction and inflammation are the most common disorders of the gallbladder. Obstruction is caused by gallstones, which are aggregates of substances in the bile. The gallstones may remain in the gallbladder or enter the cystic duct. If gallstones become lodged in the cystic duct, they obstruct the flow of bile into and out of the gall- bladder and cause inflammation. Gallstone formation is termed **cholelithiasis,** whereas inflammation of the gall- bladder or cystic duct is known as **cholecystitis.**

Cirrhosis of the Liver

Type	Cause	Manifestations
Alcoholic cirrhosis	Toxic effects of chronic and excessive alcohol intake; alcohol is oxidized by the liver to ac- etaldehyde, which damages hepatocytes	Typical; decreased sexual function
Primary biliary cirrhosis	Unknown, possibly an autoimmune mecha- nism that scars ducts	Typical; circulating IgG
Secondary biliary cirrhosis	Obstruction by neoplasms, strictures, or gall- stones scar the ducts proximally	Typical
Post-necrotic cirrhosis	Viral hepatitis due to HAV or hepatitis C, drugs or other toxins, autoimmune destruction	Typical

NOTE: Typical manifestations include hepatomegaly, splenomegaly, ascites, and jaundice. Serologic studies reveal elevated enzymes and bilirubin, de- creased albumin, and prolonged prothrombin time.

Gallstones are of two types: cholesterol and pigmented. Cholesterol stones are the most common. Cholesterol gallstones form in bile that is supersaturated with cholesterol produced by the liver. Usually within the gallbladder, supersaturation sets the stage for cholesterol crystal formation and aggregation into "macro-stones." If the stones become lodged in the cystic or common duct, they cause pain and cholecystitis. Pigmented stones occur later in life and are associated with cirrhosis. Pigmented stones are created by unconjugated bilirubin binding with calcium. Risk factors for cholelithiasis include obesity, middle age, female gender, American Indian ancestry, and gallbladder, pancreatic, or ileal disease.

Abdominal pain and jaundice are the cardinal manifestations of cholelithiasis. Vague symptoms include heartburn, flatulence, epigastric discomfort, and fatty food intolerances. Biliary colic pain is caused by the lodging of one or more gallstones in the cystic or common duct. The pain can be intermittent or steady and is located in the right upper quadrant with radiation to the mid-upper back. Jaundice indicates that the stone is located in the common bile duct.

Laparoscopic cholecystectomy is the preferred treatment for gallstones that cause obstruction or inflammation. Alternative treatments are the administration of drugs that dissolve the stones and ultrasonic lithotripsy.

Cholecystitis can be acute or chronic and is almost always caused by the lodging of a gallstone in the cystic duct. Obstruction causes the gallbladder to become distended and inflamed, followed by decreased blood flow, ischemia, necrosis, and possible perforation. Fever, leukocytosis, rebound tenderness, and abdominal muscle guarding are common findings. Serum bilirubin and alkaline phosphatase levels may be elevated.

13. Describe the pathogenesis of pancreatitis.
Study pages 1011-1012.

Pancreatitis, or inflammation of the pancreas, is a relatively rare but potentially serious disorder. It is be-

lieved that **acute pancreatitis** develops because of an injury or disruption of the pancreatic ducts or acini that permits leakage of pancreatic enzymes into pancreatic tissue. The leaked enzymes initiate autodigestion and acute pancreatitis. Bile reflux into the pancreas occurs if gallstones obstruct the common bile duct; the refluxed bile also injures pancreatic tissue. Toxic enzymes also are released into the bloodstream and cause injury to vessels and other organs such as the lungs and kidneys. **Chronic pancreatitis** is caused mostly by alcohol abuse.

Mild to severe epigastric or midabdominal pain is the cardinal symptom of acute pancreatitis. The pain is caused by distended pancreatic ducts and capsule, chemical irritation and inflammation of the peritoneum, and irritation or obstruction of the biliary tract. Fever and leukocytosis accompany the inflammatory response. Nausea and vomiting are caused by hypermotility or paralytic ileus secondary to the pancreatitis or peritonitis. Elevated serum amylase is a characteristic diagnostic feature. Hypotension and shock often occur because plasma volume is lost as enzymes and kinins released into the circulation increase vascular permeability and dilate vessels. The results are hypovolemia, hypotension, and myocardial insufficiency.

The goal of treatment for acute pancreatitis is to stop the process of autodigestion and prevent systemic complications. Parenteral fluids are given to restore blood volume and prevent hypotension and shock. Severe, unremitting pancreatitis may require peritoneal lavage or surgical drainage of the pancreas to remove toxic exudates.

14. Characterize the various cancers of the digestive system.
Study pages 1012-1019; refer to Figures 34-13 through 34-15 and Tables 34-10 and 34-11. (See box on page 252.)

Cancers of the Digestive System

Type	Risks	Manifestations
Esophagus Squamous cell carcinoma Adenocarcinoma	Malnutrition, alcohol, tobacco, chronic reflux	Chest pain, dysphagia

Stomach
  Adenocarcinoma
  Squamous cell carcinoma
	Dietary salty foods, nitrates, nitrosamines, gastric atrophy, *H. pylori* associated gastritis	Anorexia, malaise, weight loss, upper abdominal pain, vomiting, occult blood, symptoms of organ involved in metastasis from stomach

Colorectal Adenocarcinoma (left colon grows in ring; right colon grows in mass)	Chromosomal deletions, polyps, diverticulitis, ulcerative colitis, high refined CHO, low-fiber/high-fat diet	Pain, anemia, bloody stool, mass—right colon, obstruction—left colon, distention, elevated CEA

Liver
  Hepatocarcinoma
  Cholangiocarcinoma
	HBV, HCV, HDV, cirrhosis, intestinal parasites, aflatoxin	Pain, anorexia, bloating, weight loss, portal hypertension, ascites, +/− jaundice, elevated serum proteins and enzymes

Gallbladder Secondary metastases Adenocarcinoma Squamous cell carcinoma	Cholelithiasis	Steady pain, diarrhea, anorexia, vomiting, +/− jaundice
Pancreas Adenocarcinoma	Chronic pancreatitis, cigarette smoking, alcohol, diabetic women	Weight loss, weakness, nausea, vomiting, abdominal pain, depression, +/− jaundice, possible hypoglycemia if an insulin-secreting tumor

NOTE: Treatment for esophageal, stomach, gallbladder, and pancreatic cancer is essentially surgical. Liver neoplasms are treated by surgery and chemotherapy. Colorectal cancer therapy uses surgery, radiation, and chemotherapy.

Practice Examination

1. During vomiting, there is:
   a. forceful diaphragm and abdominal muscle contractions, airway closure, esophageal sphincter relaxation, and deep inspiration.
   b. deep inspiration, airway closure, forceful diaphragm and abdominal muscle contractions, and esophageal sphincter relaxation.
   c. airway closure, forceful diaphragm and abdominal muscle contractions, deep inspiration, and esophageal sphincter relaxation.
   d. esophageal sphincter relaxation, forceful diaphragm and abdominal muscle contractions, deep inspiration, and airway closure.

2. Which does *not* cause constipation?
   a. opiates
   b. megacolon
   c. sedentary lifestyle
   d. hyperthyroidism
   e. emotional depression

3. Osmotic diarrhea is caused by:
   a. lactase deficiency.
   b. bacterial enterotoxins.
   c. ulcerative colitis.
   d. Crohn disease.
   e. Both c and d are correct.

4. Melena is:
   a. bloody vomitus.
   b. gaseous bowel distension.
   c. blood in the stool.
   d. loss of appetite.
   e. black, tarry stools.

5. A common manifestation of hiatal hernia is:
   a. gastroesophageal reflux.
   b. diarrhea.
   c. belching.
   d. postprandial substernal pain.
   e. Both a and d are correct.

6. Gastroesophageal reflux is:
    a. caused by rapid gastric emptying.
    b. excessive lower esophageal sphincter functioning.
    c. associated with abdominal surgery.
    d. caused by spontaneously relaxing lower esophageal sphincter.

7. Intestinal obstruction causes:
    a. decreased intraluminal tension.
    b. hyperkalemia.
    c. decreased nutrient absorption.
    d. Both a and b are correct.
    e. a, b, and c are correct.

8. Peptic ulcers may be located in the:
    a. stomach.
    b. esophagus.
    c. duodenum.
    d. colon.
    e. a, b, and c are correct.

9. Gastric ulcers:
    a. may lead to malignancy.
    b. occur at a younger age than duodenal ulcers.
    c. always have increased acid production.
    d. exhibit nocturnal pain.
    e. Both a and c are correct.

10. Duodenal ulcers:
    a. occur four times more often in females than in males.
    b. may be complicated by hemorrhage.
    c. are associated with sepsis.
    d. may cause inflammation and scar tissue formation around the sphincter of Oddi.

11. In malabsorption syndrome, flatulence and abdominal distension are likely caused by:
    a. protein deficiency and electrolyte imbalance.
    b. undigested lactose fermentation by bacteria.
    c. fat irritating the bowel.
    d. impaired absorption of amino acids and accompanying edema.

12. The characteristic lesion of Crohn disease is
    a. found in the ileum.
    b. precancerous.
    c. granulomatous.
    d. malignant.
    e. Both a and c are correct.

13. Low-residue diets and chronic constipation play a role in the pathogenesis of:
    a. appendicitis.
    b. diverticulitis.
    c. ulcerative colitis.
    d. Crohn disease.
    e. cholecystitis.

14. A 14-year-old male has been admitted to the emergency room suffering with acute-onset abdominal pain in the lower right quadrant. Abdominal rebound tenderness is intense, and he has a fever and leukocytosis. This individual most likely is suffering from:
    a. acute appendicitis.
    b. diverticulitis.
    c. ulcerative colitis.
    d. cholelithiasis.
    e. cholecystitis.

15. Adult-onset obesity usually is:
    a. both hyperplastic and hypertrophic.
    b. dispersed over the entire body.
    c. hypertrophic.
    d. unrelated to genotype.
    e. None of the above is correct.

16. Short-term starvation involves:
    a. glycogenolysis.
    b. gluconeogenesis.
    c. proteolysis.
    d. Both a and b are correct.
    e. a, b, and c are correct.

17. The most common manifestation of portal hypertension is:
    a. rectal bleeding.
    b. cirrhosis.
    c. intestinal bleeding.
    d. duodenal bleeding.
    e. vomiting of blood from esophageal bleeding.

18. Hepatic encephalopathy is manifested by:
    a. ascites.
    b. splenomegaly.
    c. dark urine.
    d. oliguria.
    e. cerebral dysfunction.

19. Which would be consistent with a diagnosis of viral hepatitis? (More than one answer may be correct.)
    a. Elevated AST serum enzymes
    b. Decreased serum albumin levels
    c. Prolonged coagulation times
    d. Increased serum bilirubin levels
    e. Decreased ALT serum enzymes

20. Which viral hepatitis is *not* associated with a chronic state or a carrier state?
    a. Hepatitis A
    b. Hepatitis B
    c. Hepatitis C
    d. Serum hepatitis
    e. Hepatitis D

21. Which type of jaundice is due to increased destruction of erythrocytes?
    a. Obstructive
    b. Hemolytic
    c. Hepatocellular
    d. Both b and c are correct.

22. Which most often causes biliary cirrhosis?
    a. malnutrition
    b. alcoholism
    c. hepatitis A or C
    d. autoimmunity
    e. biliary obstruction

23. Symptoms of cholelithiasis include all of the following *except:*
    a. nausea and vomiting.
    b. right upper quadrant tenderness.
    c. jaundice.
    d. decreased serum bilirubin levels.
    e. abdominal distress.

24. In pancreatitis:
    a. the tissue damage likely results from release of pancreatic enzymes.
    b. high cholesterol intake is causative.
    c. diabetes is uncommon in chronic pancreatitis.
    d. bacterial infection is the etiological cause.

25. Predisposing factors in the development of colon cancer include all of the following *except:*
    a. familial polyposis.
    b. ulcerative colitis.
    c. low-fiber/high-fat diet.
    d. high-fiber diet.
    e. high refined CHO diet.

Case Study

Dr. R. is a 55-year-old male professor whose department chair is an unrelenting harasser. Dr. R.'s family investments have failed, and his early planned retirement is no longer possible. Persistent upper abdominal pain for the last 2 months has convinced him that he needs a diagnostic work-up.

At the physician's office, Dr. R. reveals a history of smoking one pack of cigarettes a day for 25 years. His eating habits are irregular. However, he indicates a pain-antacid-relief pattern. The pain is more intense right after eating. He often takes aspirin for headaches and to relieve rheumatoid stiffness while golfing. His family and remaining history are unremarkable except that he has lost 10 pounds during the last 6 weeks.

Which type of peptic ulcer do you suspect? How could your suspicion be confirmed?

35

Alterations of Digestive Function in Children

Objectives

After studying this chapter, the learner will be able to do the following:

1. **Describe the pathophysiology and treatment associated with cleft lip and palate.**
Study pages 1028-1029; refer to Figure 35-1.

   Cleft lip is caused by incomplete fusion of the nasomedial or intermaxillary process during the second month of fetal development and occurs in approximately 1 in 1000 births. The defect in cleft lip usually is beneath one or both nostrils and may involve the external nose, nasal cartilages, nasal septum, and alveolar processes. It also may be associated with a flattening and broadening of the facial features, probably due to the absence of constraining structures that are omitted by the cleft.

   Cleft palate occurs in approximately 1 in 1250 births and is often associated with cleft lip but can occur alone. The defect may affect only the uvula and soft palate but

may extend forward toward the nostrils through the hard palate. If it extends through the hard palate, open communication between the structures of the nasopharynx and the oral cavity leads to sinusitis and otitis media.

Cleft lip and cleft palate are caused by genetic and nongenetic factors; a multifactorial inheritance exists. A major difficulty seen with these defects is poor feeding. The infant with isolated cleft lip but an intact palate may feed without great difficulty. On the other hand, cleft palate may significantly interfere with feeding. Bottle feeding may require a large, soft nipple with an oversized opening. Breast feeding may be impossible for some cleft palate infants without a prosthesis for the roof of the mouth.

Treatment is surgical correction that is usually accomplished in stages. Supportive therapy may include prosthodontics, orthodontics, and speech therapy.

2. **Describe the structural defects of esophageal atresia and tracheoesophageal fistula.**
Study pages 1029-1030; refer to Figure 35-2.

   Congenital malformations of the esophagus occur in approximately 1 in 3000 to 4500 births. **Esophageal atresia** is a condition wherein the esophagus ends in a blind pouch and may be accompanied by a connection between the esophagus and the trachea called a **tracheoesophageal fistula (TEF).** These conditions develop from aberrant differentiation of the trachea at 4 to 6 weeks of embryonic development. The blind esophageal pouch in atresia fills rapidly with secretions or food and overflows; regurgitated food and fluid may enter the lungs. Thirty percent of children with this anomaly have other associated congenital defects, particularly cardiovascular defects.

Diagnosis may not be made until recurrent aspiration and pneumonias become problematic. Diagnosis is confirmed by the inability to pass a catheter into the stomach. The x-ray shows the catheter coiled at the level of the defect. Treatment is surgical correction.

3. Describe the structural defect and pathophysiology associated with pyloric stenosis.
Study page 1030.

Pyloric stenosis is an obstruction of the pylorus caused by hypertrophy of the pyloric sphincter. Obstruction becomes evident between 1 to 2 weeks and 3 to 4 months of age. Boys are affected five times more often than girls, and whites are more often affected than Asians or blacks. Pyloric stenosis is seen more often in term than in premature infants. Increased gastrin secretion in the mother tends to increase the probability of pyloric stenosis and may be linked to maternal stress. Hereditary factors also may be involved.

Generally, stenosis is manifested in a previously healthy infant who begins to have marked forceful vomiting at 3 to 4 weeks of age that does not resolve. Weight loss and fluid and electrolyte imbalances follow and may end in death without intervention. A small, movable mass at the site of the hypertrophic pylorus may be palpable in the left upper quadrant of the abdomen.

Stenosis is usually suspected by history and clinical manifestations. Sonography shows hypertrophied pyloric muscles and narrowed pyloric channel. Treatment is usually surgical release of the hypertrophic fibers or pyloromyotomy after stabilization of the infant's fluid and electrolyte balance.

4. Describe meconium ileus.
Study pages 1031-1032.

Meconium (intestinal secretions and amniotic fluid) is a substance that fills the entire intestine before birth. **Meconium ileus** is an intestinal obstruction caused by the meconium in the newborn. The cause is usually a lack of digestive enzymes during fetal life associated with cystic fibrosis. Abdominal distention usually develops during the first days of life, and the infant, unable to pass meconium, begins to vomit.

The treatment in cases without volvulus or perforation is a hyperosmolar enema performed using fluoroscopy to evacuate the meconium. If evacuation is not possible, the meconium is removed surgically.

5. Describe congenital aganglionic megacolon, or Hirschsprung disease.
Study pages 1032-1033; refer to Figure 35-3.

Congenital aganglionic megacolon, or **Hirschsprung disease,** is a condition generally associated with failure of the parasympathetic nervous system to produce intramural ganglion cells in the enteric nerve plexuses. This failed innervation causes a section of the colon to be immotile and creates a functional intestinal obstruction in the affected area. This section becomes distended with feces, thus the name "megacolon." Eighty percent of these disorders are limited to the rectal end of the sigmoid colon. Hirschsprung disease accounts for one-third of all intestinal obstructions in infants and occurs in 1 in 5000 births, with a greater incidence in males.

Clinical manifestations are mild to severe chronic constipation, although diarrhea may be the first sign because only liquid may pass the aganglionic section. Severe edema of the colon begins to obstruct blood and lymphatic flow, causing **enterocolitis** and tissue destruction. Bacteria can infiltrate the bowel wall from the lumen and may cause gram-negative sepsis. Severe fluid and electrolyte imbalance caused by diarrhea may become life-threatening.

Diagnosis is confirmed by rectal biopsy that demonstrates the aganglionic bowel. Definitive treatment consists of resection of the aganglionic segment and constant attention to bowel hygiene thereafter.

6. Describe intussusception.
Study pages 1033-1034; refer to Figure 35-5.

Intussusception is the telescoping or invagination of one portion of the intestine into another that causes an intestinal obstruction. The most commonly affected area is the ileum, which invaginates into the cecum through the ileocecal valve. Collapse is in the direction of peristaltic flow. Intussusception causes 80% to 90% of intestinal obstructions in infants and children, and boys are more commonly affected. Intussusception generally occurs between 3 and 35 months of age; 75% occur before 1 year of age.

The pathophysiology of intussusception is like that of megacolon because the telescoping bowel obstructs blood and lymphatic flow, which causes rapid edema and tissue necrosis. Gangrene may follow.

The obstruction is usually accompanied by passage of dark and gelatinous, or "currant jelly," stools. Diagnosis is made on clinical manifestations and confirmed by ultrasonography. Reduction of the intussusception must be done immediately and is often performed using hydrostatic pressure of the contrast media used for x-ray or an enema to push the invaginated bowel segment from its intussusception. This is successful 60% to 70% of the time, although some children require surgery to correct the intussusception or related complications. This condition is fatal if untreated.

7. Describe the pathophysiology and potential complications related to gastroesophageal reflux.
Study page 1034.

Gastroesophageal reflux (GER) is the return of gastric contents into the esophagus because of poor function of the lower esophageal sphincter. GER is more common in premature than in term newborn infants and usually resolves by 6 to 12 months of age without significant effect on the infant. GER has been implicated as a possible factor in sudden infant death syndrome (SIDS). The cause of GER is unknown, although delayed maturation of the sphincter or impaired hormonal response mechanisms are suspected. Other factors include location of the gastroesophageal junction and the angle of the junction and mucosal gathering.

Clinical manifestations include forceful vomiting (with an 85% occurrence within the first week of life), aspiration pneumonia in one-third of those affected, and poor weight gain. **Esophagitis** may result from exposure of the esophagus to acidic gastric contents that may cause either strictures or anemia from prolonged occult blood loss.

Diagnosis may be made from clinical manifestations or confirmed by barium swallow or esophageal pH probe studies that demonstrate an abrupt drop in esophageal pH during the reflux episodes. Mild GER resolves without treatment, although some children require elevated prone positioning after feedings to help reduce reflux. Pharmacologic therapies include medication to increase lower gastrointestinal motility and gastric emptying time in an effort to decrease the opportunity for reflux; medications that decrease gastric acidity can be used. Surgical correction or fundoplication is rarely required but may be performed if medical management is ineffective.

8. Describe the gastrointestinal and digestive abnormalities associated with cystic fibrosis.
Study pages 1035-1036; refer to Table 35-1.

Cystic fibrosis (CF) is a multisystem disease. The classic triad of pathophysiology of cystic fibrosis is pancreatic enzyme deficiency leading to maldigestion, overproduction of mucus in the respiratory tract leading to chronic obstructive pulmonary disease, and elevated levels of sodium and chloride in sweat. Very viscous exocrine secretions tend to obstruct glandular ducts. Approximately 85% of children with CF have pancreatic insufficiency. The lack of pancreatic enzymes results in maldigestion of proteins, carbohydrates, and fats, leading to chronic malnutrition. Pancreatic ducts also may be blocked with viscous secretions that eventually may damage pancreatic cells and lead to diabetes mellitus. Maldigestion of fats causes steatorrhea

or fatty stools. Other complications include anemia, biliary cirrhosis, vitamin K deficiency, and rectal prolapse because of the passage of large, bulky stools.

Pancreatic enzyme function may be estimated by 72-hour fecal fat measurement; fecal content of trypsin and chymotrypsin also may be measured. Pancreatic enzyme replacement may be administered with meals, and a high-calorie/high-protein diet is usually prescribed.

9. Describe gluten-sensitive enteropathy.
Study pages 1036-1037; refer to Figure 35-6.

Gluten-sensitive enteropathy, formerly called *celiac sprue* or *celiac disease,* is the loss of mature villous epithelium caused by ingestion of gluten, the protein components of cereal grains. The gluten is toxic to the intestinal epithelial cells. Pathogenesis appears to involve dietary, genetic, and immunologic factors. The disease occurs mostly in whites.

Diarrhea is an early sign in most infants. The stools are pale, bulky, greasy, and foul-smelling; they may contain oil droplets. Vomiting and abdominal pain are prominent in infants but unusual in older children. Anorexia is prevalent and growth is usually diminished. Consequences of malabsorption such as rickets, tetany, frank bleeding, or anemia may be obvious. The child may bleed easily.

An intestinal biopsy is required to detect the classic mucosal changes caused by gluten-sensitive enteropathy. Serum gluten antibodies also may be measured.

Treatment requires immediate and permanent institution of a diet free of wheat, rye, barley, oats, and malt. Lactose (milk sugar) is also excluded because lactose intolerance is presumed. Infants are given vitamin D, iron, and folic acid supplements to treat deficiencies.

10. Compare kwashiorkor to marasmus.
Study pages 1037-1038.

Kwashiorkor and **marasmus** are types of malnutrition in children. They are collectively known as **protein energy malnutrition (PEM).** Both are states of long-term starvation. Kwashiorkor is a severe protein deficiency, and marasmus is a severe deficiency of all nutrients. Both are problems in impoverished populations; the conditions are less common in the United States.

In kwashiorkor, protein synthesis is reduced in all tissues. Physical and mental growth are stunted. The lack of sufficient plasma proteins results in generalized edema. The liver swells with stored fat because no hepatic proteins are synthesized to form and release lipoproteins. Kwashiorkor also causes malabsorption, reduced bone density, and impaired renal function.

In marasmus, metabolic processes including liver function are preserved, but growth is severely retarded. Caloric intake is too low to support protein synthesis for growth or the storage of fat. Muscle and fat wasting occur. Anemia is common and may be severe. The presence of subcutaneous fat, hepatomegaly, and fatty liver distinguishes kwashiorkor from marasmus.

11. Describe physiologic jaundice of the newborn.
Study page 1040.

Physiologic jaundice of the newborn is usually a transient, benign icterus that occurs during the first week of life in otherwise healthy, full-term infants. It is caused by mild unconjugated (indirect reacting) hyperbilirubinemia. A high level of indirect hyperbilirubinemia (15 mg/dl) is considered pathologic. There is a risk of brain damage (kernicterus) as the bilirubin passes into brain cells and is toxic with persistent high indirect hyperbilirubinemia.

Physiologic jaundice is usually treated by ultraviolet light. Pathologic jaundice requires an exchange transfusion.

12. Identify common metabolic disorders injurious to the liver.
Refer to Table 35-2.

The three most common metabolic disorders that cause liver damage in children are galactosemia, (galactose cannot be converted to glucose), fructosemia (fructose, sucrose, or honey cannot be metabolized), and Wilson disease (impaired copper transport in blood). All three are inherited as genetic traits and permit the accumulation of toxins in the liver.

Practice Examination

True/False

_____ 1. Pyloric stenosis is caused by the prolapse of gastric tissue into the pylorus and results in edema and obstruction.

_____ 2. Tracheoesophageal fistula is often associated with esophageal atresia.

_____ 3. Poor weight gain associated with gastroesophageal reflux may be ignored because it is a self-limiting disorder.

_____ 4. Intussusception involves a blind pouch in the esophagus.

_____ 5. Kernicterus is present in physiologic jaundice of the newborn.

_____ 6. Increased gastrin secretion in pregnant women may contribute to pyloric stenosis in their infants.

_____ 7. Diabetes mellitus may be a complication of cystic fibrosis.

_____ 8. The pharmacologic approach to gastroesophageal reflux includes pancreatic enzyme replacement.

_____ 9. Congenital aganglionic megacolon is the result of faulty innervation of the colon.

_____10. The pharmacologic approach to cystic fibrosis includes the administration of medications that increase lower gastrointestinal motility in an effort to aid passage of large, bulky stools.

_____11. Rectal manometry is useful in the diagnosis of aganglionic megacolon.

Fill-In-the-Blanks

12. _____ has been implicated as a possible factor in sudden infant death syndrome.

13. Congenital aganglionic megacolon is diagnosed by rectal manometry and rectal _____.

14. A pH probe will demonstrate a _____ in esophageal pH during a period of reflux.

15. Cleft palate is often complicated by communication

between the _____ and _____

_____ cavities.

16. _____ may be a complication of

cystic fibrosis secondary to passing large stools.

Match the description with the alteration.

_____17. involves the rectal segment of the sigmoid colon   a. congenital aganglionic megacolon

_____18. acute onset of abdominal pain and distention   b. tracheoesophageal fistula

_____19. accompanying cardiovascular defects   c. intussusception

_____20. may initially present with diarrhea   d. gastroesophageal reflux

_____21. food regurgitation   e. esophageal atresia

_____22. may contribute to aspiration pneumonia

_____23. incompetent lower esophageal sphincter

_____24. "currant jelly" stools

_____25. enema may be treatment

Case Study

Baby B. is a male term infant born vaginally to a 21-year-old white woman; he is her first child. Three weeks after birth, he began to vomit without apparent reason. At the pediatrician's office, it is determined that the infant had fed well and gained weight until now. The vomiting occurs immediately after eating, and the vomitus consists of the bulk of the feeding.

What is Baby B's likely problem, and what can be done?

36

Structure and Function of the Musculoskeletal System

Objectives

After reviewing this chapter, the learner will be able to do the following:

1. **Identify the structural elements and function of bone.**
   Review pages 1048-1051; refer to Figure 36-1 and Tables 36-1 through 36-3.

2. **Describe the features of compact and spongy bone; classify bones.**
   Review pages 1051 and 1053; refer to Figures 36-2 and 36-3.

3. **Describe the process of bone remodeling and healing.**
   Review pages 1053-1054; refer to Figure 36-5.

4. **Classify joints structurally and functionally.**
   Review pages 1054-1055 and 1059; refer to Figures 36-6 through 36-10.

5. **Describe the arrangements of muscle fiber in a skeletal muscle; explain the structure and function of a motor unit.**
   Review pages 1059-1063; refer to Figures 36-12 through 36-14 and Tables 36-4 and 36-5.

6. **Describe skeletal muscle contraction at the molecular level.**
   Review pages 1063-1065; refer to Figure 36-15.

7. **Identify the energy sources for muscular contraction.**
   Review pages 1065-1066; refer to Table 36-6.

8. **Indicate the types of skeletal muscle contractions and the interaction between groups of muscles.**
   Review pages 1066-1067; refer to Figure 36-16.

9. **Describe the changes in the musculoskeletal system that accompany normal aging.**
   Review pages 1067-1068.

Practice Examination

1. The skeletal system (more than one answer may be correct):
   a. supports tissues.
   b. binds organs together.
   c. protects CNS structures.
   d. participates in blood cell formation.
   e. lines body cavities.

2. Sialoprotein:
   a. promotes resorption.
   b. binds calcium.
   c. stabilizes the basement membrane of bones.
   d. promotes calcification.

Match the microscopic feature of bone with its description.

_____ 3. Volkmann's canals

_____ 4. trabeculae

_____ 5. lamellae

a. small canals that connect bone cells

b. concentric rings

c. cavities where bone cells are housed

d. contains blood vessels

e. irregular meshwork

---

6. The diaphysis is the:
   a. rounded end of long bones.
   b. shaft of long bones.
   c. lattice framework of spongy bones.
   d. surface of a synovial cavity.

7. A function of the epiphyseal plate that is *not* a function of the articular cartilage is to:
   a. enable articulation of bones.
   b. enable bone to increase in length.
   c. repair damaged bone tissue.
   d. provide sensory nerves to bone.

8. The remodeling of bone is done by basic multicellular units that consist of bone precursor cells. Precursor cells:
   a. differentiate into osteoclasts and osteoblasts.
   b. are located on free surfaces of bone and along vascular channels.
   c. Neither a nor be is correct.
   d. Both a and b are correct.

9. Identify the sequence of bone healing in fractures and surgical injuries.
   a. 2, 1, 3, 4, 5   1. procallus formation
   b. 3, 1, 2, 4, 5   2. callus formation
   c. 3, 2, 1, 4, 5   3. hematoma formation
   d. 1, 2, 3, 4, 5   4. callus replacement with lamel
   e. 1, 2, 3, 5, 4   lar or trabecular bone
                         5. periosteum and endosteum
                            remodeling

10. Joints are classified functionally and structurally. Which is a proper function and structural relationship?
    a. amphiarthrosis/fibrous
    b. diarthrosis/synovial
    c. synarthrosis/synchondrosis
    d. diarthrosis/fibrous
    e. synarthrosis/cartilaginous

11. In older individuals, the bone remodeling cycle:
    a. is faster because osteoclastic activity is enhanced.
    b. is enhanced because mineralization increases.
    c. has more precursor cells.
    d. has fewer bone cells because the bone marrow becomes infiltrated with fat.
    e. Both a and b are correct.

12. Which is *not* included in a motor unit?
    a. muscle fibers
    b. motor nerve axons
    c. anterior horn cell
    d. upper motor neuron

13. The perimysium is to a fasciculus as the:
    a. periosteum is to a bone.
    b. muscle is to epimysium.
    c. myofibril is to a muscle fiber.
    d. epimysium is to the endomysium.
    e. muscle cell is to the endomysium.

Match the microscopic feature of muscle fibers with its description.

_____14. sarcomere

_____15. sarcolemma

_____16. sarcoplasmic reticulum

a. membrane covering the muscle cell

b. flattened, tubelike network

c. unit of contraction

d. calcium transport

e. tubules that run perpendicular to muscle myofibrils

---

17. Which is *not* a characteristic of type I muscle fibers?
a. sparse capillary supply
b. slow contraction speed
c. high resistance to fatigue
d. profuse capillary supply
e. oxidative metabolism

18. Which protein is found in the thick myofilaments?
a. actin
b. myosin
c. troponin
d. tropomyosin
e. a, c, and d are correct.

19. An important function of the transverse tubules is to:
a. provide organic nutrients to muscle fibers.
b. initiate fiber contraction.
c. enable regeneration of muscle fibers.
d. allow for intracellular calcium uptake.

20. The ion necessary for coupling is:
a. sodium.
b. calcium.
c. potassium.
d. magnesium.
e. phosphate.

21. Aerobic respiration:
a. permits the body brief periods during which it does not require oxygen.
b. causes an increase in the amount of lactic acid.
c. yields more molecules of ATP than anaerobic respiration.
d. uses more glycogen to produce ATP than anaerobic respiration.
e. leads to oxygen debt.

22. Repayment of oxygen debt:
a. converts lactic acid to glycogen.
b. replenishes ATP stores.
c. replenishes phosphocreatine stores.
d. Both b and c are correct.
e. a, b, and c are correct.

23. The strength of muscle contraction depends on the:
a. extent of the load.
b. initial length of muscle fibers.
c. recruitment of additional motor units.
d. nerve innervation ratios.
e. All of the above are correct.

24. Attempting to push an object that is too heavy to move is an example of a(n) _____ contraction.
a. isotonic
b. concentric
c. flaccid
d. tetanic
e. isometric

25. Which does *not* happen with muscle as individuals grow older?
a. Type II fibers may decrease.
b. Mitochondrial volume decreases.
c. The amount of RNA increases to compensate for decreased size of motor units.
d. All of the above occur with advancing age.

37

Alterations of Musculoskeletal Function

Foundational Objectives

a. Describe the processes that maintain bone integrity.
Review pages 1053-1054; refer to Figure 36-5.

MEMORY CHECK!

- In the first phase of the remodeling cycle, a stimulus such as hormone, drug, vitamin, or physical stressor activates the bone cell precursor to become osteoclasts. In phase two, the osteoclasts resorb bone and leave in its place an elongated cavity termed a *resorption cavity*. The resorption cavity in compact bone follows the longitudinal axis of the haversian system; in spongy bone the resorption cavity parallels the surface of the trabeculae. In phase three, new bone or secondary bone is laid down by osteoblasts lining the walls of the resorption cavity. In compact bone, successive layers are laid down until the resorption cavity is reduced to a narrow haversian canal around a blood vessel. This process destroys old haversian systems and forms new haversian systems. New trabeculae are formed in spongy bone.

- The remodeling process is capable of repairing microscopic bone injuries, but gross injuries such as fractures and surgical wounds heal by a different process. In bone wound healing, the stages are as follows:

  1. Hematoma formation
  2. Procallus formation
  3. Callus formation
  4. Osteoblasts continue to replace the callus with either lamellar bone or trabecular bone.
  5. The periosteal and endosteal surfaces are remodeled to the size and shape of the bone before injury.

Copyright ©2004 Mosby, Inc. All rights reserved.

263

b. Describe the types of joints.

Review pages 1054-1055 and 1059; refer to Figures 36-6 through 36-10.

MEMORY CHECK!

- Joints are classified by the degree of movement they permit or by the connecting tissues that hold them together. Based on movement, a joint is classified as (1) a synarthrosis or an immovable joint, (2) an amphiarthrosis or a slightly movable joint, or (3) a diarthrosis or a freely movable joint. On the basis of connective structures, joints are classified as fibrous, cartilaginous, or synovial.

- A joint united directly to bone by fibrous connective tissues is called a fibrous joint. Generally, fibrous joints are synarthrotic, or immovable, but many fibrous joints allow some movement. The degree of movement depends on the distance between the bone and the flexibility of the fibrous connective tissue.

- There are two types of cartilaginous joints, or amphiarthroses. A symphysis is a cartilaginous joint in which bones are united by a pad or disk of fibrocartilage. The articulating surfaces are usually covered by a thin layer of hyaline cartilage and a thick pad of fibrocartilage, which acts as a shock absorber and stabilizer. Examples of symphyses are the symphysis pubis and the intervertebral discs. A synchondrosis is a joint in which hyaline cartilage connects the two bones. The joints between the ribs and the sternum are synchondroses. Slight movement at the synchondroses between the ribs and the sternum allows the chest to move outward and upward during breathing.

- Synovial joints or diarthroses are the most movable and complex joints in the body. A synovial joint consists of a fibrous joint capsule or articular capsule, a synovial membrane, a joint cavity or synovial cavity, synovial fluid, and an articular cartilage. The joint capsule consists of parallel, interlacing bundles of dense, white fibrous tissue. It has a rich supply of nerves, blood vessels, and lymphatic vessels. The nerves are sensitive to the rate and direction of motion, compression, tension, vibration, and pain.

- The synovial membrane is the smooth, delicate inner lining of the joint capsule. It lines the nonarticular portion of the synovial joint and any ligaments or tendons that traverse the joint cavity. The synovial membrane is capable of rapid repair and regeneration.

- The joint cavity or synovial cavity is an enclosed, fluid-filled space between the articulating surfaces of the two bones that enables the two bones to move "against" one another. Synovial fluid within the cavity lubricates the joint surfaces, nourishes the pad of the articular cartilage, and contains free-floating synovial cells and various leukocytes that phagocytose joint debris and microorganisms.

- Articular cartilage is a layer of hyaline cartilage that covers the end of each bone. The function of articular cartilage is to reduce friction and to distribute the weight-bearing forces.

c. **Define terms associated with muscle fibers.**
   Review pages 1059-1063; refer to Figures 36-12 through 36-15 and Tables 36-4 and 36-5.

MEMORY CHECK!

- Each anterior horn cell, its axon, and the innervated muscle fibers is called a *motor unit*. The motor unit behaves as a single entity and contracts as a whole when it receives an adequate electrical impulse. A muscle fiber is a single muscle cell. This long cell is cylindrical in structure and surrounded by a membrane capable of excitation and impulse propagation. The muscle fiber contains bundles of myofibrils in a parallel arrangement along the longitudinal axis of the muscle. The myofibrils contain sarcomeres that are the actual contracting units. The sarcomeres consist of actin and myosin, which are the contractile proteins.

- Besides the myofibrils, the major components of the muscle fiber include the muscle membrane, sarcotubular system, sarcoplasm, and mitochondria. The muscle membrane is a two-part membrane. It includes the sarcolemma, which contains the plasma membrane of the muscle cell, and the cell's basement membrane. At the motor nerve endplate, where the nerve impulse is transmitted, the sarcolemma forms the highly convoluted synaptic cleft. The protein systems of the sarcolemma transport nutrients and synthesize proteins. They also provide the sodium-potassium pump and include the cell's cholinergic receptor. The basement membrane serves as the cell's microskeleton and maintains the shape of the muscle cell.

- The sarcoplasm is the cytoplasm of the muscle cell and contains numerous enzymes and proteins that are responsible for the cell's energy production, protein synthesis, and oxygen storage. Unique to the muscle is the sarcotubular system, which includes the transverse tubules and the sarcoplasmic reticulum. The sarcoplasmic reticulum is involved in calcium transport, which initiates muscle contraction at the sarcomere. The sarcoplasmic reticulum is composed of tubules that run parallel to the myofibrils and are termed *sarcotubules*. The transverse tubules are closely associated with the sarcotubules and run across the sarcoplasm and communicate with the extracellular space. Both tubules allow for intracellular calcium uptake, regulation, release during muscle contraction, and storage of calcium during muscle relaxation.

d. **Identify the major events of muscle contraction and relaxation.**
   Review pages 1063-1065; refer to Figure 36-15.

MEMORY CHECK!

MAJOR EVENTS OF MUSCLE CONTRACTION AND RELAXATION

Excitation and Contraction

A nerve impulse reaches the end of a motor neuron and releases acetylcholine

↓

Acetylcholine diffuses across the neuromuscular junction and binds to acetylcholine receptors on the muscle fiber

↓

Stimulation of acetylcholine receptors initiates an impulse that travels along the sarcolemma, through the transverse tubules, and to the sarcoplasmic reticulum

↓

Calcium is released from the sarcoplasmic reticulum into the sarcoplasm; calcium binds to troponin molecules on the thin myofilaments

↓

Tropomyosin molecules shift to expose actin's active engagement sites

↓

Energized myosin cross-bridges of the thick myofilaments bind to actin and use their ATP energy to pull the thin myofilaments toward the center of each sarcomere

↓

As the thin myofilaments slide past the thick myofilaments, the entire muscle fiber shortens

↓

After the impulse passes, the sarcoplasmic reticulum begins actively pumping calcium back into the sarcoplasm

↓

As calcium leaves the troponin molecules of the thin myofilaments, tropomyosin returns to its position and blocks actin's active engagement sites

↓

Myosin cross-bridges cannot bind to actin and can no longer sustain the contraction

↓

The thick and thin myofilaments are no longer connected, so the muscle fiber returns to its longer, resting length

Objectives

After studying this chapter, the learner will be able to do the following:

1. **Compare the types of fractures; describe the causes, manifestations, and treatment of fractures.**
   Study pages 1072-1075; refer to Figure 37-1 and Table 37-1.

Fractures are classified as complete or incomplete and open or closed. In a **complete** fracture, the bone is broken all the way through; in an **incomplete** fracture, the bone is damaged but remains in one piece. Complete or incomplete fractures also are considered **open** if the skin is broken or **closed** if it is not. A fracture wherein the bone breaks into two or more fragments is termed a **comminuted** fracture. Fractures also are classified according to the direction of the fracture line.

The signs and symptoms of a fracture include unnatural alignment, swelling, muscle spasm, tenderness, pain, and impaired sensation. The immediate pain of a fracture is severe and usually caused by the traumatic injury. Subsequent pain often is produced by muscle spasm. Numbness is caused by the pinching of a nerve by the trauma or by bone fragments. Pathologic fractures are not usually associated with trauma or trauma-related pain. Stress fractures are painful because of accelerated remodeling and are usually relieved by rest. Range of motion in the joint is limited, and movement may evoke audible clicking sounds or crepitus.

Fracture treatment involves realigning the bone fragments to their normal or anatomic position and holding the fragments in place so that bone union can occur. Several methods are available to reduce or align a fracture, including closed manipulation, traction, and open surgical reduction. Splints and plaster casts are used to immobilize and hold a reduction in place. Improper reduction or immobilization of a fractured bone may result in nonunion, delayed union, or malunion. (See box on page 268.)

2. **Define terms associated with skeletal system stress.**
   Study pages 1075-1080; refer to Figures 37-5 through 37-8 and Table 37-2.

Dislocation is the temporary displacement of two bones in which the two bone surfaces lose contact entirely. If the contact between the surfaces is only partially lost, the injury is called **subluxation.** Dislocations and subluxations are often accompanied by fracture. As the bone separates from the joint, it may bruise or tear adjacent nerves, blood vessels, ligaments, supporting structures, and soft tissue.

A tear in a tendon is a **strain.** Major trauma or excessive stress can tear a tendon at any site in the body. The tendons of the hands, feet, knee, upper arm, thigh, ankle, and heel are often injured sites. Ligament tears are known as **sprains.** Ligament tears and ruptures can occur at any joint but are most common in the wrist, ankle, elbow, and knee joints. A complete separation of a tendon or ligament from its attachment is an **avulsion.** An avulsion is the result of abnormal stress on the ligament or tendon and is commonly seen in young athletes, especially sprinters, hurdlers, and runners.

Trauma also can cause painful inflammation of tendons, or **tendinitis,** and bursae, or **bursitis.** Besides trauma, causes of tendinitis include crystal deposits, postural misalignment, and hypermobility in a joint. **Epicondylitis** is inflammation of a tendon where it attaches to a bone. Examples of epicondylitis include tennis elbow, which is an inflammation of the lateral epicondyle of the humerus, and medial epicondylitis, which is referred to as *golfer's elbow.* Acute **bursitis** occurs primarily in the middle years and is caused by repeated trauma. Septic bursitis is caused by wound infection or bacterial infection of the skin overlying the bursae. The shoulder is the most common site of bursitis.

Muscle strain is often the result of sudden, forced motion causing the muscle to become stretched beyond its normal capacity. Muscles are injured more often than tendons in young people; the opposite is true in older populations. Regardless of the cause of trauma, muscle cells usually are able to regenerate, although regeneration may take up to 6 weeks.

Myositis ossificans is thought to be caused by scar tissue calcification and subsequent ossification. An example is seen in football players after injury to thigh muscles.

Myoglobinuria can be a life-threatening complication of severe muscle trauma manifested by excess myoglobin, an intracellular muscle protein, in the urine. Muscle damage releases the myoglobin. The most severe form is often called *crush syndrome.* Less severe and more localized forms are called *compartment syndromes,* which can lead to Volkmann ischemic contracture in the forearm or leg. Crush syndrome first gained notoriety in injuries seen following the London air raids in World War II. More recently, it has been reported in individuals found unresponsive because of drug overdoses and those who are immobile for long periods of time. Myoglobinuria also can be seen following viral infections, administration of certain anesthetic agents, strychnine poisoning, tetanus, excessive muscular activity, heatstroke, electrolyte disturbances, fractures, status epilepticus, electroconvulsive therapy, and high-voltage electrical shock.

Types of Fractures

Type	Characteristic	Cause
Common Complete Fractures		
Open fracture	Communicating wound between bone and skin	Moderate to severe energy that exceeds tissue tolerance
Oblique fracture	Fracture line at 45-degree angle to long axis of bone	Angulation and compressive energy
Spiral fracture	Fracture line encircling bone	Twisting energy with distal part unable to move
Transverse fracture	Fracture line perpendicular to long axis of bone	Energy directly toward bone
Impacted fracture	Fracture fragments pushed into one another	Compressive energy directly to distal fragment
Pathologic fracture	Fracture occurs at any point in the bone	Minor energy to already weakened bone
Common Incomplete Fractures		
Greenstick fracture	Break of the cortical bone on the convex side of a bent bone only with spongy bone splintering	Minor direct or indirect energy in children or elderly
Stress fracture	Microfracture	Bone is subjected to repeated stress beyond its strength; muscles are stronger than bone

3. **Differentiate between osteoporosis, osteomalacia, Paget disease, and osteomyelitis.**
   Study pages 1080-1090; refer to Figures 37-9 through 37-16 and Table 37-3. (See box on next page.)

4. **Compare noninflammatory osteoarthritis to inflammatory rheumatoid arthritis; characterize other inflammatory joint diseases.**
   Study pages 1090-1102; refer to Figures 37-17 through 37-25 and Table 37-4.

Ankylosing spondylitis is a chronic, inflammatory joint disease characterized by stiffening and fusion or ankylosis of the spine and sacroiliac joints. Like rheumatoid arthritis, ankylosing spondylitis is a systemic, immune inflammatory disease. The disease is strongly associated with the presence of histocompatibility antigen HLA-B27 on the chromosomes of affected individuals; this suggests a genetic predisposition to the disease. In ankylosing spondylitis, the primary pathologic site is at the point where ligaments, tendons, and the joint capsule are inserted into bone rather than in the synovial membrane as in rheumatoid arthritis. The end result of ankylosing spondylitis is fibrosis, ossification, and fusion of the joint.

Ankylosing spondylitis begins with inflammation of fibrocartilage in cartilaginous joints, particularly in the vertebrae. As inflammatory cells infiltrate and erode fibrocartilage in joint structures, repair begins to occur. Repair begins with the proliferation of fibroblasts. The collagen synthesized by fibroblasts becomes organized into fibrous scar tissue. Eventually, the scar tissue calcifies and ossifies. With time, all the cartilaginous structures of the joint are replaced by ossified scar tissue and the joints fuse or lose flexibility.

The most common symptoms of early ankylosing spondylitis are low back pain and stiffness. The pain initially is insidious but progressively becomes persistent. Forward flexion, rotation, and lateral flexion of the spine are restricted and painful. As the disease progresses, the individual becomes increasingly stooped. The thoracic spine becomes rounded, the head and neck are flexed. Along with low back pain, many individuals may have peripheral joint involvement, uveitis or inflammation of eye structures, fibrotic changes in the lungs, cardiomegaly, aortic incompetence, amyloidosis, and Achilles tendonitis.

Common Disorders of Bone

Disorder	Cause	Pathophysiology	Manifestations	Treatment
Osteoporosis	Decreased levels of estrogen and testosterone, reduced physical activity lessens muscle stress on bone, inadequate vitamins C and D, insufficient dietary magnesium and calcium, corticosteroid use	Reduced bone mass or density, imbalance in bone resorption and formation	Pain and bone deformity, fracture, increased radiolucency	Weight-bearing exercise, dietary supplements, selective estrogen receptor modulators, intranasal calcitonin, possible PTH and testosterone
Osteomalacia (adult) Rickets (children)	Deficiency of vitamin D lowers absorption of calcium from intestines	Inadequate and delayed mineralization, osteoid tissue is not mineralized.	Pain, bone fractures, vertebral collapse, radiolucent bands perpendicular to bone surface, pseudofracture	Serum calcium and phosphorus adjustments, vitamin D supplements, renal dialysis
Paget disease	Unknown	Excessive resorption of spongy bone followed by accelerated formation of softened bone	Thickening of bones, radiographic findings of irregular bone trabeculae with thickened and disorganized patterns	Infrequently required—bisphosphonates and calcitonin surgery if neurologic complications
Osteomyelitis	Most often a staphylococcal infection, contaminated open wound or hematogenous bone infection	Acute inflammation of marrow and cortex, necrosis	Acute and chronic inflammation, fever, pain, lymphadenopathy, necrotic bone by radiographic imaging	Antibiotics and debridement, surgical removal of exudates, hyperbaric oxygen therapy

Treatment of individuals with ankylosing spondylitis consists of physical therapy to maintain skeletal mobility and prevent the natural progression of contractures. Antiinflammatory and analgesic medications are prescribed to suppress some of the pain and stiffness and to facilitate exercise. Surgical procedures and radiotherapy are sometimes used to provide relief for individuals with end-stage disease or intolerable deformity.

Gout is a metabolic disorder that disrupts the body's control of uric acid production or excretion. High levels of uric acid accumulate in the blood and in other body fluids, including synovial fluid. When the uric acid reaches a certain concentration in fluids, it crystallizes. The crystals are deposited in connective tissues throughout the body.

When crystallization occurs in synovial fluid, painful *inflammation* of the joint develops. This condition is known as **gouty arthritis.** With time, crystal deposition in subcutaneous tissues causes the formation of small, white nodules or **tophi** and their inflammatory sequelae. Crystal aggregates deposited in the kidneys can form urate renal stones and lead to renal failure. In classic gouty arthritis, inflammation of the joint is caused by the formation of monosodium urate crystals. In **pseudogout,** the crystals are of calcium pyrophosphate-dihydrate. Either crystal causes the onset of acute inflammatory response.

Approximately 95% of affected individuals, almost always men, have **primary gout** wherein the hyperuricemia is due to an overproduction of uric acid. The defect in primary gout is unknown but is likely an inherited enzyme defect. In **secondary gout,** the hyperuricemia is the result of an acquired chronic disease or a drug that interferes with balance between production and excretion of uric acid. Hyperuricemia from overproduction of uric acid can be due to increased metabolic processes such as leukemia, increased cellular breakdown like hemolytic anemia, neoplastic processes, and genetic metabolic disorders in which hyperuricemia is just one of many clinical manifestations. Diuretics are thought to cause secondary gout because they decrease the renal tubular excretion of urate. Chronic renal disease, hypertension, and starvation also decrease uric acid excretion.

Noninflammatory Osteoarthritis and Inflammatory Rheumatoid Arthritis

	Osteoarthritis (OA)	Rheumatoid arthritis (RA)
Pathologic feature	Noninflammatory (enzymatic lysis), loss of proteoglycans from articular cartilage in synovial joints, bone sclerosis, bone spurs	Inflammatory; damage or destruction of synovial membrane, extends to articular cartilage joint capsule and surrounding ligaments and tendons; pannus
Onset age	>40, increases with age, equal sex distribution	Middle age, prevalence in females
Cause	Primary: autosomal recessive Secondary: joint stress, congenital abnormalities, joint instability	Genetics, environmental microbes, autoimmunity, estrogen, released TNF-α and IL-1
Joints affected	Peripheral and central, weight-bearing	Phalangeal, wrists, knee
Joint fluid	Proteoglycans/fragments, normal mucin, few cells	Inflammatory exudates, poor mucin
Manifestations	Pain, stiffness, enlargement, tenderness, limited motion, muscle wasting, dislocation, deformity	Same as OA with systemic involvement, subcutaneous nodules, deviation of joints, rheumatoid factor (RF) and circulating immune complexes

NOTE: Conservative treatment for OA includes rest and support for weight-bearing joints. For RA, conservative treatment includes disease-modifying antirheumatic drugs (DMARDs) and biologic response modifiers (BRMs), and antiinflammatory drugs. Surgery for RA can correct deformities or create new joints.

The pathophysiology of gout is closely linked to purine metabolism, cellular metabolism of purines, and kidney function. Uric acid is a breakdown product of purine nucleotides. Some individuals with gout have an accelerated rate of purine synthesis and other individuals break down purine nucleotides at an accelerated rate. Both conditions result in an overproduction of uric acid. Kidney function is involved in the pathophysiology of gout because most uric acid is eliminated from the body through the kidneys. Urate undergoes both reabsorption and excretion within the renal tubules. Sluggish urate excretion by the kidney may be caused by decreased glomerular filtration of urate or an acceleration in urate reabsorption.

The presence of urate crystals anywhere triggers the acute inflammatory response as the neutrophils are attracted to phagocytose the crystals. Tissue damage occurs when the phagocytizing neutrophils release the contents of their digestive lysosomes.

Attacks of gouty arthritis occur abruptly, usually in a peripheral joint. The primary symptom is severe pain. Approximately 50% of the initial attacks occur in the metatarsophalangeal joint of the great toe. Other involved joints are the heel, ankle, instep of the foot, knee, wrist, or elbow.

Tophaceous gout, the chronic stage of disease, can begin as early as 3 years or as late as 40 years after the initial attack of gouty arthritis. Progressive inability to excrete uric acid expands the urate pool until tophi appear in cartilage, synovial membranes, tendons, and soft tissue. The helix of the ear is the most common site of tophi, which are the diagnostic lesions of chronic gout. Each tophus consists of a deposit of urate crystals surrounded by a granuloma made of mononuclear phagocytes that have developed into epithelial giant cells. Tophaceous deposits appear in other areas and produce irregular swellings of the fingers, hands, knees, and feet. Though the tophi themselves are painless, they often cause progressive stiffness and persistent aching of the affected joint.

Acute gouty arthritis is treated with antiinflammatory drugs. The individual should have a low purine diet and high fluid intake to increase urinary output. Antihyperuricemic drugs can be given to reduce serum urate concentrations.

5. **Describe examples of secondary muscular dysfunction.**
   Study page 1102.

Muscular symptoms arise from causes unrelated to the muscle itself. These secondary muscular phenomena include contracture, stress-related muscle tension, and immobility.

Several conditions cause the muscle fibers to shorten without contracting; this is called a **contracture.** A physiologic muscle contracture occurs without muscle action potential in the sarcolemma and is explained as failure of the calcium pump even in the presence of plentiful adenosine triphosphate (ATP). A physiologic contracture is seen in McArdle disease, which is an enzyme deficiency, and malignant hyperthermia. The contracture is usually temporary if the underlying pathology can be corrected.

A pathologic contracture is considered a permanent muscle shortening caused by muscle spasm or weakness. It is associated with plentiful ATP and will occur in spite of a normal action potential. The most common form of contracture is seen in muscular dystrophy and central nervous system (CNS) injury. Contractures also may develop secondary to scar tissue contraction in the flexor tissues of a joint.

Stress-induced muscle tension has been associated with chronic anxiety as well as a variety of stress-related muscular symptoms, including neck stiffness, back pain, and headache. The underlying pathophysiology presumably is caused by increased activity of the reticular-activating system and increased firing of the efferent loop of the gamma fibers, which produce further muscle contraction and increased muscle tension.

Progressive relaxation training and biofeedback are possible ways to treat muscle tension. The hope is to enhance the individual's ability to relax specific muscle groups in order to relieve tension. This could reduce CNS and ANS arousal.

The term **disuse atrophy** describes the pathologic reduction in normal size of muscle fibers following inactivity due to bed rest, trauma, casting, or local nerve damage. Atrophy may be prevented by frequent forceful isometric muscle contractions and passive lengthening exercises.

6. **Describe fibromyalgia.**
   Study pages 1103-1104; refer to Figures 37-26 and 37-27 and Table 37-5.

Fibromyalgia is a chronic musculoskeletal syndrome characterized by increased sensitivity to touch, the absence of systemic or localized inflammation, and fatigue and sleep disturbances. Because the symptoms are vague, fibromyalgia has often been misdiagnosed or completely dismissed by clinicians.

The etiology of fibromyalgia is likely multifactorial. The most common precipitating factors include viral illnesses, physical traumas, or emotional trauma. Certain rheumatic diseases, such as rheumatoid arthritis (RA) or systemic lupus erythematosus (SLE), may coexist if not initially present with fibromyalgia.

Studies have documented lower ATP, lower ADP, and higher concentrations of AMP and more alterations in the number of capillaries and the fiber area in individuals with fibromyalgia than in study control subjects. Most studies have demonstrated that increased muscle tenderness in fibromyalgia is a result of generalized pain intolerance that is possibly related to functional abnormalities within the CNS. The prominent symptom of fibromyalgia is chronic pain. The majority of individuals experience pain and fatigue during more than 90% of their wakefulness. Fatigue is most notable when arising from sleep and during mid afternoon. Headaches, symptoms of irritable bowel syndrome, and sensitivity to cold are reported in 50% of individuals. Almost 25% of individuals seek psychologic support for depression. Anxiety, particularly in regard to diagnosis and future, is almost universal. The only finding on examination is the presence of multiple tender points.

No one regimen of medication has proved successful for fibromyalgia. Amitriptyline can significantly improve pain tolerance, morning stiffness, and sleep quality but not tender points.

7. **Distinguish between muscle membrane abnormalities.**
   Study pages 1104-1105.

The hyperexcitable membrane seen in myotonic disorders and the intermittently unresponsive membrane seen in the periodic paralyses are defects in the plasma membrane of the muscle fiber. **Myotonia** is a delayed relaxation after voluntary muscle contraction such as gripes, eye closure, or muscle percussion. It is due to the prolonged depolarization of the muscle membrane. Myotonia is seen mostly in inherited disorders. Its symptoms are mild except in myotonic muscular dystrophy. Myotonia is treated by drugs that reduce muscle fiber excitability.

In **periodic paralysis,** the muscle membrane is unresponsive to neural stimuli. Periodic paralysis is triggered by exercise and any process or medication that alters serum potassium. The disorder is often inherited in an autosomal dominant pattern. Oral and intravenous potassium can relieve acute attacks. A low-salt diet and drugs are useful for long-term therapy.

8. **Compare the metabolic, inflammatory, and toxic myopathies.**
   Study pages 1105-1108; refer to Figure 37-28.

Myopathies

Myopathy	Causes	Manifestations
Metabolic Myopathy		
	Altered thyroid hormone levels change muscle protein synthesis and electrolyte balance	
	Thyrotoxicosis	Proximal weakness, paresis of extraocular muscles
	Hypothyroidism	Flabby and weak muscles, sluggish movements
McArdle disease	Absence of muscle phosphorylase, inability to catabolize glycogen or produce lactic acid	Exercise intolerance, fatigue, painful muscle cramps, muscle weakness and wasting
Acid maltase deficiency	Autosomal recessive; absence of acid maltase, accumulation of glycogen in lysosomes of muscle and other cells	Adult: similar to muscular dystrophy or polymyositis, severe respiratory muscle weakness
Pompe disease (infantile form of acid maltase deficiency)		Infant: hypotonia; areflexia; enlarged heart, tongue, and liver; early death
Myoadenylate deaminase deficiency	Absence of myoadenylate deaminase, inability to form phosphocreatine and ATP during exercise	Exercise intolerance
Carnitine palmitoyl transferase (CPT) and carnitine deficiency	Absence of CPT and carnitine; fatty acid byproducts and energy are not transported to myofibrils	CPT: mild muscular symptoms, episodes of renal failure because of myoglobinuria. Carnitine: progressive muscle weakness
Inflammatory Myopathy		
	Infectious	
	Tuberculosis and sarcoidosis	Granulomas in muscle and other tissues
	Trichinosis	Larvae from infected pork migrate to host lymphatics: pain, rash, and muscle stiffness
	Viral infections	Muscle pain and tenderness similar to symptoms of influenza
Polymyositis (generalized muscle inflammation) Dermatomyositis (polymyositis with skin lesions)	Cell-mediated, immune system abnormalities, human leukocyte antigen (HLA) genetic markers	Necrosis of muscle fibers; malaise; fever; muscle swelling, pain, and tenderness; lethargy; symmetric proximal muscle weakness; both diseases show dysphagia, vasculitis, Raynaud phenomenon, cardiomyopathy, fibrosis, coexisting pulmonary collagen disorders; dermatomyositis exhibits skin rash, calcinosis, and eyelid edema
Toxic Myopathy		
	Alcohol abuse; direct toxic effect and nutritional deficiency cause necrosis of muscle fibers	Benign cramps and pain, severe weakness, myoglobinuria and renal failure
	Antimalarial and amebicidal agents impair lysosomal processes	Generalized muscle weakness
	Sedatives and narcotics	Myoglobinuria
	Repeated therapeutic drug injection	Local muscle fiber necrosis, fibrotic bands

9. **Classify bone tumors by tissue of origin, whether benign or malignant, and their pattern of bone destruction.**
   Study pages 1108-1110; refer to Figure 37-29 and Tables 37-6 and 37-7.

Bone tumors may originate from bone cells, cartilage, fibrous tissue, marrow, or vascular tissue. On the basis of mesodermal tissue of origin, bone tumors are classified as osteogenic, chondrogenic, collagenic, or myelogenic. The mesoderm contributes to primitive fibroblasts and reticulum cells. The fibroblast is the progenitor of the osteoblast, the chondroblast, and the fibrous connective tissue cell.

Benign bone tumors destroy small areas of bone, tend to be limited to the anatomic confines of the host bone, and have a well-demarcated border. Benign bone tumors push against neighboring tissue, have a symmetrical, controlled growth pattern, and tend to compress and displace neighboring normal bone tissue, which weakens the bone's structure until it leads to pathologic fracture.

The geographic pattern, the moth-eaten pattern, and the permeative pattern are patterns of bone destruction in bone tumors. Tumors exhibiting the geographic pattern have well-defined margins that can be easily separated from the surrounding normal bone. There is a uniform and well-defined lytic area in the bone of these benign lesions.

In the moth-eaten pattern, the cancerous lesion has a less-defined or demarcated margin that cannot be easily separated from normal bone. Areas of partially destroyed bone adjacent to completely lytic areas are found. This pattern of bone destruction is characteristic of rapidly growing, **malignant bone tumors.** An aggressive, malignant tumor causes the permeative pattern of bone destruction. The margins of the tumor are poorly demarcated, and abnormal bone merges with surrounding normal bone tissue. Malignant bone tumors tend to be large and aggressive in their bone destruction, to invade surrounding tissue, and to metastasize. (See flow chart below.)

10. **Characterize the common types of bone tumors.**
   Study pages 1110-1113; refer to Figures 37-30 and 37-31.

Osteosarcoma is a malignant bone-forming tumor that is large and destructive and most often is found in bone marrow; it has a moth-eaten pattern of bone destruction. Osteosarcomas always contain osteoid and callus and also may contain chondroid and fibrinoid tissue. The osteoid is deposited between the trabeculae of the callus. The "streamers" of osteoid infiltrate the normal compact bone, destroy it, and replace it with dense callus and masses of osteoid. The bone tissue never matures to compact bone. Ninety percent of osteosarcomas are located in the metaphyses of long bones. Fifty percent of osteosarcomas occur around the knee area. The tumor breaks through the cortex, lifts the periosteum, and forms a soft tissue mass that is not covered by new bone.

Origin of Benign and Malignant Bone Tumors

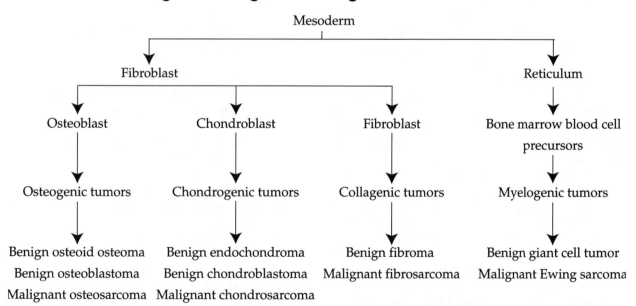

NOTE: Diagnosis depends on serum metabolite and enzyme levels, radiologic studies, CT scans, MRI, blood counts, and biopsy.

Common initial symptoms are pain and swelling; pain is usually worse at night. Systemic symptoms are uncommon. Preoperative chemotherapy has improved the treatment for localized osteosarcoma. Chemotherapy can be given both preoperatively and postoperatively. Combination treatment includes radiation therapy and surgery.

Chondrosarcoma, a chondrogenic tumor, is a large, ill-defined malignant tumor that infiltrates trabeculae in spongy bone. It occurs most often in the metaphysis or diaphysis of long bones. The tumor contains large lobules of hyaline cartilage separated by bands of fibrous tissue and anaplastic cells. It expands and enlarges the contour of the bone, causes extensive erosion of the cortex, and expands into the soft tissues.

Symptoms associated with the chondrosarcoma have an insidious onset. Local swelling and pain are usual symptoms. At first, the pain is intermittent; then, it gradually intensifies and becomes constant. Surgical excision is generally regarded as the treatment of choice; however, individuals demonstrate recurrences and so amputation is considered.

Fibrosarcoma, a malignant collagenic tumor, is a solitary tumor that most often affects the metaphyseal region of the femur or tibia. The tumor is composed of a firm, fibrous mass of tissue containing collagen, malignant fibroblasts, and occasional osteoclast-like giant cells.

Pain and swelling are the usual symptoms and indicate that the tumor has broken through the cortex. Local tenderness, a palpable mass, limitation of motion, or a pathologic fracture are other symptoms and signs. Radical surgery and amputation are the treatments of choice for fibrosarcoma.

Giant cell tumors are common primary bone tumors. The giant cell tumor is a solitary, circumscribed tumor that causes extensive bone resorption because of its osteoclastic origin. The tumor is rich in osteoclast-like giant cells and anaplastic stromal cells and is found in the center of the epiphysis in the femur, tibia, radius, or humerus. The tumor has a slow, relentless growth rate and is usually contained within the original contour of the affected bone. It may extend into the articular cartilage. It has recurrence rates as high as 80%.

The most common symptoms associated with the giant cell tumor are pain, local swelling, and limitation of movement. Cryosurgery and resection of the tumor decrease recurrence and are more successful treatments than curettage and radiation; amputation may be necessary.

Myeloma is a malignant neoplastic proliferation of plasma cells. Myelomas cause cortical and medullary bone lysis and infiltrate the bone marrow. The bone lesions occur next to the myeloma cells and not in areas of normal bone marrow.

The most common symptom of myeloma is pain that is initially aching, intermittent, and aggravated by weight bearing. As the disease progresses, the pain becomes severe and prolonged. Myeloma has a poor prognosis and the treatment is generally palliative. Radiotherapy and chemotherapy have limited success. Marrow transplant is an option. For drug resistant individuals, a thalidomide derivative that acts as a potent immune modulating agent and increases cell death (apoptosis) is being studied.

11. **Identify the incidence, manifestations, treatment, and prognosis of rhabdomyosarcoma.**
    Study page 1113.

The malignant tumor of striated muscle is a **rhabdomyosarcoma.** The incidence of rhabdomyosarcoma is extremely rare, but it is highly malignant because of its rapid metastasis. These tumors are located in the muscle tissue of the head, neck, and genitourinary tract 75% of the time. The remainder are in the trunk and extremities.

The diagnosis of rhabdomyosarcoma is made by incisional biopsy and histologic examination of the specimen. Pleomorphic, embryonal, and alveolar types can be differentiated. The pleomorphic type is a highly malignant tumor of the extremities of adults.

Treatment consists of a combination of surgical excision, radiation therapy, and systemic chemotherapy. Cure in cases with distant metastasis is unlikely.

Practice Examination

1. In a complete fracture:
   a. the fracture crosses or involves the entire width or thickness of the bone.
   b. more than two bone fragments are present.
   c. separation of ligaments exists.
   d. posttraumatic infection is always present.
   e. the surface opposite the break is intact.

2. In an oblique fracture, the energy or force is:
   a. twisting with the distal part unable to move.
   b. compressive and at an angle.
   c. directly to an already weakened bone.
   d. directly to the distal fragment.

3. Which is a definite sign of a fracture?
   a. abrasion
   b. shock
   c. muscle spasm
   d. unnatural alignment
   e. All of the above are correct.

Match the term with its characteristic.

_____ 4. subluxation

_____ 5. sprain

a. articular cartilages lose contact entirely

b. articular cartilages are partially separated

c. complete separation of a tendon or a ligament

d. a ligament tear

6. Secondary muscular dysfunctions:
    a. involve large compartments of hemorrhage.
    b. can display contractures.
    c. result from failure of calcium pump.
    d. are related to the muscle itself.
    e. Both b and c are correct.

7. The most common cause of osteomyelitis is:
    a. hematogenous spread of infection.
    b. rheumatoid disease.
    c. direct contamination of an open wound.
    d. deficiency of calcium.
    e. deficiency of vitamin D.

8. Osteoporosis is:
    a. inadequate mineralization.
    b. impaired synthesis of bone organic matrix.
    c. reduced bone mass or density.
    d. formation of sclerotic bone.
    e. None of the above is correct.

9. Osteomalacia causes:
    a. loss of bone matrix.
    b. inadequate mineralization.
    c. radiolucency.
    d. All of the above are correct.
    e. Both b and c are correct.

10. Bone tumors may originate from all of the following *except:*
    a. epithelial tissue.
    b. cartilage.
    c. fibrous tissue.
    d. vascular tissue.
    e. mesoderm.

11. In benign bone tumors, there is:
    a. a uniform and well-defined lytic area.
    b. a moth-eaten pattern of bone destruction.
    c. abnormal bone merging with surrounding normal bone tissue.
    d. an area of partially destroyed bone adjacent to completely lytic areas.

12. An osteosarcoma is a(n):
    a. collagenic, malignant bone tumor.
    b. myelogenic, benign tumor.
    c. myelogenic, malignant tumor.
    d. osteogenic, benign bone tumor.
    e. osteogenic, malignant tumor.

13. A major symptom of bone cancer is a:
    a. faltering gait.
    b. persistent pain that worsens at night.
    c. lack of sensation.
    d. general swelling over a bone.
    e. coolness over a bone.

14. Giant cell tumors:
    a. are collagenic tumors.
    b. are located in the diaphysis of a long bone.
    c. have extensive osteoblastic activity.
    d. have high recurrence rates.
    e. are multifocal.

15. Myeloma:
    a. is a malignant proliferation of plasma cells.
    b. has a poor prognosis.
    c. infiltrates the bone marrow.
    d. Both a and c are correct.
    e. a, b, and c are correct.

16. Rheumatoid arthritis begins with:
    a. destruction of the synovial membrane and subsynovial tissue.
    b. inflammation of ligaments.
    c. destruction of the articular cartilage.
    d. softening of the articular cartilage.
    e. destruction of the joint capsule.

17. The causes of osteoarthritis include which of the following? (More than one answer may be correct.)
    a. enzymatic breakdown
    b. proteoglycan destruction
    c. rheumatoid factor
    d. circulating immune complexes
    e. infections

18. Ankylosing spondylitis (more than one answer may be correct):
    a. is a systemic immune inflammatory disease.
    b. is characterized by stiffening or fusion of the spine.
    c. causes instability of synovial joints.
    d. begins with inflammation of fibrocartilage.
    e. is manifested early by low back pain and stiffness.

19. In gout:
    a. the pathogenesis is formation of monosodium urate crystals in joints and tissues.
    b. purine metabolism is altered.
    c. affected individuals likely have an inherited enzyme defect.
    d. the hyperuricemia can be the result of acquired chronic disease or a drug.
    e. All of the above are correct.

20. A muscle contracture is:
    a. likely caused by increased activity in the reticular activating system and the gamma loop in the muscle fiber.
    b. muscle shortening possible because of CNS injury.
    c. often helped by relaxation training and biofeedback.
    d. a consequence of reduced muscle protein synthesis.
    e. All of the above are correct.

21. Myotonia is all of the following *except:*
    a. delayed relaxation after voluntary muscle contractions.
    b. prolonged depolarization of the muscle membrane.
    c. mostly inherited.
    d. unresponsiveness to neural stimulation.
    e. progressive atrophy of skeletal muscle.

Match the myopathy with its cause.

_____22. McArdle disease

_____23. acid maltase deficiency

_____24. polymyositis

a. hypothyroidism

b. hyperparathyroidism

c. accumulation of glycogen in lysosomes

d. inability to catabolize glycogen

e. immune system abnormality

25. Rhabdomyosarcomas have:
    a. a poor prognosis.
    b. aggressive invasion.
    c. early, widespread dissemination.
    d. pleomorphic types.
    e. All of the above are correct.

Case Study

Mrs. B. is a 52-year-old homemaker who has complained of bilateral knee and hand pain for 7 years. The pain has progressively worsened and persists during rest and limits her walking, climbing stairs, and weight bearing. Her physical examination showed slight ulnar deviation of the digits and swelling of the metacarpal, phalangeal, and proximal interphalangeal joints with limited range of motion and some instability of both knees.

Laboratory studies revealed the following:

    CBC = normal, except for mild anemia

    Rheumatoid factor = high titer

    Synovial fluid analysis = turbid appearance

    Radiographic examination of knees = joint narrowing on both knees, thinning of the articular cartilage, cystic areas, and bony spurs

Which arthritis is Mrs. B. experiencing? Explain your answer.

38

Alterations of Musculoskeletal Function in Children

Objectives

After studying this chapter, the learner will be able to do the following:

1. **Describe congenital musculoskeletal defects in children.**
   Study pages 1118-1120; refer to Figures 38-1 through 38-4 and Table 38-1.

Clubfoot, or congenital equinovarus, describes a deformity in which the forefoot is twisted inward toward the floor and the heel is in equines, or pointing down. The clubfoot deformity can be positional, idiopathic, and teratologic (due to another syndrome, such as spina bifida). The idiopathic clubfoot occurs in 1:1000 live births with males twice as likely as females to be affected. The deformity involves not only the forefoot adduction and supination but also hindfoot equines (pointed downward) and varus (heel in toward the midline).

In the idiopathic clubfoot, manipulation and casting above the knee, begun soon after birth, can often correct the forefoot deformity. The hindfoot equines may require lengthening of the Achilles tendon, which can be performed in a clinic under local anesthetic at about 6 to 8 weeks of age. Bracing may be required until age 2. Idiopathic feet recalcitrant to these procedures require a posteromedial release (PMR), a much larger surgical intervention. Teratologic feet are usually stiffer and a higher percentage require PMR.

Developmental dysplasia of the hip (DDH) describes imperfect development of the hip that can affect the femoral head, the acetabulum, or both. Although most often present at birth, it may occur at any time in the newborn or infant period. Like clubfoot, DDH can be idiopathic or teratologic. Teratologic hips are much more difficult to treat and often need operative intervention. For the idiopathic hip, 70% are on the left, girls are more commonly affected, and certain antenatal events, such as breech position and oligohydramnios (low fluids) and positive family history predispose to DDH. Variants of idiopathic DDH are **dislocated hip** (no contact between femoral head and acetabulum), **subluxated hip** (partial contact only), and **acetabular dysplasia** (the femoral head is located properly but the acetabulum is shallow).

Clinical examination is the mainstay of diagnosis. The examination must be performed in a relaxed infant for accuracy. A positive Ortolani sign (hip out but reductive) or Belaris sign (hip in but dislocatable) are absolute indications for treatment. Other indicators for further evaluation are imitation of abduction or apparent shortening of the femur (Galeazzi sign).

In children less than 6 months old, bracing with a Pavlik harness is successful in 90% of DDH. With advancing age, closed reduction of the hip and spica (body) casting under general anesthesia is required. The spica cast is worn for 3 months. Children over 18 months of age require surgery either on the joint, the femur, or all three.

Osteogenesis imperfecta (OI) (brittle bone disease) is a spectrum of disease caused by genetic mutation in the gene that encodes for type I collagen, the main component of bone and blood vessels. Classification defines four types. Types I and IV are milder forms and inherited in an autosomal dominant pattern; Types II and III are more severe and inherited in a recessive pattern. Children with type II often die during infancy.

The classic clinical manifestations of osteogenesis imperfecta (OI) are osteopenia (decreased bone mass) and an increased rate of fractures. With recurrent fractures, bone deformity (bowing) often occurs. The children are of short stature, have triangular faces, possibly blue sclera, and poor dentitions.

Treatment is a combination of medical and surgical approaches. For fractures and deformity, often utilized is intramedullary rodding of the bone to help hold position and splint new fractures. Telescoping rods, which grow with the child, have been used but mechanical failure limits efficacy. Unfortunately, these children may undergo multiple surgeries and re-roddings with growth. The medical treatment, classically involving increased calcium and vitamin D, is under study.

2. **Describe bony infections.**
   Study pages 1120-1122; refer to Figures 38-5 and 38-6.

Osteomyelitis, or bone infection, is caused by either bacterial or granulomatous (i.e., tuberculosis) infective processes. **Acute hematogenous osteomyelitis** is the most common form in children.

Osteomyelitis usually begins as a bloody abscess in the metaphysis of the bone. The abscess ruptures under the periosteum and spreads along the bone shaft or into the bone marrow cavity if untreated. Debris accumulates, causing the periosteum to separate and form a shell of new bone around the infected portion of the shaft. Because the periosteum is separated from an adequate blood supply, sections of the bone die, becoming **sequestrum.** The periosteum that maintains a blood supply generates new bone, or **involucrum.** The presence of the sequestra and involucrum indicates that the disease has progressed to subperiosteal abscess formation.

Treatment consists of appropriate antibiotic coverage for 6 weeks (all IV or a combination of IV and oral dos-

ing) and surgical debridement of dead bone (sequestrum) or if there is no response to medication alone. Bone aspiration is required to identify the microorganism if blood cultures are negative.

Septic arthritis can occur de novo or secondary to osteomyelitis at locations where the metaphysis is still located within the joint capsule (hip, proximal humerus, proximal radius, and distal lateral tibia). The most common sites for septic arthritis are knees, hips, ankles, and then elbows. These children present with severe joint pain, inability to bear weight or move the affected joint, and severe malaise. Anorexia, fever, and elevated CBC, ESR, and CRP are more common than in osteomyelitis, and these laboratory findings can be very helpful in distinguishing between pyogenic and nonpyogenic arthritis. Plain radiographs are often normal, but a bone scan is helpful, especially with pelvis, scapula, and ankle sites.

Septic arthritis is a surgical emergency. Blood cultures taken at time of aspiration and debridement of the joint are 75% positive, and a cell count of the joint fluid shows a left shift (immature white blood cells [WBCs]) with greater than 50,000 WBCs. As with osteomyelitis, *Staphylococcus aureus* is the most common microorganism. In neonates, Group B streptococcus may be causative and gonococcus may occur in the adolescent population. Bacterial and host enzymes can cause rapid destruction of articular cartilage, which is irreparable and can cause a lifetime of pain and disability. After definitive surgical intervention, antibiotics are required for 2 to 4 weeks. Long-term follow-up to assess articular or physeal damage is required.

3. **Describe the features of juvenile rheumatoid arthritis.**
   Study page 1122; refer to Table 38-2.

The basic pathophysiology of **juvenile rheumatoid arthritis (JRA)** is the same as that of adult rheumatoid arthritis, but JRA differs in the following points:

a. Mode of onset has three distinct forms:
   • Arthritis in fewer than five joints (pauciarticular)
   • Arthritis in more than five joints (polyarthritis)
   • Systemic disease (most common)
b. The large joints are predominantly affected.
c. Subluxation and ankylosis of the cervical spine are common.
d. Joint pain is not as severe as the adult type.
e. Chronic uveitis is common.
f. JRA continuing through adolescence can affect growth and adult morbidity.
g. Serologic tests seldom detect rheumatoid factor.

Treatment for children with JRA is supportive but not curative—its aims being to control inflammation and other clinical manifestations of the disease and to minimize deformity.

4. **Describe the pathophysiology, evaluation, and treatment of the osteochondroses and Legg-Calve-Perthes disease.**
   Study pages 1123-1125; refer to Figures 38-7 through 38-9.

The **osteochondroses** are a series of childhood diseases involving areas of significant tensile or compromise stress (i.e., tibial tubercle, Achilles insertion, hip) which undergo partial but insufficient blood supply, death of bone (osseous necrosis), progressive bony weaknesses, and then microfracture. The cause of the decreased blood supply is controversial; this could be due to trauma, change in clotting sensitivity, vascular injury, or a combination. Reparative processes by neovascularization is the rule, although years may be required for full healing. All osteochondroses present as pain in active children.

Legg-Calve-Perthes disease (LCP) is a process of interrupted blood supply to the femoral head. It commonly occurs between 3 and 10 years of age with a peak incidence at 6 years of age. It is self-limiting in nature, running its course in 2 to 5 years. Interruption of blood flow to the femoral head results in necrosis of the femoral head. Inflammation and new bone formation follow over time with a resultant flattening of the femoral head. The first necrotic stage lasts only a short time; however, the healing phase lasts from 2 to 4 years. The etiology of LCP is a history of antecedent trauma. It is probable that an antecedent synovitis causes increased hydrostatic pressure within the joint and interferes with blood flow. Birth weight tends to be low in children with LCP disease, and skeletal maturation is delayed as well.

Presentation of LCP disease may be fairly incipient, with the child complaining of lower extremity pain for weeks to months. A limp known as the antalgic abductor lurch then follows. The child often demonstrates pain when the hip is externally rotated while in extension. Treatment is accomplished by antiinflammatory medications, crutches for episodes of synovitis, avoiding activities that stress the hip, bracing the legs in abduction or by surgical intervention if necessary.

Osgood-Schlatter disease consists of osteochondrosis of the tubercle of the tibia and often tendonitis of the patella. The mildest form of Osgood-Schlatter disease causes ischemic (avascular) necrosis in the region of the bony tibial tubercle, with hypertrophic cartilage formation during the stages of repair. In more severe cases the abnormality involves a true apophyseal separation of the tibial tubercle with avascular necrosis. The child complains of pain and swelling in the region around the patellar tendon and tibial tubercle, which becomes prominent and is tender to direct pressure.

The goal of treatment for Osgood-Schlatter disease is to decrease the stress at the tubercle. Often a period of 4 to 8 weeks of restriction from strenuous physical activity, especially activities requiring deep knee bending, is sufficient. If relief from pain is not achieved, a cast or knee immobilization is required, a situation that is particularly difficult if the condition is bilateral.

5. **Describe scoliosis.**
   Study page 1125; refer to Figure 38-10.

There are three main types of **scoliosis:** idiopathic; congenital, due to bony deformity such as hemivertebrae; and teratologic, due to another systemic syndrome such as cerebral palsy. Eighty percent of all scoliosis is idiopathic, which may have a genetic component. True structural scoliotic deformity involves not only a side-to-side spinal curve but also rotation; curves without rotation may be nonstructural or due to another cause such as limb length inequity.

Idiopathic curves progress while a child is growing and progression can be very rapid during growth spurts. When idiopathic curves progress to 25 degrees or greater, and the child is skeletally immature, bracing is required. Curves over 50 degrees will progress after skeletal maturity and, therefore, spinal fusion is required to stop progression. Early diagnosis is therefore necessary so that bracing can be attempted in the hopes of halting progression before surgical indicators are reached. Children are required to wear the brace 16 hours per day and full compliance can be difficult to attain. Nevertheless, bracing is the only nonoperative measure known to slow scoliotic progression. Bracing is less successful in teratologic or congenital curves; unfortunately, these conditions often require surgical intervention.

6. **Describe the pathophysiology, evaluation, and treatment of Duchenne muscular dystrophy.**
   Study pages 1125 and 1127; refer to Figure 38-11 and Table 38-3.

Duchenne muscular dystrophy is an X-linked inherited disorder that is caused by a deletion of a segment of DNA. This deletion results in an absence of dystrophin, which is found in normal muscle cells. The lack of dystrophin apparently causes loss of muscle bulk and fibers. In the late stages, interstitial connective tissue and fat may replace muscle fibers.

The disease is often diagnosed at approximately 3 years of age when parents notice slow motor development, problems with coordination and walking, and generalized weakness. Weakness always begins in the pelvic girdle, and hypertrophy is present in the calf muscles of approximately 80% of affected children. Gower sign, a peculiar manner of standing up from a sitting position by climbing up the legs, is often evident. Within 3 to 5 years, the shoulder girdle muscle becomes involved with constant progression of the illness. Pulmonary and cardiac failure may follow and, eventually, death usually results by age 20.

Diagnosis is confirmed by serum enzyme studies and electromyelography. Creatine phosphokinase (CPK) may be 10 times normal, and histologic examination of biopsied muscle fibers will be abnormal as well. Treatment is chiefly supportive, with the goal being to preserve function of remaining muscle groups for as long as possible.

7. Characterize common benign bone tumors of childhood.

Study pages 1127-1128.

Osteochondromas (exostoses) can occur as a solitary lesion or an inherited syndrome of **hereditary multiple exostoses (HME)**. HME is an autosomal dominant condition. Osteochondromas appear as bony protuberances either sessile or pedunculated lesions appearing in the periphyseal area. They are most common near active growth plates of the proximal humerus, distal femur, or proximal tibia. The most common presentation is a palpable mass that is painful when traumatized. Rarely, the lesion may cause neurologic, vascular, or tendon excursion anomalies because of local compression on nearby structures. HME is a type of systemic skeletal dysplasia with tens to hundreds of lesions throughout the body. The lesions can lead to growth disturbance and mildly short stature. Knee valgus (knock knee), ankle valgus, and hip problems are common. Upper extremity lesions can lead to a pronounced deformity in the forearm with a very short ulna bone. Three genetic loci have been identified on chromosomes 8, 11, and 19. Two of these loci (8 and 11) have been associated with the very rare (1%) but serious complication of malignant degeneration to chondrosarcoma after skeletal maturity.

Treatment involves minimizing growth disturbance, local tissue compression, and pain by resection of symptomatic lesions. Regrowth rate is 30% when lesions are removed in early childhood; therefore, only symptomatic lesions should be surgically addressed.

Nonossifying fibroma or fibrous cortical defect is 50% of all benign bone tumors. **Nonossifying fibromas** are sharply demarcated, cortically-based lesions of fibrocytes that have replaced normal bone. The lesion can oc-

cur in any bone, at any age. Nonossifying fibromas are discovered in 20% to 30% of all children as an incidental finding.

Microscopically, these benign nonmetastasizing lesions appear as whorled bundles of fibroblasts and osteoclast-like giant cells. As the tumor grows, lipids make the fibroblasts foamy in appearance and are known as foam cells.

Treatment is observational only. If these lesions grow too large, however, they will compromise the biomechanical strength of the bone causing pathologic features. Curettage and bone grafting is suggested when fractures occur or when fractures are impending.

8. Characterize childhood osteosarcoma and Ewing sarcoma.

Study pages 1128-1129; refer to Figures 38-12 and 38-13.

Osteosarcoma accounts for 60% of the bone tumors in children and originates in bone-producing mesenchymal cells. Three-fourths of these neoplasms occur between the ages of 10 and 25.

Osteosarcoma can be induced by ionizing radiation or by therapeutic radiation for other forms of cancer. It is more likely to occur if an individual has bilateral retinoblastoma. The link between retinoblastoma and subsequent osteosarcoma occurs whether or not radiation has been part of the treatment for retinoblastoma.

The most common complaint is pain. Symptoms also may include cough, dyspnea, and chest pain when lung metastasis occurs.

Surgery and chemotherapy are the primary treatments for osteosarcoma. Chemotherapy is an important component of treatment because children treated with surgery alone eventually develop metastatic disease. The tumor is resistant to radiation.

Ewing sarcoma is the second most common but most lethal malignant bone tumor of childhood. It probably originates from cells within the bone marrow space and does not involve bone-forming cells. Its incidence is greatest between 5 and 15 years of age; it is rare after age 30. The most common site of this tumor is the marrow of the femur. Followed by the marrow of the pelvis and then of the humerus.

The most common symptom is pain that increases in severity. A soft-tissue mass is often present. Ewing sarcoma metastasizes early to nearly every organ. The most common sites are the lung, other bones, lymph nodes, liver, spleen, and central nervous system.

Treatment is preoperative chemotherapy followed by radiation or surgical resection or both and continued chemotherapy for 12 to 18 months afterward. Involved sites with the best prognosis are the extremities; the worst prognosis involves tumors of the trunk and the pelvis.

Practice Examination

True/False

_____ 1. In clubfoot, the entire foot points upward.

_____ 2. Osteosarcoma is responsive to radiotherapy.

_____ 3. Osteogenesis imperfecta is a disease related to overcalcification of the bone that causes it to be brittle and easily broken.

_____ 4. Septic arthritis can involve sites where the metaphysis still is located within the joint capsule.

_____ 5. Osgood-Schlatter disease consists of osteochondrosis of the tubercle of the fibula and tendonitis of the patella.

_____ 6. Osteomyelitis is an infection of bone that can be spread to the site through the blood.

_____ 7. Juvenile rheumatoid arthritis predominately affects small joints.

_____ 8. True structural scoliosis involves spinal rotation.

_____ 9. Muscular dystrophies are characterized by defective creatine metabolism.

_____ 10. Nonossifying fibromas are poorly demarcated.

Fill-In-the-Blanks

11. The process of Legg-Calve-Perthes disease is presumably produced by interruption of the blood supply to the _____ head.

12. A risk factor in developmental dysplasia of the hip may be _____ in utero.

13. Duchenne muscular dystrophy results from a lack of _____ in muscle cells.

14. DDH is treated by bracing the hips in a _____.

15. Congenital equinovarus is also known as _____.

Match the outcome or circumstance with the alteration.

_____ 16. fractures present at birth

_____ 17. hypertrophied calf muscles

_____ 18. chronic uveitis

_____ 19. Gower sign

_____ 20. antalgic abductor lurch

_____ 21. large joints affected

_____ 22. pain in external rotation with affected limb

_____ 23. long-term antibiotics required

_____ 24. defect in collagen synthesis

_____ 25. lateral curvature of the spine

a. scoliosis

b. osteogenesis imperfecta

c. osteomyelitis

d. Legg-Calve-Perthes disease

e. JRA

f. Duchenne muscular dystrophy

Case Study

Bobby B. is a 3-year-old white male visiting a pediatrician's office because of his mother's concern regarding his clumsiness, frequent falls, and difficulty in climbing stairs. On physical examination, Bobby B. tends to walk on his toes, exhibits a positive Gower sign, and appears to have hypertrophy of calf muscles.

What disease is suspected? How could the diagnosis be confirmed?

Structure, Function, and Disorders of the Integument

a. Describe the skin and its layers.
Review pages 1134-1135; refer to Figure 39-1 and Table 39-1.

MEMORY CHECK!

- The skin has two major layers: a superficial epidermis and a deeper layer, the dermis. The subcutaneous tissue, or hypodermis, is an underlying layer of connective tissue that contains macrophages, fibroblasts, and fat cells.

- The dermal appendages include the nails, hair, sebaceous glands, and the eccrine and apocrine sweat glands. The nails are protective keratinized plates that appear at the ends of fingers and toes. Hair follicles arise from the matrix located deep in the dermis. Hair growth begins in the bulb, with cellular differentiation occurring as the hair progresses up the follicle. Hair is fully cornified by the time it emerges at the skin surface. The sebaceous glands open onto the surface of the skin through a canal and secrete sebum composed primarily of lipids, which oil the skin and hair and prevent drying.

- The eccrine sweat glands are distributed over the body and are important in cooling of the body through evaporation. The apocrine sweat glands are fewer in number and are located in the axillae, scalp, face, abdomen, and genital area.

- The blood supply to the skin is by the papillary capillaries or plexus of the dermis. Arteriovenous anastomoses in the dermis facilitate the regulation of body temperature. Heat loss can be regulated by varying blood flow through the skin by opening or closing the arteriovenous anastomoses to modify evaporative heat loss through sweat. The sympathetic nervous system regulates both vasoconstriction and vasodilation as there are only adrenergic receptors in the skin. The lymphatic vessels of the skin arise in the dermis and drain into larger subcutaneous trunks; these vessels remove cells, proteins, and immunologic mediators.

b. **Identify the changes that occur in skin during aging.**
   Review page 1135.

• The skin becomes thinner, dryer, and wrinkled, and pigmentation changes during aging. Fewer melanocytes decrease the protection against ultraviolet radiation. Fewer Langerhans cells decrease the skin's immune response during aging. The thickness of the dermis decreases and the skin becomes translucent and assumes a paper-thin quality. Loss of the rete pegs gives the skin a smooth, shiny appearance. Atrophy of eccrine, apocrine, and sebaceous glands causes the skin to become drier with age. Loss of elastin fibers is associated with wrinkling. The collagen fibers become less flexible and decrease the ability of the skin to stretch and regain shape. Decreased cell generation and blood supply delay wound healing in aging skin. Graying of hair color is due to loss of melanocytes. Barrier function of the stratum corneum is reduced. There is increased permeability and decreased clearance of substances from the dermis. The accumulation of such substances can cause skin irritation. Temperature regulation is less effective in the elderly, and there is increased risk for both heatstroke and hypothermia. The pressure and touch receptors and free nerve endings all decrease in number and reduce sensory perception.

Objectives

After studying this chapter, the learner will be able to do the following:

1. **Distinguish between skin lesions.**
   Refer to Tables 39-2 and 39-3.

Basic Lesions of the Skin

Type	Characteristics	Example/Disease
Flat Lesions		
Macule	A flat, circumscribed, discolored lesion of any size	Hyperpigmentation, erythema, telangiectasia, purpura
Patch	A flat, irregular lesion larger than a macule	Vitiligo
Petechiae	A circumscribed area of blood less than 0.5 cm in diameter	Thrombocytopenia
Purpura	A circumscribed area of blood greater than 5.0 cm in diameter	Bruises
Telangiectasia	Dilated, superficial blood vessels	Rheumatoid arthritis, hepatitis
Elevated Characteristics		
Papule	A lesion 1 cm or less in diameter because of infiltration or hyperplasia of the dermis	Verrucae (warts), lichen planus, nevus
Plaque	A lesion with a large surface area, larger laterally than in height	Psoriasis, eczema
Nodule	A palpable, circumscribed lesion 1-2 cm in diameter located in the epidermis, dermis, or hypodermis; smooth to ulcerated	Benign or malignant tumors, foreign body inflammation, calcium deposits
Wheal	A transient lesion with well-defined and often changing borders caused by edema of the dermis	Hives, angioedema

Basic Lesions of the Skin *(cont'd)*

Type	Characteristics	Example/Disease
Vesicle and bulla	A fluid-filled, thin-walled lesion; a bulla is a vesicle greater than 0.5 cm in diameter	Herpes zoster, impetigo, pemphigus, second-degree burns
Pustule	A lesion containing an exudate of white blood cells	Acne, pustular psoriasis
Comedo	Plugged hair follicle	Blackhead, whitehead
Scale	Accumulation of loose stratum corneum from cellular retention or cellular overproduction	Psoriasis
Crust	Accumulation of dried blood or serum; size varies	Eczema, impetigo
Lichenification	Thickening, toughening of the skin with accentuation of skin lines caused by scratching	Chronic dermatitis
Cyst	An encapsulated mass of dermis or subcutaneous layers, solid or fluid-filled	Sebaceous cyst
Tumor	A well-demarcated solid lesion greater than 2 cm in diameter	Fibroma, lipoma, melanoma, hemangioma
Scar	Thin or thick fibrous tissue	Healed laceration, burn, surgical incision

Depressed Lesions

Atrophy	Thinning of the epidermis or dermis caused by decreased connective tissue	Thin facial skin of the elderly, striae of pregnancy
Ulcer	Loss of epidermis and dermis	Pressure sores, basal cell carcinoma
Excoriation	Loss of epidermis with exposed dermis	Scratches
Fissure	Linear crack or break exposing dermis	Athlete's foot, cheilosis
Erosion	Moist, red break in epidermis, follows rupture of vesicle or bulla, larger than fissure	Chickenpox, diaper dermatitis

2. **Describe keloids; identify stimuli for pruritus.**
   Study page 1142; refer to Figure 39-3.

Keloids are sharply elevated, irregularly shaped scars that progressively enlarge. They are caused by trauma to the skin and the excessive accumulation of collagen in the corneum during connective tissue repair. Burns incite this reaction more commonly than other types of injury. Even minor trauma may result in a keloidal reaction in blacks and Asians. A familial tendency for keloid formation exists, with both autosomal recessive and autosomal dominant inheritance patterns present.

Keloids begin as pink or red, firm, well-defined, rubbery plaques that persist for several months after trauma. The fibrous tissue that accumulates in keloids is associated with increased cellularity and metabolic activity of fibroblasts. Injection of corticosteroids into the lesion is the treatment of choice.

Pruritus, or itching, is a symptom associated with many primary skin disorders and systemic diseases. The condition may be localized or generalized and may move from one location to another.

Multiple stimuli can produce itching, including substance P, histamine, heat, and electrical stimulation. Substance P, a neurotransmitter, causes histamine release and wheal formation with itching when injected into the skin. Lymphocytes present in itching skin may be involved in the pathogenesis of itching. Unmyelinated nociceptor fibers may be involved in itching.

Management of pruritus depends on the cause; the primary condition must be treated. Symptomatic relief can be obtained from antihistamines and topical steroids in some cases. Some pruritus is resistant to any type of therapy.

3. **Compare pemphigus with erythema multiforme.**
   Study pages 1147-1148; refer to Figure 39-14.

4. **Identify the causes and lesions of inflammatory and papulosquamous disorders of the skin.**
   Study pages 1143-1147; refer to Figures 39-4 through 39-13. (See box on page 287.)

Pemphigus is a rare, chronic, blister-forming disease of the skin and oral mucous membranes with several different types that include pemphigus vulgaris, pemphigus foliaceus, and pemphigus erythematosus. The blisters form in the epidermis and occur deeply in pemphigus vulgaris and superficially in pemphigus foliaceus and pemphigus erythematosus.

Pemphigus is an autoimmune disease caused by circulating IgG autoantibodies. Serum autoantibodies are formed, which react with the intracellular cement of substance that holds the epidermal cells together. The antibody reaction likely causes the intraepidermal blister formation and acantholysis, or loss of cohesion between epidermal cells.

Pemphigus vulgaris is the most common form of the disease and begins with the formation of a blister in the mouth or on the scalp. Within 6 months to 1 year, flaccid bullous lesions appear that rupture easily and leave crusty, denuded skin. Pressure on the blister may cause it to spread to adjacent skin; this is the *Nikolsky sign.* In **pemphigus foliaceus** and **pemphigus erythematosus,** oral lesions are usually absent and erythema with localized crusting, scaling, and occasional bullae develop. **Paraneoplastic pemphigus** exhibits intractable cutaneous lesions, distinct autoantibodies, and associated hematologic malignancies.

In the diagnosis of pemphigus, immunofluorescence demonstrates the presence of antibodies at the site of blister formation. The primary treatment for pemphigus is systemic corticosteroids usually in high doses to suppress the immune response during acute episodes or when there is widespread involvement.

Erythema multiforme is an acute, recurring, inflammatory disorder of the skin and mucous membranes. It is associated with allergic or toxic reactions to drugs or microorganisms such as *Mycoplasma pneumoniae* and herpes simplex. Immune complex formation and deposition of C3, IgM, and fibrinogen around the superficial dermal blood vessels, basement membrane, and keratinocytes can be observed in most individuals with erythema multiforme. The characteristic "bull's eye" lesion occurs on the skin surface with a central erythematous region surrounded by concentric rings or alternating edema and inflammation. A vesiculobullous form is characterized by mucous membrane lesions and erythematous plaques on the extensor surfaces of the extremities.

The most common form expressed in children and young adults is **Stevens-Johnson syndrome,** wherein there are numerous erythematous, bullous lesions on both the skin and mucous membranes. The bullous lesions form erosions and crusts when they rupture. The mouth, air passages, esophagus, urethra, and conjunctiva may be involved. Mild forms of the disease require no treatment because they are self-limiting; underlying infections should be treated.

Inflammatory and Papulosquamous Skin Disorders

Disorder	Cause	Lesion
Inflammatory Disorders		
Allergic contact dermatitis	Allergen binds to carrier protein to form a sensitizing antigen, T cell hypersensitivity, IgE	Pruritic (itching) vesicles
Irritant contact dermatitis	Nonimmunologic inflammation due to chemicals	As above
Atopic dermatitis	Mast cell and IgE, T lymphocytes, and monocytes interact	Red, weeping crusts, lichenification
Stasis dermatitis	Venous stasis and edema	Initial erythema and pruritus; then scaling, petechiae, and hyperpigmentation
Seborrheic dermatitis	Unknown	Scaly plaques with mild pruritus
Papulosquamous Disorders		
Psoriasis	Unknown, genetic or immunologic	Thick, silvery, scaly, erythematous plaque surrounded by normal skin; rapid shedding of epidermis
Pityriasis rosea	Unknown (virus?)	Pruritus, demarcated salmon-pink scale within a plaque
Lichen planus	Unknown (exposure to drugs?)	Nonscaling, violet-colored pruritic papules
Acne vulgaris	Increased activity of sebaceous glands or sebum inability to escape through the narrow opening	Comedones
Acne rosacea	Unknown, associated with chronic flushing and sensitivity to sun	Erythema, papules, pustules, and telangiectasis
Discoid lupus erythematosus	Immune response to unknown antigen	Cutaneous manifestations of elevated red plaque with brown scale, hair loss, urticaria (hives), telangiectasis

5. **Identify the causes and lesions of cutaneous infections.**
   Study pages 1148-1151; refer to Figures 39-15 through 39-19 and Tables 39-4 and 39-5.

Cutaneous Infections

Infection	Cause	Lesion
Folliculitis	Bacterial infection of hair follicles usually by *Staphylococcus aureus*	Pustules with surrounding erythema
Furuncle	Infection from folliculitis spreading into dermis	Deep, red, firm, painful nodule changes to fluctuant and tender cystic nodule
Carbuncle	Collection of infected hair follicles	Erythematous, painful mass that drains through many openings
Cellulitis	Infection of dermis and subcutaneous tissue; extension from skin wound, ulcer, furuncle, or carbuncle	Erythematous, swollen, and painful area
Erysipelas	Group A streptococci	Systemic manifestations, red spots progress to pruritic vesicles
Impetigo	Coagulase-positive staphylococci; beta-hemolytic streptococci	Serous and purulent vesicles that rupture and crust
Herpes simplex virus (HSV-1)	Primary and secondary infections (sensory nerve ganglion latency) on nongenital sites such as cornea, mouth, and labia	Clusters of vesicles on an erythematous base that become purulent and crusty ("cold sores" or "fever blisters")
(HSV-2)	Primary and secondary infection (sensory nerve ganglion latency) genital herpes	Vesicles that progress to painful ulceration, pruritus, and weeping
Varicella (chickenpox) primary	Varicella-zoster virus	Varicella: pink papules with reddened halo that is dry and crusty
Herpes zoster (shingles) secondary		Zoster: erythema followed by grouped vesicles along a unilateral dermatome that later crust
Warts (verrucae)	Human papillomavirus	Round, elevated with a rough, grayish surface
Tinea capitis (scalp)	Dermatophytes (fungi) that invade and thrive on keratin	Scaling and erythema, vesicles and fissures
Tinea pedis (athlete's foot)		
Tinea corporis (ringworm)		
Tinea cruris ("jock itch")		
Candidiasis	*Candida albicans* (yeastlike fungus) changes from a skin and mucous membrane commensal to a pathogen	Thin-walled pustule with inflammatory pruritic base

6. Differentiate among vasculitis, urticaria, and scleroderma.
Study pages 1151-1152; refer to Figure 39-20.

Vasculitis, or angiitis, is an inflammation of the blood vessels. Cutaneous vasculitis develops from the deposit of immune complexes in small blood vessels as a response to drugs, allergens, or streptococcal or viral infection. The deposit of immune complex likely activates complement, which is chemotactic for polymorphonuclear leukocytes. The lesions appear as palpable purpura and progress to hemorrhagic bullae with necrosis and ulceration because of occlusion of the vessel. Identifying and removing the antigen is the first step in treatment. Prednisone may be used if symptoms are severe.

Urticarial lesions are most commonly associated with type I hypersensitivity reactions to drugs, certain foods, intestinal parasites, or physical agents. The lesions are mediated by histamine release, which causes the endothelial cells of skin blood vessels to contract and increase their permeability. Individuals with chronic urticaria have histamine-releasing autoantibodies; this entity is known as autoimmune urticaria.

The fluid from the vessel appears as wheals, welts, or hives. Antihistamines usually reduce the hives and provide relief from itching. Corticosteroids may be required for treatment of severe attacks.

Scleroderma is sclerosis of the skin, which may remain localized to the skin or affect the visceral organs. If systemic, scleroderma involves the connective tissue and affects the kidneys, gastrointestinal tract, and lungs. The cutaneous lesions can cover the entire skin but are most often on the face and hands, the neck, and the upper chest.

The lesions exhibit massive deposits of collagen with fibrosis, inflammatory reactions, vascular changes in the capillary network with decreased capillary loops, and dilation of the remaining capillaries. Autoimmunity and an immune reaction to toxic substances are possible initiating mechanisms of the disease. Autoantibodies often can be recovered from the skin and serum of individuals with scleroderma. Growth factors or failure of apoptosis of myofibroblasts may be causative mechanisms.

The skin is hard, hypopigmented, taut, and tightly connected to the underlying tissue. An immobile masklike appearance with incomplete opening of the mouth is due to the tightness of facial skin. The fingers become tapered and flexed and lose fingertips from atrophy. Calcium deposits develop in the subcutaneous tissue and erupt through the skin. When progression to body organs occurs, death is caused by subsequent respiratory failure, renal failure, cardiac dysrhythmias, or obstructions or perforations of the esophagus or intestine. There is no specific treatment, and 50% of individuals die within 5 years of the onset of scleroderma. Trials with photopheresis, plasma pheresis, and stem cell treatment are in progress.

7. Identify diseases caused by insect bites.
Study page 1153.

Ticks are significant vectors of transmitted diseases, including Rocky Mountain spotted fever and other rickettsial diseases, tularemia, and Lyme disease. Ticks embed their heads in the skin to obtain blood. If mouth parts remain in the skin after tick removal, a persistent nodule may develop. As ticks feed, they enlarge to many times their normal size and may release toxins or transmit microorganisms. In most instances, tick bites cause only a papular urticaria.

Lyme disease is a multisystem inflammatory disease caused by *Borrelia burgdorferi* transmitted by tick bites. The disease occurs in stages. Soon after the bite, a rash with or without flulike illness occurs. Nine months later, secondary erythema migrans, arthralgias, meningitis, neuritis, and carditis develop. Persistent infection continues for years with arthritis, encephalopathy, and polyneuropathy. Serologic tests may confirm the diagnosis subsequent to presence or history of tick bite. Antibiotics are used for treatment with good success in early stages, but the response may be slow.

Mosquitoes are responsible for malaria, yellow fever, dengue fever, filariasis, and St. Louis encephalitis. Mosquitoes can bite through thin, loose clothing and are attracted by warmth and perspiration. The edema, pruritus, and papular lesions are caused by insertion of a blood tube by a female mosquito. Irritating salivary secretions also contain anticoagulants. Reactions vary depending on the sensitivity of the victim.

Several species of flies are bloodsuckers. The bite of a small female fly produces immediate pain, erythema, and vesicles. Itching and vesicular reactions may persist for weeks. The fiercest bloodsuckers are the larger types such as the horseflies and deerflies. These produce painful, bleeding bites because of their large mouth parts. The bites produce urticaria that may be accompanied by weakness, dizziness, and wheezing.

8. Compare the benign tumors of the skin.
   Study pages 1153-1154; refer to Figure 39-21.

Seborrheic keratosis is a benign proliferation of basal cells that produces elevated smooth or warty lesions. Multiple lesions are seen on the chest, back, and face in older people. The color varies; it may be tan to waxy yellow, flesh-colored, or dark brown-black, and the lesions are often oval and greasy-appearing with a hyperkeratotic scale. Lesion size varies from a few millimeters to several centimeters. Cryotherapy with liquid nitrogen is an effective treatment, and the lesions usually slough in 2 or 3 weeks after treatment.

A **keratoacanthoma** is a benign, self-limiting tumor that arises from hair follicles. It usually occurs on sun-exposed surfaces and develops in individuals between 60 and 65 years of age. The lesion develops in stages. The proliferative stage produces a rapid-growing, dome-shaped nodule with a central crust. In the mature stage, the lesion is filled with whitish-colored keratin. The mature lesion requires differentiation from squamous cell carcinoma. The involution stage usually occurs over a 3-to 4-month period as the lesion regresses. Although the lesion will resolve spontaneously, it can be removed surgically.

Actinic keratosis is a premalignant lesion found on skin surfaces exposed to ultraviolet radiation of the sun. The lesions can progress to squamous cell carcinoma. The prevalence is highest in individuals with unprotected, light-colored skin. The lesions appear as pigmented patches of rough, adherent scale, and surrounding areas may have telangiectasia. Freezing with liquid nitrogen provides quick, effective treatment. Excisions provide tissue for biopsy.

Nevi, or moles, are pigmented or nonpigmented lesions that form from melanocytes beginning at ages 3 to 5 years. During early development, the melanocytes accumulate at the junction of the dermis and epidermis and become macular lesions. Over time, the cells move into the dermis and become nodular and palpable. Nevi may appear anywhere on the skin singly or in groups and vary in size. Nevi may undergo transition to malignant melanoma; if irritated, they can be excised.

9. **Describe malignant skin lesions.**
   Study pages 1154-1157; refer to Figures 39-22
   through 39-25 and Table 39-6. (See box below.)

Cancerous Skin Lesions

Lesion	Cause	Growth Rate/Metastasis	Appearance
Basal cell carcinoma	Sunlight-exposed skin; alterations in *p53* tumor supressor gene	Slow growth; lesions almost never metastasize; invasive destruction	Smooth surface with rolled border, depressed center, telangiectasis
Squamous cell carcinoma	Sunlight-exposed skin; arise from premalignant lesions; activation of proto-oncogenes or inactivation of tumor-supressor genes	Moderate growth; some lesions metastasize	Rough, firm nodule with an indurated base; ulceration, bleeding
Malignant melanoma	Genetic predisposition, solar radiation and steroid hormones, precursor nevi	Fast growth; highly invasive; rapid metastasis	Nevi that change color, size, or margins; pruritus, bleeding, nodule formation or ulceration
Kaposi sarcoma	Immunodeficient states; genetics and gender—black, Jewish, or Italian males	Slow spread through skin, some aggressive change	Multifocal purplish, brown vascular macules that develop into plaques and nodules that may be painful and pruritic (may affect gastrointestinal and respiratory tracts)

NOTE: Treatment consists of surgery, electrodesiccation, radiation, or cryosurgery. For basal cell and squamous cell skin cancers, cure is virtually ensured with early detection and treatment. For malignant melanomas, wide and deep excisions and removal of lymph nodes is required. Early recognition of malignant melanomas by the ABCD rule (*A*ssymetry, *B*order irregularity, *C*olor variation, and *D*iameter larger than 6 mm) affects the surgical cure of these lesions. The survival is poor for malignant melanoma because it metastasizes quickly. The general response to treatment of Kaposi sarcoma is poor.

10. Classify burns according to the extent of injury.
Study pages 1157-1159; refer to Figures 39-26
through 39-31, 39-33, and 39-34 and Table 39-7.
(See box below.)

Burn Injury

| Feature | First-Degree | Second-Degree | | Third-Degree |
		Superficial Partial-Thickness	Deep Partial-Thickness	Full-Thickness
Morphology	Destruction of epidermis only	Destruction of epidermis and some dermis	Destruction of epidermis and dermis	Destruction of epidermis, dermis, and subcutaneous tissue
Skin function	Yes	No	No	No
Tactile and pain sensors	Yes	Yes	Diminished	No
Blisters	Present after 24 hours	Present within minutes	May not appear; a flat dehydrated layer lifts off in sheets	Rare; a flat dehydrated layer lifts off easily
Appearance of wound after initial debridement	Skin peels after 24 to 48 hours, normal or slightly red	Red to pale ivory, moist surface	Mottled with areas of waxy white, dry surface	White, cherry red, or black; may contain visible thrombosed veins; dry, hard leathery surface
Healing time	3 to 5 days	21 to 28 days	30 days to many months; excision and grafting	Will not heal; may close from edges as secondary healing if wound is small; excision and grafting
Scarring	None	May be present, influenced by genetic predisposition	Highest incidence; influenced by genetic predisposition	Scarring minimized by early excision and grafting; influenced by genetic predisposition

11. Characterize the edematous, cardiovascular, and cellular response to burn injury.
Study pages 1159-1161; refer to Figure 39-32.

Hypovolemic shock develops quickly after major burn injury. Within minutes of a major burn injury, the capillary bed opens not only in the burn area but also in the entire capillary system. This increased capillary permeability is the mechanism for fluid, electrolyte, and protein loss into the interstitium; this leads to the ensuing hypovolemic shock and massive edema. The fluid and protein movement from the vascular compartment result in decreased cardiac output, elevated hematocrit and WBC count, and hypoproteinemia. If the profound hypovolemic shock is not treated with fluid resuscitation, irreversible shock and death may occur within a few hours.

Burn shock resuscitation involves infusion of intravenous fluid at a rate faster than the loss of circulating volume fluid for 24 hours after burn injury. The most reliable criterion to determine adequate resuscitation of burn shock is the urine output. If the individual does not have adequate urine output, sufficient fluid is not being administered. As burn shock ends, fluid administered remains in the circulating volume and is reflected as increased urine output.

The cellular response to burn injury has a metabolic response and an immunologic response. Burn injury induces an immediate **hypermetabolic state** related to an increase and resetting of the thermal regulatory set-point. As core body temperature increases, tachycardia, hypercapnia, and body wasting develop. In individuals surviving burn shock, **immunosuppression** and increased susceptibility to potentially fatal systemic burn wound sepsis develop. Phagocytosis is impaired and cellular and humoral immunity is abnormal. The burned individual has decreased opsonization of bacteria and less polymorphonuclear neutrophil chemotaxis. Individuals with altered immunocompetence who are burned are at additional risk for complications.

12. Characterize frostbite.
Study pages 1161-1162.

Frostbite is an injury to the skin caused by exposure to extreme cold. The mechanism of injury appears to be direct cold injury to cells, indirect injury from ice crystal formation, or impaired circulation from anoxia to the exposed area.

Frozen skin becomes white or yellowish, is waxy, and has no sensation of pain. With mild frostbite during rewarming, there is redness and discomfort followed by a return to normal in a few hours. Cyanosis and mottling develop, followed by redness, swelling, and burning pain on rewarming in more severe cases. The most severe cases result in gangrene and loss of the affected part. Frostbite may be classified by depth of injury. Superficial frostbite includes partial skin freezing and is known as *first-degree;* full-thickness skin freezing is called *second-degree;* full-thickness skin and subcutaneous freezing is known as *third-degree.*

Immersion in a warm water bath until frozen tissue is thawed is the best treatment. Pain during the thawing period is severe and should be treated with potent analgesics. Gentle cleansing and avoidance of pressure on the skin should be maintained during healing. Amputation of necrotic tissue is delayed until a clear line of demarcation appears.

13. Define terms used in disorders of the hair and nails.
Study pages 1162-1163.

Male-pattern alopecia is an inherited form of irreversible baldness in which hair is lost in the central scalp and recession of the temporofrontal hairline occurs. **Female-pattern alopecia** is a thinning of the central hair of the scalp that begins in women at 20 to 30 years of age. **Alopecia areata** is patchy loss of hair usually associated with stress or metabolic diseases; it is usually reversible. **Hirsutism** is a male pattern of hair growth in women; it may be normal or the result of excessive secretion of androgenic hormones. **Paronychia** is an inflammation of the cuticle that can be acute or chronic and is usually caused by staphylococci or streptococci or occasionally by Candida. **Onychomycosis** is a fungal infection of the nail plate; the plate turns yellow or white and accumulates hyperkeratotic debris.

Practice Examination

1. Which stratum of the epidermis contains dead keratinocytes?
   a. corneum
   b. lucidum
   c. granulosum
   d. spinosum
   e. germinativum

2. The dermis is composed of all of the following *except:*
   a. melanocytes.
   b. collagen.
   c. elastin.
   d. apocrine sweat glands.
   e. sebaceous glands.

3. Which does *not* occur as the skin ages?
   a. more melanocytes
   b. decreased Langerhans cells
   c. loss of rete pegs
   d. loss of elastin fibers
   e. depressed immune response

4 Arteriovenous anastomoses in the dermis:
   a. prevent skin drying.
   b. regulate vasoconstriction.
   c. oppose evaporative heat loss.
   d. facilitate the regulation of body temperature.
   e. None of the above is correct.

Match the lesion with its descriptor.

_____ 5. macule

_____ 6. nodule

_____ 7. scale

_____ 8. wheal

a. hardened, adherent

b. changed color; not raised or depressed

c. accentuated skin lines caused by scratching

d. palpable, elevated solid lesion

e. flaky, accumulated stratum corneum

f. ridgelike, reddened elevation caused by edema and congestion

---

9. The cause of atopic dermatitis is:
   a. unknown.
   b. venous stasis.
   c. increased activity of sebaceous glands.
   d. mast cell degranulation, T cells, and monocyte interaction.
   e. nonimmunologic inflammation to chemicals.

10. The skin lesion of psoriasis is a:
    a. nonscaling, violet-colored pruritic papule.
    b. comedo.
    c. pruritic vesicle.
    d. erythematous, butterfly-shaped rash.
    e. thick, scaly, erythematous plaque.

11. A circular, demarcated, salmon-pink scale within a plaque is characteristic of:
    a. psoriasis.
    b. seborrheic dermatitis.
    c. acne rosacea.
    d. pityriasis rosea.
    e. lichen planus.

12. The Nikolsky sign is seen in:
    a. herpes simplex.
    b. pemphigus.
    c. erythema multiforme.
    d. Stevens-Johnson syndrome.
    e. Both c and d are correct.

13. The cause of impetigo in the adult is:
    a. *Streptococcus aureus.*
    b. group A streptococci.
    c. coagulase-positive staphylococci.
    d. beta-hemolytic streptococci.
    e. Both c and d are correct.

14. The usual manifestation of herpes simplex virus is a:
    a. painful nodule.
    b. pustule.
    c. cold sore or fever blister.
    d. wheal.

15. Of the benign tumors of the skin, keratoacan-thomas are characterized by:
    a. proliferation of basal cells.
    b. hyperkeratotic scales.
    c. origination from hair follicles.
    d. a proliferative stage that produces a nodule with a central crust.
    e. Both c and d are correct.

16. Which are most likely to undergo malignant transition?
    a. Seborrheic keratosis and keratoacanthoma
    b. Seborrheic keratosis and actinic keratosis
    c. Nevi and keratoacanthoma
    d. Nevi and actinic keratosis
    e. None of the above is correct.

17. The cause of Kaposi sarcoma likely is:
    a. solar radiation.
    b. steroidal hormones.
    c. precursor nevi.
    d. immunodeficiency.
    e. keratinization.

18. Squamous cell carcinoma of the skin is manifested as:
    a. irregular pigmentation.
    b. elevated, firm lesions.
    c. a smooth, pearly lesion with multiple telangiectasia.
    d. multifocal purplish, brown macules.

19. An untreated basal cell carcinoma:
    a. metastasizes frequently.
    b. often involves regional lymphatics.
    c. ulcerates and involves local tissue.
    d. grows rapidly.
    e. will eventually require removal of nearby lymph nodes.

20. Which malignant skin lesion metastasizes the earliest?
    a. basal cell carcinoma
    b. squamous cell carcinoma
    c. malignant melanoma
    d. Kaposi sarcoma

21. In which type of burn does skin function continue?
    a. first-degree
    b. superficial partial-thickness
    c. deep partial-thickness
    d. full-thickness

22. A burn that destroys the epidermis and dermis is a:
    a. first-degree burn.
    b. superficial partial-thickness burn.
    c. deep partial-thickness burn.
    d. full-thickness burn.

23. Hypovolemic shock in severely burned individuals is the result of:
    a. dilation of capillaries.
    b. increased capillary permeability.
    c. increased peripheral resistance.
    d. Both a and b are correct.
    e. a, b, and c are correct.

24. In individuals surviving burn shock, increased wound sepsis is due to:
    a. released inflammatory cytokines.
    b. fewer opsonins.
    c. inability of phagocytes to migrate to the site of infection.
    d. All of the above are correct.
    e. Both b and c are correct.

25. Onychomycosis is:
    a. a fungal infection of the nail plate.
    b. caused by staphylococci or streptococci.
    c. an inflammation of the cuticle.
    d. None of the above is correct.

Case Study

Mr. E. is a 26-year-old white male who sustained severe burns while welding an automobile gasoline tank that had been removed from a truck. Mr. E.'s friend, for whom the welding was being done, took him immediately to a regional burn center located 20 miles away.

Initial assessment reveals that Mr. E. has received full-thickness burns on his face, to both arms and hands bilaterally and circumferentially, and to the anterior trunk.

What are the immediate and major concerns of the burn unit?

Alterations of the Integument in Children

Foundational Objective

a. **Identify the structures of the integumentary system and describe their functions.**
Review pages 1134-1135; refer to Figures 39-1 and 39-2 and Table 39-1.

MEMORY CHECK!

- See *Workbook's* narrative for Foundational Objective **a** in Chapter 39.

Objectives

After studying this chapter, the learner will be able to do the following:

1. **Differentiate between atopic and diaper dermatitis in infants and children.**
Study pages 1170-1171; refer to Figures 40-1 and 40-2.

Atopic dermatitis, or eczema, is an inflammation of the skin of unknown etiology. There is, however, an increased incidence of 75% to 80% in individuals who have allergies and reactive airways. Onset usually is in infancy, with 85% of cases occurring by 5 years of age. Positive allergy tests, increased serum IgE levels, and eosinophilia are common findings. The face, scalp, trunk, and extensor surfaces of the extremities are commonly affected in younger children; the neck, hands, feet, and flexor surfaces are commonly affected in older children. In the infant, the characteristic rash is erythematous with weeping and crusting lesions. In older children, the rash is often erythematous with scaling and thick, leather-like lesions. Pruritus or itching leads to rubbing and scratching and more damage to the skin. Scratching causes microscopic cracking in the skin that allows water loss and exposes the lower layers to irritants which, in turn, lead to increased pruritus and scratching.

Treatment includes avoiding known irritants, hydration of the skin, antihistamines to relieve pruritus, and topical steroids to decrease inflammation. Antibiotics or antifungal agents may be necessary for secondary skin infections.

Diaper dermatitis is an inflammation of the skin in the diaper area that is caused by many factors, including lengthy exposure to wet and soiled diapers. It mostly is localized in the perineal area but may extend from the abdomen to the thighs and usually affects infants and young children. Diaper dermatitis is characterized by an erythematous rash of varying degrees of severity and often is complicated by a secondary fungal infection caused by the microorganism *Candida albicans.* The characteristic rash of *C. albicans* is very erythematous and papular and is associated with **papulovesicular satellite lesions.**

The best treatment is preventive by keeping the perineal area clean and dry with frequent diaper changes and routine hygiene. Topical barriers may become necessary once the rash develops. If *C. albicans* is present, a topical antifungal agent should be included in the treatment.

2. Describe acne vulgaris.
Study page 1171; refer to Figure 40-3.

Acne vulgaris is the most common of the skin diseases and affects 85% of the population between the ages of 12 and 25. The incidence of acne is the same in both genders; severe disease affects males more often. Genetics may determine the susceptibility and severity of the disease.

Acne develops primarily on the face and upper parts of the chest and back from sebaceous follicles. The follicles have many large sebaceous glands, a small vellus hair, and a dilated follicular canal that is visible on the skin surface as a pore. In **noninflammatory acne,** the comedones are open (blackheads) and closed (whiteheads) and the accumulated material causes follicular distension and thinning of follicular canal walls. **Inflammatory acne** develops in closed comedones when follicular walls rupture and expel sebum into the surrounding dermis and initiate inflammation.

The causes are abnormal keratinization of follicular epithelium, excessive sebum production, and proliferation of *Propionibacterium acnes.* Androgenic hormones increase the size and productivity of the sebaceous glands. Sebum and bacterial accumulation produce inflammation of the dermis as the follicle ruptures.

Topical treatment, including benzoyl peroxide, salicylic acid, and tretinoin, is used because it is the least invasive. Use of systemic therapies, including antibiotics, sex hormones, and corticosteroids, may be limited because of side effects.

3. Categorize and characterize the infectious processes of impetigo.
Study page 1171; refer to Figure 40-4.

Impetigo is a common bacterial skin infection in children and is either bullous or vesicular. (See box below.)

4. Describe the etiology and pathophysiology of staphylococcal scalded-skin syndrome.
Study page 1172; refer to Figure 40-5.

Staphylococcal scalded-skin syndrome is a serious infection caused by group II staphylococci. The primary site of infection often is in the throat or chest, with the onset of lesions usually preceded by an upper respiratory infection characterized by fever, rhinorrhea, and malaise. This severe infection is often seen in newborns because their immune systems are immature.

Manifestations are caused by an epidermolytic toxin produced by the staphylococcal microorganisms at the primary site of infection; the toxin circulates to the skin where it produces the classic effects. The toxin splits the epidermis away from the underlying layers. The first sign of skin involvement is the acute onset of generalized erythema and tenderness over the entire body except the palms, soles of the feet, and mucous membranes. Blisters and bullae form over the next several days, which rupture and denude the skin, leaving the child at risk for dehydration and secondary infection. In severe cases, generalized skin sloughing may occur.

Diagnosis is confirmed by culture and histologic studies. Lesions are treated like severe burns, and the primary infection is treated with oral or parenteral antibiotics. Healing in uncomplicated cases usually requires 10 to 14 days.

5. Compare tinea capitis with tinea corporis; describe thrush.
Study pages 1172-1173; refer to Figure 40-6.

Candida albicans is part of the normal skin flora in certain individuals that invades susceptible tissue sites if the predisposing factors are not eliminated. This organism penetrates the epidermal barrier because of its keratolytic proteases and other enzymes. *C. albicans* attracts

Impetigo

Feature	Bullous	Vesicular
Etiologic agent	*Staphylococcus aureus*	*Streptococcus pyogenes* or combined with staphylococci
Source	Other infected individuals or contaminated objects	Other infected individual, contaminated objects, insect bites
Regional lymphadenitis	Uncommon	Common
Treatment	Systemic antibiotics	Systemic antibiotics
Potential complications	Uncommon	Acute glomerulonephritis

neutrophils to skin sites of invasion and generates inflammation by activation of the complement system.

Thrush is the presence of *Candida* in the mucous membranes of the mouth of infants and, less often, adults. Thrush is characterized by white plaques or spots in the mouth that lead to shallow ulcers. The underlying mucous membrane is red and tender and may bleed when the plaques are removed.

Treatment is with oral antifungal washes. Simultaneous treatment of nipple infection or vaginitis in the mother is helpful in reducing *C. albicans* surface colonization of the infant. (See box below.)

6. **Describe the infections in children caused by poxviruses, papovaviruses, and herpes-viruses.**
   Study pages 1173-1176; refer to Figures 40-7 through 40-9 and Table 40-1.

Molluscum contagiosum is a contagious (via skin-to-skin contact or by contact with contaminated fabrics) viral disease characterized by a pearlescent, dome-shaped lesion that may appear anywhere on the body but most often affects the face, trunk, and extremities. The lesions are not inflamed. No specific treatment is recommended because it is self-limiting, although recurrence is common.

Rubella, or 3-day measles, is a communicable disease of children and young adults caused by an RNA virus that enters the bloodstream through the respiratory tract. The incubation period is between 14 and 21 days. A faint-pink to red coalescing maculopapular rash develops on the face and spreads to the trunk and extremities 1 to 4 days after the prodromal symptoms. Women of childbearing age are immunized if their antibody titers are low, and pregnancy should be avoided for 3 months after vaccination because the attenuated virus may remain for this time period. A fetus of a pregnant woman who has rubella early in the first trimester may develop congenital

defects. There is no specific, only supportive, treatment. Recovery is spontaneous.

Rubeola, or red measles, is a contagious disease of children transmitted by direct contact with droplets from infected persons. Rubeola is caused by an RNA paramyxovirus having an incubation period of 7 to 12 days. Prodromal symptoms are followed within three to four days by an erythematous maculopapular rash over the head that spreads distally over the trunk, extremities, hands, and feet. Early lesions blanch with pressure, but do not do so as the rash fades. Pinpoint white spots surrounded by an erythematous ring develop over the buccal mucosa and are known as Koplik spots. Most children recover completely, but measles encephalitis occurs in about 1 in 800 cases. There is no specific treatment for measles.

Roseola likely is a viral infection; it is seen most often in infants between the ages of 6 months and 2 years. There is a sudden onset of fever that lasts for 3 to 5 days. After the fever, an erythematous macular rash lasts for about 24 hours; it is primarily over the trunk and neck. Usually, there is no treatment.

Chickenpox is a highly contagious disease of early childhood and is primarily spread by droplet transmission from an infected person to others. Household infection rates approach 90% in susceptible individuals. The incubation period is approximately 14 days, with infected persons contagious for approximately 24 hours before the onset of the rash and for 5 to 6 days after the rash appears. Chickenpox is usually an illness of late winter or early spring. The first signs of illness are pruritus or itching or the appearance of vesicles. There may be no prodromal symptoms.

Characteristically, the rash undergoes a process of maturation with lesions starting as macules that progress to superficial papules and vesicles, which then rupture and heal. The rash lasts for 4 to 5 days and may consist of up to 300 lesions distributed over the body. Complica-

Fungal Infections

Feature	Tinea Capitis	Tinea Corporis
Etiologic agent	*Microsporum canis, Trichophyton tonsurans*	*Microsporum canis, Trichophyton mentagrophytes*
Source	*M. canis* from cats, dogs, or rodents *T. tonsurans* from humans	*M. canis* and *T. mentagrophytes* from kittens or puppies
Lesion	Circular, slight erythema, scaling raised border	Oval or round with scale, central clearing, mild erythema, or ringworm
Diagnostic test	KOH examination	KOH examination
Treatment	Oral antifungals (topicals do not penetrate hair bulb)	Topical antifungals

tions from chickenpox are fairly rare but may include pneumonia due to the varicella virus. Treatment is symptomatic and consists of cool baths, wet dressings, and oral antihistamines.

Herpes zoster (shingles) occurs mainly in adults, but approximately 5% of cases are in children younger than 15 years of age. The chickenpox virus persists for life in sensory nerve ganglia and reactivates to cause herpes zoster. The zoster consists of groups of vesicles situated on an inflammatory base that follows the course of a sensory nerve. The base of the lesion appears hemorrhagic, and some may become necrotic and ulcerative. In children, the thorax is the site of distribution of the lesions. Therapy is similar to that for chickenpox unless it is disseminated zoster or there is ophthalmic involvement; then, acyclovir is indicated.

7. **Compare and contrast the infestations of scabies and lice; note other lesions from insects and parasites.**
   Study pages 1176-1177; refer to Figure 49-10. (See box below.)

Insect Infestations

Feature	Scabies (Mite)	Pediculosis (Lice)
Etiologic agent	*Sarcoptes scabiei*	*Pediculus capitis* (head), *Pediculus corporis* (body), *Phthirus pubis* (pubic)
Transmission	Contact with infested person	Contact with infested person or object (hat, clothing)
Symptoms	Burrows, papules, and vesicles	Pruritus, ova (nits) may be seen on hair shafts; mature lice may be seen
Cause of symptoms	Sensitization to larva buried in the skin	Irritation from toxic saliva from louse bites
Treatment	Permethrin/lindane, treatment of exposed persons and infested objects	Permethrin/lindane, treatment of exposed persons and infested objects

NOTE: Flea bites produce a pruritic wheal with a central puncture site and occur as clusters in areas of tight-fitting clothing. Bedbugs are blood-sucking parasites that live in cracks of floors, furniture, or bedding and feed at night. They produce pruritic wheals and nodules.

8. **Compare and contrast the congenital vascular disorders.**
   Study pages 1178-1179; refer to Figures 40-12 through 40-14. (See box below.)

Vascular Disorders

Feature	Strawberry Hemangioma	Cavernous Hemangioma	Salmon Patches	Portwine Stain
Description	Raised vesicular	Raised vesicular with larger mature vessels	Macular; most common	Flat; becomes papular and cavernous
Manifestation	At birth or in 3 to 5 weeks	At birth	At birth	At birth or in a few days
Color	Bright red (capillary projections)	Bluish, indistinct borders	Pink, distended dermal capillaries	Pink to dark reddish-purple
Location	One lesion on head, neck, or trunk	Head, neck	Nape of neck, forehead, upper eyelid	Face and other body surfaces
Growth	Initially rapid, then at child's rate of growth	Rapid first six months, matures at one year	Fades in one year	Does not fade
Involution	Begins by 12 to 16 months, complete by 5 to 6 years	Begins by 6 to 12 months, complete by 9 years	N/A	N/A
Treatment	None	May require surgery, laser surgery, or liquid nitrogen depending on location of lesion	None	Cryosurgery, laser surgery

Practice Examination

True/False

_____ 1. Diaper dermatitis is caused by *Candida albicans.*

_____ 2. Impetigo is contracted only by human-to-human contact.

_____ 3. Molluscum contagiosum is a very painful viral infection.

_____ 4. Atopic dermatitis is also called *eczema.*

_____ 5. Staphylococcal scalded-skin syndrome is a contagious disease of the skin.

_____ 6. Tinea capitis must be treated with systemic antifungal agents.

_____ 7. Salmon patches are commonly called *stork bites* and fade over time.

_____ 8. Portwine stains will involute by adulthood.

_____ 9. Acute glomerulonephritis is a complication of bullous impetigo.

_____10. The microorganism that causes bullous impetigo is *Streptococcus pyogenes.*

Match the description with the alteration.

_____11. viral skin infection contracted during the first
            decade of life

_____12. positive allergy tests, increased IgE, and
            eosinophilia

_____13. erythematous lesions in the perineal area with
            secondary papulovesicular satellites

_____14. raised, erythemic, scaling lesions on the scalp

_____15. dome-shaped lesions ranging from 1 mm to
            5 mm on the extremities without pruritus

_____16. macules, fever, itching, papules, and rupturing
            and healing vesicles

_____17. crusted lesion

_____18. mite burrowing in the stratum corneum

_____19. present at birth or shortly after birth

_____20. entire skin sloughing

_____21. nits on hair shaft

_____22. chronic condition with acute exacerbations, pruritus

_____23. oval or circular lesions, peripheral spreading,
            central clearing (ringworm)

_____24. action of an epidermolytic toxin

_____25. parasitic in nature, acquired by personal contact
            and sharing combs or hair brushes

a. staphylococcal scalded-skin syndrome

b. tinea capitis

c. atopic dermatitis

d. pediculosis

e. diaper dermatitis complicated with
    Candida albicans

f. chickenpox

g. vascular disorders

h. impetigo

i. molluscum contagiosum

j. scabies

k. tinea corporis

Case Study

Lance D. is a 5-year-old white male who visits the nurse practitioner's office with a "runny" nose that started about 1 week ago but has not resolved. He has been blowing his nose quite frequently, and "sores" have developed on his face. His mother states that the sores started as "big blisters" that rupture; sometimes, a scab forms with a crust that looks like "dried maple syrup" but continues to weep and drain. She is worried because the lesions are now also on his forearm. Lance's past medical and family histories are normal. He has been febrile but is otherwise asymptomatic. The physical examination is unremarkable except for moderate, purulent rhinorrhea and weeping lesions 0.5 to 1 cm in diameter around the nose and mouth and on the radial surface of the right forearm. There is no regional lymphadenopathy.

What is the likely name and cause of these lesions? Why have these lesions spread to Lance's arm?

Answers to Practice Examinations

Chapter 1

1. c	6. a	11. g	16. b	21. a, b, c, d, e
2. a, c, e	7. d	12. e	17. b, d	22. a, b, c, d
3. a	8. d	13. f	18. b	23. b
4. e	9. h	14. j	19. c	24. c
5. d	10. d	15. e	20. d	25. d

Chapter 2

1. a	6. b	11. d	16. f	21. h
2. b	7. b	12. d	17. h	22. d
3. d	8. c	13. b	18. g	23. f
4. c	9. c	14. c	19. i	24. g
5. d	10. a	15. a	20. b	25. c

Chapter 3

1. d	6. b	11. d	16. c	21. c
2. c, d	7. d	12. b	17. b	22. a
3. d	8. a	13. a	18. d	23. d
4. e	9. c	14. d	19. a	24. b
5. d	10. e	15. d	20. e	25. e

Chapter 4

1. e	6. e	11. d	16. c	21. e
2. b	7. b	12. d	17. e	22. b
3. b	8. b	13. a, b, e	18. b	23. a
4. c	9. a	14. b	19. d	24. c
5. d	10. c	15. e	20. a	25. b

Chapter 5

1. c	6. e	11. d	16. d	21. c
2. a	7. b	12. e	17. a	22. a
3. d	8. d	13. d	18. b	23. a
4. e	9. d	14. e	19. c	24. b
5. f	10. a	15. d	20. f	25. a

Chapter 6

1. e	6. a	11. d	16. d	21. b
2. b	7. a	12. a	17. d	22. d
3. d	8. b	13. e	18. e	23. e
4. b	9. e	14. b	19. e	24. g
5. d	10. d	15. c	20. e	25. f

Chapter 7

1. b	6. b	11. d	16. a	21. e
2. c	7. d	12. e	17. d	22. e
3. a	8. c	13. c	18. e	23. d
4. c	9. d	14. d	19. c	24. a
5. d	10. d	15. a	20. b	25. d

Chapter 8

1. c	6. a	11. c	16. a	21. c
2. f	7. b	12. a	17. c	22. e
3. d	8. c	13. d	18. a	23. g
4. e	9. b	14. a	19. c	24. h
5. g	10. d	15. a	20. a	25. i

Chapter 9

1. c	6. a	11. c	16. b	21. e
2. e	7. d	12. d	17. e	22. c
3. f	8. e	13. e	18. e	23. d
4. e	9. b	14. c	19. a	24. a
5. c	10. f	15. e	20. c	25. f

Chapter 10

1. e	6. e	11. c	16. d	21. g
2. c	7. b	12. d	17. d	22. c
3. d	8. e	13. a	18. b	23. e
4. e	9. d	14. e	19. c	24. f
5. e	10. c	15. c	20. e	25. a

Chapter 11

1. False	6. True	11. e	16. c	21. True
2. False	7. True	12. f	17. True	22. True
3. True	8. False	13. a	18. False	23. False
4. True	9. True	14. d	19. False	24. False
5. False	10. True	15. b	20. False	25. False

Chapter 12

1. c	6. a	11. a	16. c	21. a
2. d	7. c	12. c	17. a	22. b
3. c	8. a	13. a	18. d	23. a
4. b	9. b	14. c	19. c	24. d
5. e	10. b, d	15. a	20. a	25. c

Chapter 13

1. b	6. b	11. e	16. c	21. c
2. a	7. e	12. b	17. a	22. j
3. e	8. e	13. d	18. e	23. i
4. b	9. c	14. b	19. d	24. h
5. c	10. c	15. b	20. e	25. g

Case Study Discussion

Her history and response to medication were typical of *depression*. Depression causes sleep disturbances characterized by insomnia, early morning awakenings, or multiple awakenings during the night. The improvement in the quality of sleep following antidepressants often occurs before other appropriate behavioral changes are seen. It seems likely that her insomnia may return, and an appropriate course of action might involve seeking assistance from a sleep disorder center.

Chapter 14

1. c	6. c	11. c	16. c	21. l
2. e	7. e	12. b	17. a	22. b
3. b	8. d	13. a	18. e	23. e
4. a	9. e	14. b	19. j	24. f
5. b	10. d	15. c	20. k	25. g

Case Study Discussion

Normal laboratory values and the normal CSF likely exclude the possibility of an infection such as meningitis and other causes known to precipitate seizures. The skull x-ray ruled out the possibility of a skull fracture. A normal EEG likely excludes intracranial pressure from brain masses. Since an EEG may be normal between seizures, the episodal pattern suggests a *generalized grand mal seizure*. A judicious administration of anticonvulsant medications likely is indicated.

Chapter 15

1. d	6. d	11. a	16. d	21. b
2. b	7. e	12. b	17. b	22. d
3. e	8. a	13. c	18. c	23. g
4. c	9. b	14. e	19. b	24. c
5. b	10. e	15. c	20. a, c	25. f

Case Study Discussion

Mrs. B. exhibits risk factors for a CVA. She smokes cigarettes, is overweight, and is hypertensive. Her mother and siblings have histories of diabetes, CVA, and hypertension; all of these indicate a family history that increases the risk for CVA.

Her symptoms and signs suggest a *thrombotic stroke* with ischemia rather than a hemorrhagic or embolic stroke. The absence of blood in CSF rules out a hemorrhagic stroke. Since there was no fibrillation on the electrocardiogram, the heart was an unlikely source for emboli, thus ruling out an embolic stroke. Mrs. B.'s elevated blood pressure likely is caused by atherosclerosis, which can lead to a thrombus formation.

Chapter 16

1. False	6. True	11. False	16. Craniosynostosis	21. e
2. False	7. True	12. Reye, hepatic	17. i	22. d
3. False	8. True	13. posterior	18. h	23. c
4. True	9. False	14. anterior	19. g	24. b
5. False	10. False	15. meningitis	20. f	25. a

Case Study Discussion

X-rays reveal an absence of spinal processes on the vertebrae from L3 to L5. A *meningomyelocele* at the same level with tethering of the cord is revealed. A neurosurgical consultation is ordered, and surgery is likely.

Chapter 17

1. a	6. e	11. b	16. d	21. a
2. e	7. a	12. d	17. e	22. c
3. c	8. c	13. e	18. b	23. e
4. b	9. d	14. c	19. d	24. d
5. d	10. c	15. d	20. e	25. f

Chapter 18

1. c	6. a	11. a	16. c	21. a, b, c
2. a	7. d	12. b	17. a	22. c
3. a	8. a	13. b	18. e	23. e
4. d	9. a	14. b	19. c	24. d
5. b	10. d	15. c	20. e	25. b

Case Study Discussion

Scott's symptoms, signs, and laboratory values are classic for *diabetes ketoacidosis*. The serum values indicated metabolic acidosis with some accompanying respiratory compensation. His elevated glycosylated hemoglobin showed that he likely had been hyperglycemic for several months. This diabetes is type 1 (IDDM) and will require insulin administration and personal instructions regarding recognition of future signs and symptoms of hyperglycemia and hypoglycemia, self-blood glucose monitoring, insulin therapy, diet, and exercise.

Chapter 19

1. e	6. c	11. d	16. b	21. e
2. b	7. c	12. e	17. c	22. e
3. e	8. c	13. e	18. a	23. b
4. d	9. d	14. d	19. a	24. d
5. a	10. e	15. d	20. b	25. d

Chapter 20

1. e	6. a	11. e	16. c	21. a
2. d	7. b	12. c	17. e	22. b
3. d	8. a	13. b	18. c	23. a
4. a	9. b	14. c	19. b	24. d
5. b	10. b	15. d	20. a	25. e

Case Study 1 Discussion

Three anemias have erythrocytes that are microcytic and hypochromic: iron deficiency, sideroblastic anemia, and thalassemia. Ann's history has some factors that could contribute to anemia from blood loss. The menorrhagia causes more iron loss than is normal with each menstrual period, and excessive aspirin intake irritates the gastrointestinal mucosa and can precipitate chronic mucosal microhemorrhage.

Iron deficiency anemia is most likely and can be verified by providing oral iron replacement and checking her hemoglobin values in one month. If the hemoglobin deficit is corrected, it is likely that the correct diagnosis was made. The source of bleeding should be corrected, if possible; a substitute for aspirin should be used; and iron supplementation should be used for at least one year.

Ann's homeostatic mechanisms are trying to compensate in several ways, including shunting blood to more critical organs, increasing erythropoiesis, increasing the heart rate to handle increased venous return, and increasing the respiratory rate to make oxygen available to the remaining erythrocytes. The last two signs are relevant compensation efforts in Ann's circumstance.

Case Study 2 Discussion

The physician likely would conclude that L.L. has *acute lymphocytic leukemia*. The pale skin with petechiae and ecchymoses is abnormal, as is the gingival bleeding from minor trauma. Although the abnormal values for RBCs, hemoglobin, total leukocyte count, and platelet count have many possible causes, the presence of leukocytic blasts in peripheral blood indicates a bone marrow dysfunction. At this time, the physician likely will refer L.L. to a pediatric oncologist for extensive diagnostic tests and treatment.

Chapter 21

1. False	6. False	11. d	16. b	21. e
2. True	7. False	12. c	17. e	22. c
3. True	8. a	13. e	18. e	23. d
4. False	9. b	14. d	19. a	24. c
5. True	10. e	15. e	20. b	25. d

Case Study Discussion

Steven has the typical manifestations of *idiopathic thrombocytopenic purpura* (ITP), although it has come to medical attention in a very circuitous manner.

Chapter 22

1. b	6. b	11. a	16. b, d, e	21. a
2. b	7. e	12. a	17. c	22. d
3. b	8. a	13. c	18. b	23. b
4. c	9. c	14. d	19. d	24. b
5. b, c	10. e	15. a	20. a	25. b

Chapter 23

1. d	6. b	11. e	16. f	21. a, b, c
2. e	7. d	12. a	17. b, d	22. d
3. c	8. e	13. b	18. c	23. e
4. b	9. c	14. c	19. a, c	24. c
5. a	10. b, d, e	15. e	20. b, d	25. b

Case Study Discussion

Alterable myocardial infarction risk factors for W.S. are essential hypertension and cigarette smoking. Unalterable risk factors for W.S. include advancing age, male sex, and family history of early cardiac death. Atherosclerosis in the anterior descending branch of the left coronary artery was the beginning process leading to this infarction. The location of infarction was verified by the electrocardiogram.

The precipitating event in this myocardial infarction was complete occlusion of the coronary artery. The history of hypertension also supports occlusion of the coronary artery as the cause for this myocardial infarction.

Pulmonary thromboembolism is a common cause of death from myocardial infarction as emboli disseminate from debris or clots from the infarcted endocardium. Prophylactic heparin therapy decreases the risk of pulmonary embolism by interfering with the conversion of prothrombin to thrombin so that thrombi are less likely to form.

Chapter 24

1. False	7. left, right	12. first weeks	15. coarctation of	20. c
2. True	8. right, left	13. pulonary	the aorta	21. c
3. False	9. oxygenated,	stenosis	16. e	22. e
4. True	unoxygenated	14. afterload,	17. a	23. d
5. False	10. equal	congestive heart	18. a	24. d
6. shunt	11. left, right	failure	19. b	25. a

Case Study Discussion

Following the consultation, the echocardiogram demonstrates a moderate *coarctation of the aorta* in the aortic arch. This discrepancy in the quality of upper and lower extremity pulses is due to well-developed collateral circulation to the descending aorta; the femoral pulses will be decreased as blood fills the collateral vessels.

Chapter 25

1. d	6. e	11. c	16. d	21. a
2. d	7. d	12. a	17. a	22. a
3. c	8. c	13. c	18. b	23. a
4. d	9. a	14. d	19. e	24. b
5. d	10. b	15. b	20. e	25. a

Chapter 26

1. g	6. d	11. c	16. a, b, c, d	21. a, b, d
2. c	7. e	12. e	17. e	22. d
3. h	8. f	13. d	18. b, c	23. e
4. l	9. j	14. e	19. b	24. b
5. i	10. m	15. a	20. a, b, d	25. a

Case Study Discussion

Mr. S. presents the classic symptoms and signs of *emphysema*. His long-term, extensive smoking is consistent with most cases of emphysema, as is his dyspnea on exertion progressing to dyspnea even at rest. Hyperinflation of lungs causes the anteroposterior chest diameter to increase. The chest radiograph is consistent with findings in emphysema. Prolonged forced expiratory volume, decreased tidal volume, and increased total lung capacity are also present in emphysema. These tests indicate that the walls of alveoli have been destroyed and the lungs have become more distended or less compliant and have less elastic recoil. Therefore, air is trapped and expiration flow is diminished.

Chapter 27

1. False	6. True	11. c	16. d	21. e
2. False	7. e	12. d	17. a	22. c
3. False	8. e	13. c	18. b	23. d
4. True	9. d	14. e	19. f	24. c
5. False	10. e	15. d	20. f	25. a

Case Study Discussion

Tyler has classic manifestations of *bronchiolitis*. The most likely etiologic agent in Tyler's illness is respiratory syncytial virus to which his parents likely exposed him during their "colds." He is displaying the classic signs of respiratory distress in an infant and is unable to feed due to this respiratory distress. His lethargy is probably due to mild hypoxia and hypercapnia, and his general fatigue is from prolonged ventilatory effort. He may suffer respiratory failure if left untreated. Hospitalization for rehydration and respiratory therapy should support him through the worst of his illness, and he should improve within a few days.

Chapter 28

1. c	6. b	11. e	16. d	21. b
2. a	7. b	12. b	17. a	22. c
3. d	8. c	13. b	18. c, d, e	23. c
4. a	9. d	14. d	19. d	24. c
5. d	10. d	15. b	20. a	25. d

Chapter 29

1. d	6. d	11. d	16. b	21. c
2. b	7. a, b, c	12. e	17. d	22. b
3. a	8. b	13. d	18. c	23. d
4. a	9. b	14. d	19. a	24. a
5. e	10. b, c, d	15. a, e	20. d	25. e

Case Study Discussion

Eddie's history of sore throat and back pain and his laboratory values suggest *poststreptococcal glomerulonephritis.* Proteinuria is a sensitive indicator of glomerular dysfunction. In glomerulonephritis, the glomerulus is injured and its permeability increased enough to permit protein to enter into the filtrate and urine. Blood and RBC casts also are seen in glomerulonephritis. BUN and creatinine are excreted entirely by the kidneys and therefore are directly related to renal excretion. Eddie's pediatrician most likely will place him on penicillin and may prescribe an antihypertensive medication and monitor his blood pressure, electrolyte balance, and BUN and creatinine levels.

Chapter 30

1. False	6. False	11. e	16. d	21. b
2. True	7. d	12. d	17. e	22. c
3. False	8. a	13. d	18. e	23. c
4. False	9. d	14. d	19. d	24. a
5. True	10. c	15. d	20. f	25. g

Case Study Discussion

The laboratory values reveal an anemia and thrombocytopenia; the child is losing red blood cells and platelets. Since she has not voided any urine, acute renal failure is very likely. These results suggest the diagnosis of *hemolytic uremic syndrome.* She will require hospitalization for blood transfusions and dialysis.

Chapter 31

1. b, d	6. d	11. a	16. c	21. a
2. a	7. a	12. e	17. e	22. c
3. e	8. b	13. b	18. c	23. c
4. d	9. e	14. c	19. e	24. e
5. c	10. b	15. a	20. a	25. a

Chapter 32

1. d	6. b	11. d	16. d	21. c
2. c	7. d	12. d	17. b	22. e
3. e	8. a	13. d	18. a	23. f
4. d	9. e	14. a	19. b	24. h
5. e	10. b	15. d	20. b	25. i

Case Study Discussion

Mrs. B.'s history and examination are indicative of *breast cancer* in her left breast. A positive familial history of breast cancer has a strong, confirmed causal link to breast cancer. A chromosome 17 defect has been implicated as a genetic causal factor in breast cancer as well. Other associated risk factors for breast cancer that Mrs. B. exhibits include late age at first delivery, early menarche, birth control pills, and benign breast tumors.

The cardinal manifestation of breast cancer was a hard, fixed mass palpable in Mrs. B.'s left breast. The freely movable, soft masses of the right breast are likely benign, since they display fluctuating patterns of tissue proliferation different from those of the left breast. The palpation of the axillary lymph node indicated that cancer cells have metastasized through the lymphatic channels surrounding the breast.

Chapter 33

1. d	6. d	11. d	16. d	21. b
2. d	7. d	12. b	17. a	22. c
3. b	8. a	13. a	18. b	23. e
4. e	9. d	14. c	19. a	24. c
5. e	10. b	15. c	20. c	25. a

Chapter 34

1. b	6. d	11. b	16. d	21. b
2. d	7. c	12. e	17. e	22. e
3. a	8. e	13. b	18. e	23. d
4. e	9. a	14. a	19. a, b, c, d	24. a
5. e	10. b	15. c	20. a	25. d

Case Study Discussion

A *gastric ulcer* is likely. Factors associated with these ulcers include smoking, stress, and use of aspirin or other ulcerogenic drugs. Although the clinical manifestations of gastric ulcers are similar to those of duodenal ulcers, the pain of gastric ulcers is more likely to occur immediately after eating. Also, gastric ulcers tend to be chronic rather than alternate between periods of remission and exacerbation. An upper gastrointestinal study using barium sulfate as a contrast medium and endoscopy can detect the location of the ulcer and confirm that Dr. R. has a gastric ulcer.

Chapter 35

1. False	7. True	12. Gastroesopha-geal reflux	17. a	23. d
2. True	8. False		18. c	24. c
3. False	9. True	13. biopsy	19. b	25. c
4. False	10. False	14. decrease	20. a	
5. False	11. True	15. nasal, oral	21. e	
6. True		16. Rectal prolapse	22. d	

Case Study Discussion

A *pyloric stenosis* is diagnosed on the basis of clinical manifestations. The standard treatment is a pyloromyotomy to separate the muscles of the pylorus.

Chapter 36

1. a, c, d	6. b	11. d	16. d	21. c
2. d	7. b	12. d	17. a	22. e
3. d	8. d	13. a	18. b	23. e
4. e	9. b	14. c	19. d	24. e
5. b	10. b	15. a	20. b	25. c

Chapter 37

1. a	6. e	11. a	16. a	21. d
2. b	7. c	12. e	17. a, b	22. d
3. d	8. c	13. b	18. a, b, d, e	23. c
4. b	9. e	14. d	19. e	24. e
5. d	10. a	15. e	20. b	25. e

Case Study Discussion

The presenting symptoms of Mrs. B. are compatible with either osteoarthritis or rheumatoid arthritis. The laboratory studies support a diagnosis of *rheumatoid arthritis*. The presence of rheumatoid factor is helpful in the diagnosis of rheumatoid arthritis. It is positive in about 80% of individuals who have rheumatoid arthritis. Although other diseases may show a positive test, osteoarthritis will not. Synovial fluid analysis showing inflammatory exudates satisfies the diagnostic criteria for rheumatoid arthritis. The radiograph is more representative of rheumatoid arthritis than osteoarthritis. In osteoarthritis, deformity of articular cartilage, bone sclerosis, cystic areas, and bony spurs would be likely observations.

Chapter 38

1. False	6. True	11. femoral	16. b	21. e
2. False	7. False	12. breech position	17. f	22. d
3. False	8. True	13. dystrophin	18. e	23. c
4. True	9. True	14. Pavlik harness	19. f	24. b
5. False	10. False	15. clubfoot	20. d	25. a

Case Study Discussion

Bobby B. displays the clinical manifestations of *Duchenne muscular dystrophy*. The diagnosis can be confirmed by measurement of serum creatine phosphokinase (CPK) levels, electromyography, and muscle biopsy. The CPK level in Duchenne muscular dystrophy will be increased more than ten times normal. Histologic examination of the biopsy will show muscle degeneration, with fat and connective tissue replacing muscle fibers.

Chapter 39

1. a	6. d	11. d	16. d	21. a
2. a	7. e	12. b	17. d	22. c
3. a	8. f	13. e	18. b	23. d
4. d	9. d	14. c	19. c	24. d
5. b	10. e	15. e	20. c	25. a

Case Study Discussion

Adults with burns involving large surface areas require cardiovascular support through intravenous fluid since *hypovolemic shock* develops quickly following major burn injury. Within minutes of a major burn injury, the capillary bed not only at the site of the burn but throughout the entire body becomes more permeable to water, sodium, and proteins. This leads to fluid loss from the intravascular spaces into the interstitial spaces and massive edema; the blood volume and cardiac output diminish. The infusion of intravenous fluid or burn shock resuscitation for the first 24 hours must be faster than the rate of loss of circulatory volume. To determine adequate levels of infusion, urine output must be measured, so Mr. E. will require placement of a catheter into his bladder.

Although hypovolemic shock is the immediate concern for major burn patients, other alterations are very important; monitoring and maintenance of electrolytes are required. The hypermetabolic rate of burned individuals requires adequate nutrition. Finally, early excision and grafting procedures are required.

Chapter 40

1. False	6. True	11. f	16. f	21. d
2. False	7. True	12. c	17. h	22. c
3. False	8. False	13. e	18. j	23. k
4. True	9. False	14. b	19. g	24. a
5. False	10. False	15. i	20. a	25. d

Case Study Discussion

This is a fairly classic case of *bullous impetigo* caused by a *Staphylococcus aureus* infection in Lance's nasopharynx. Abrasion from blowing and wiping his nose frequently has opened the skin and allowed the bacteria to enter the skin and cause the lesions. The infection spread to his arm because he has been wiping his nose on his arm.